SURGERY, SKIN AND SYPHILIS
DANIEL TURNER'S LONDON
(1667–1741)

Philip K. Wilson

THE WELLCOME INSTITUTE SERIES IN THE HISTORY OF MEDICINE

Forthcoming Titles
Medicine and Modern Warfare
Roger Cooter, Mark Harrison and Steve Sturdy (eds)

Pathologies of Travel
Richard Wrigley and George Revill (eds)

Academic enquiries regarding the series should be addressed to the editors C. J. Lawrence, V. Nutton, and Roy Porter at the Wellcome Institute for the History of Medicine, 183 Euston Road, London NW1 2BE, UK

SURGERY, SKIN AND SYPHILIS
DANIEL TURNER'S LONDON
(1667–1741)

Philip K. Wilson

Mike –
In hopes that you might
enjoy this historical glimpse
at the skin through the
practice of Daniel Turner.
with every best wish –
Philip

Amsterdam – Atlanta, GA 1999

First published in 1999
by Editions Rodopi B. V., Amsterdam – Atlanta, GA 1999.

Design and Typesetting by Alex Mayor, the Wellcome Trust.
Printed and bound in The Netherlands by Editions Rodopi B. V.,
Amsterdam – Atlanta, GA 1999.

British Library Cataloguing in Publication Data
A catalogue record for this book is available from the British Library
ISBN 90-420-0516-5 (Paper)
ISBN 90-420-0526-2 (Bound)

Surgery, Skin and Syphilis:
Daniel Turner's London (1667-1741) –
Amsterdam – Atlanta, GA:
Rodopi. – ill.
(Clio Medica 54 / ISSN 0045-7183;
The Wellcome Institute Series in the History of Medicine)

Front cover:
Collage of Daniel Turner, Johan Faber mezzotint set within Devonshire
Square, Bishopsgate Ward, London (Yale University Library, New Haven,
Connecticut, and Guildhall Library, London). Design by A. Mayor.

Printed in The Netherlands

Contents

Dedicated to my father
with love, admiration, and respect

Acknowledgements

I am grateful to the many individuals who offered their assistance, comments, suggestions, and support throughout the preparation of this work. Foremost, I wish to thank the Wellcome Trust for funding a three-year studentship during which time much of this material was researched and written. Truman State University also provided research funds which allowed me to continue this project throughout the 1996-97 academic year.

Fellow historians at the Wellcome Institute have generously provided intellectual stimulation and encouragement. I appreciate the suggestions of Roy Porter, Bill Bynum, Christopher Lawrence, Andrew Wear, Sandra Cavallo, Luca Ciancio, Helen Power, Joy Harvey, Holger Maehle, Antonio Poza, Molly Sutphen, John Thearle, Estelle Cohen, Denis Gibbs, and especially Akihito Suzuki. Research would be impossible without the able assistance of librarians, archivists, and other members of the research staff. In particular, I wish to thank Lyndsay (Wilson) Lardner, Caroline (Peck) Rock, Sue Gold, and Janice Wilson for their exemplary reference assistance at the Wellcome. Keith Moore, Gerald Beasley, John Symons, Andy Foley, Clare Dunne, Chris Carter, William Schupbach, Caroline Overy, Catherine Draycott, Brenda Sutton, and David Brady have also helped fulfil a variety of research needs.

Expert assistance from the following is also greatly appreciated: Andrew Baster (archivist, United Medical Schools of Guy's and St Thomas' Hospitals); Ian G. Murray (archivist, The Worshipful Company of Barbers of London); Ferenc Gyorgyey and Toby Appel (librarians, The Historical Library, Yale Medical Library); Geoffrey Davenport (librarian, Royal College of Physicians); Kevin Flude (director, St Thomas' Old Operating Theatre and Herb Garrett); Susan Case (previous rare book librarian, Clendening Medical History Library, Kansas City), and Carol Lockhart and Sheila Swafford (Pickler Memorial Library, Truman State University). I am grateful for the help from librarians, archivists, and support staff at the British Library, the Guildhall Library (London), the University of London Library, University College London Library, the London

Library, the Public Record Office, the Greater London Record Office, the Hertfordshire County Record Office, the Essex Record Office, the Royal College of Surgeons of England, the Royal Society, the Society of Genealogists, the University of Leiden, Yale University Library, the Huguenot Society, Hereford Cathedral, Hawaii Medical Library, and Truman State University. I extend my gratitude to Professor John A.A. Hunter and Dr G.W. Beveridge (Dermatology Department, Royal Infirmary, Edinburgh), Mrs B.H. Mary Hare (Bath), The Revd and Mrs Ronald A. Thomson (Watton-at-Stone), The Revd Alan Tanner (St Botolph Without Bishopsgate, London), The Revd Peter J. Beech (St Mary-at-Latton), R.S. Morton (Sheffield University), Milton Lewis (University of Sydney), Anthony Lawrence (Coventry University), Ann Dally (Wellcome Institute), Peter Earle (London School of Economics), Michael Hunter (Birkbeck College), Richard Staughton (Daniel Turner Clinic, Chelsea and Westminster Hospital, London) and Aloys Henning (Freie Universität, Berlin). John Burrows and fellow members of our "History Through Biography" class at Wansfell College helped me remember why biographical writing remains widespread as a popular as well as an academic pursuit. I appreciate the insight my colleagues Fritz Rehbock, David Morens, and George Simson at the University of Hawai'i at Manoa provided as well as the discussions on Daniel Turner before the membership of the Hawaii Society for the History of Medicine and Public Health and at Brown Bag Biography sessions at the Center for Biographical Research.

Andrew Wear, Harold Cook, Bill Bynum, Stephen Pumfrey, and John Harley Warner have taken the time to read and make extensive comments on various chapters in this work. I truly appreciate their efforts and critical insight. This book would not have progressed as it did without the continued support of Christopher Lawrence and Roy Porter. Cheers, Chris and Roy! I also appreciate the constructive criticism from the two anonymous reviewers. Alex Mayor provided splendid assistance throughout the design stage of this volume. I am grateful for my colleagues at Truman State University who have made this a conducive environment for intellectual exchange. I have been particularly privileged to have assembled a skillful group of young research scholars who have assisted in the production of this work through various ways. Undergraduates Lisa Fagnani, Gretchen Krueger, Erin Loos, Chris Wolf, Brian Yochim and Sarah Zapf have each read, discussed and copy-edited several sections of earlier drafts of this work as well as helped me procure needed sources and information. Gwendolyn Habel and Patrick Reed provided expert computer assistance. Above all, Robert Wood has been my extra right hand on this project. Without his selfless dedication, diligence, and dependability, this book could not have been completed in such a timely manner.

Commentary provided by attendees at the 1997 Honolulu Academy of Arts gathering dedicated to 'Imaging the Human Body: Artistic and Medical Representations through Western History' and the Taniguchi Symposium on 'Medical Expressions of the Body' provided stimulating ideas about ways in which Turner's surgical view of the body dovetails into modern scholarship on the body. I treasure the comments I received at these monumental gatherings together with those of fellow Enlightenment enthusiasts, Paul Child and Wayne Wilde. Janet Davis has been a delightful team-teaching colleague and sounding board for all 'Rhetoric and Medicine' matters.

I offer my esteemed gratitude to Tony and Helen Lawrence (Edinburgh and Coventry), Hank and Barbara McCloughan (Brooke and Loddon, Norfolk), Lyndsay and Mark Lardner (Blackheath), and Ann Dally and Philip Egerton (Wiblings Farm, Graffam) for repeatedly providing luxurious hospitality and an exhilarating atmosphere in which to think, work, and reflect during my stays in Britain. My personal thanks to Peter W. M. Copeman, Richard and Clare Staughton, and 'friends' of the Daniel Turner Clinic (Chelsea and Westminster Hospital, London) for their continued interest and encouragement of this project.

I remain most grateful to my parents, Robert and the late Margaret Guyot Wilson, and to Bill and Marge Franklin for their steadfast love and staunch support. I am also thankful that my boys, James and Douglas, accepted my reply to their regular question, "Why must you go back to work tonight?" Above all else, it has truly been a personal pleasure to research alongside my wife, Janice Wilson, when she worked as a reference librarian at the Wellcome Institute Library, the Yale Medical Library, the Hawaii Medical Library, and Pickler Memorial Library. Not only has she been an astute critic of each chapter of this book, but she has answered innumerable queries about bibliographical sources throughout my research. She has tolerated my biographical obsession with Daniel Turner without question. I remain indebted to Janice for her unflagging patience, assistance, encouragement, and love.

List of Figures and Tables

Brief Chronology of Daniel Turner's Life and Writings

1667	Born, 20 September, baptised October 17
1684	Began surgical apprenticeship under Charles Bateman
1686	'Turned over' to Thomas Lichfield to complete apprenticeship
1691	Completed customary seven-year surgical apprenticeship
1694	Case studies of 'Remarks, taken upon Dissecting ... a Maid ... who dyed of an Ascites', 'Woman hydropical in the ... Uterus', and 'Child bit by Mad Dog', published in the *Philosophical Transactions of the Royal Society of London*
1695	*Apologia Chyrurgica. A Vindication of the Noble Art of Surgery*
1700	Admitted as Freeman into the Barber-Surgeons' Company of London, 15 October
1703	*The Present State of Chyrurgery*
1707	Compiled private devotions, 'Religio Medici'
1709	*A remarkable case in Surgery ... of an uncommon Fracture ... of the Skull*
1711	Discharged from Barber-Surgeons' Company, 16 August
	Examined and admitted as Licentiate of the Royal College of Physicians, 22 December
1712	Married Elizabeth Altham of Mark Hall, Latton (Essex), 20 December
	Received imprimatur from the Royal College of Physicians to prepare *De Morbis Cutaneis* for publication
1714	*De Morbis Cutaneis. A Treatise of Diseases Incident to the Skin*

1717	*Syphilis. A Practical dissertation on the Venereal Disease*
1718	*The Modern Quack, or the Physical Imposter Detected*
1722	*The Art of Surgery*
	Sent parcel of books to Yale College, 24 September
1723	Conferred honorary Doctor of Medicine degree by Yale College, 11 September
1724	'Insects voided by urinary passages', *Philosophical Transactions of the Royal Society of London*
	Remarks on Dr Willoughby's translation of Monsieur Chicoyneau's Method of Cure
1725	'Some modest Animadversions on Dr Harris's *Dissertationes Medicae,* especially his thirteenth, *de Errotibus Chirurgorum*'
1726	'On the Force of the Mother's Imagination on the foetus in utero'
1727	*Discourse Concerning Fevers*
	'A Short Account of the Pulse and Urine, as Affording Signs both Diagnostic and Prognostic; as Also of Crises, and Critical Days in Fevers'
1729	*A Discourse Concerning Gleets*
	'A Defence of the XIIth Chapter of the First Part of a treatise *De Morbis Cutaneis*'
	'An Answer to a pamphlet on the Power of Imagination in Pregnant Women'
	'Prefatory Account of Professor Boerhaave's New Comments on the Venereal Disease; and Some Animadversions thereon'
1730	*De Morbo Gallico*
	'The Force of the Mother's Imagination upon the Foetus in Utero ... by Way of Reply to Dr Blondell's Work'
	'A Letter to Mr James Ferne, Surgeon, Concerning a Very Singular Suppos'd Infection'
1733	*The Ancient Physician's Legacy Impartially Survey'd*
	'A Discourse on Quicksilver'
	'Some Historical Memoirs of Quicksilver ['Case of Barton Booth

... as Communicated by Alexander Small', 'A Particular account of M. Bellost's Pill Compared with the Authors']

1735 *The Drop and Pill of Mr Ward Consider'd*

1736 Preface to Aloysius Luisini's *Aphrodisiacus, Containing a Summary of the Ancient Writers on the Venereal Disease*

1739 *Syphilis. The Second Part*

1740 Composed will, 10 July

1741 Died, 13 March, buried Church of St Andrew and St Mary, Watton-at-Stone, Hertfordshire

1743 *Traite des Maladies de la Peau en General; avec un Court Appendix sur l'Efficacite des Remedes Topiques dans les Maladies Internes, & leur Maniere d'Agir sur le Corps Humain*

1754 *Syphilis; oder, Practische Adhandlung von der Venusseuche, in zweyen Theilen*

1766 *Adhandlung von den Krankheiten dr Haut: nebst einem kurzen Anhang von den ausserlichen Mitteln, und der Art, wie sie wirken*

1767 *Dissertation sur les maladies venerienne*

1

Surgery in History

Historians have neglected London's surgeons and their practices during the Enlightenment. Those who envision history as a series of advancements typically skip from seventeenth-century heroic accounts of the military practice of Richard Wiseman to the late eighteenth-century surgical establishment centred around John Hunter.[1] Fenwick Beekman, an early twentieth-century practitioner, argued that 'improvements' in surgery, like those in medicine, occurred in Scotland rather than in England during the early Enlightenment, thereby directing historical attention away from London. Only after John Hunter imported an Edinburgh-style of surgical thinking and practice to London does Beekman acknowledge that progress occurred in the English capital.[2] Historians who appreciate a more socially constructed view of surgery have typically explored the activities within the field after the formation of London's Company of Surgeons in 1745. Susan Lawrence's prodigious research into the ways London hospitals produced and legitimized surgical know-how primarily focuses upon the last half of the 1700s.[3] These accounts convey the general impression that the early eighteenth century was, to use William Le Fanu's term, a 'lost half-century' of London surgery.[4] This historical lacuna is particularly surprising for it was during the first half of the century that London's Barber-Surgeons' Company, the contemporary organization responsible for licensing practitioners and regulating their practice in Europe's second largest city, underwent recurrent struggles from within and without its ranks, culminating in the surgeons' separation from the barbers in 1745.[5]

A thorough search of British and American libraries has uncovered nearly ninety editions of surgical treatises in the English vernacular which were first printed between 1685 and 1745 (see Appendix 1).[6] Thus, despite the lack of historical attention, early eighteenth-century England was not an 'unproductive' period of surgical writing.[7] Using these writings, particularly the descriptive case histories and suggested measures of occupational reform by the surgical author Daniel Turner (1667-1741), this book begins to reconstruct the 'lost' half-century of London surgery.

Characterizing a 'Surgical Point of View'

Historians have offered a variety of accounts of surgeons and surgery from disparate perspectives. For example, revisionist historians have begun to examine England's surgical past with aims other than identifying triumphant surgical heroes and explaining their practices only in terms of struggles towards progress. Lucinda Beier has constructed a profile of the types of patients and diseases the seventeenth-century London surgeon Joseph Binns encountered based upon his extant casebook.[8] Margaret Pelling has explained how the public perception of surgical conditions in Tudor London was, to a large extent, determined by contemporary social concerns over ugliness and deformity.[9] Christopher Lawrence has offered a promising 'theoretical model' for redirecting the writing of surgical history.[10] Specifically, Lawrence has drawn upon Owsei Temkin's suggestion of thinking about surgical 'theory' in order to construct an historical account from the 'surgical point of view'.[11] For example, surgical 'theory' of the late Enlightenment may be perceived as the integration of a surgeon's interest in localized anatomy and pathology with an understanding and treatment of 'surgical' diseases.

Other models are found in works of Continental surgical and anatomical history. Vivian Nutton has helpfully redirected the traditional view of surgery as a trade, totally subordinate to medicine and unable to advance upon its own, toward representing surgery as an art which benefited at least as much as medicine from the Renaissance zeal for humanist anatomy.[12] Andrew Cunningham's recent provocative work on anatomy leads one to consider that just as 'anatomists of the past may have seen different bodies' than their present-day counterparts, the surgeons' viewpoints of the body may also have changed over time.[13] By using records from sixteenth-century Florentine hospitals, Katherine Park has shown that particular surgical skills developed as surgeons learned to better manage diseased hospital patients, particularly plague patients.[14] Toby Gelfand has represented the professionalization and related academic institutionalization of Paris surgery by focussing upon the socio-political climate in which Paris surgeons and physicians worked in pre- and post-revolutionary France.[15] Roger Cooter convincingly argued that interrelationships between surgery and war were also essential components in the organization of 'modern' medical practice in the twentieth century.[16]

Women's historians also commonly describe surgical practices, particularly gynaecological surgery, in their writings. Some, like Jean Donnison, have represented male surgical practice as a form of 'controlling' women's bodies.[17] Following a similar argument, Ornella Moscucci developed the socio-economic background of the formulation of a British 'science of woman', (i.e., gynaecology), and relatedly, gynaecological surgery.[18] Ludmilla Jordanova has analysed present-day discourse in which abdominal surgery, sexual pleasure, power, and danger have become integrated.[19] Ann Dally produced an historically acceptable account of women's surgery by balancing the over-rhetorical, ahistorical accounts of many feminist authors with abundant historical cases as factual evidence.[20] More recently, Dally has argued that surgeons' fantasies actually created what they perceived to be necessary conditions for surgical operations.[21]

Developing a better understanding of the 'surgical point of view' has also been the aim of many authors outside the realm of history. Social constructivists like Stefan Hirschauer have argued that the anatomical body may be seen as an 'accomplishment of the sculptural practice of surgical operations'.[22] Charles Anderson has analysed the rhetorical structure of surgeon Richard Seltzer's writings. Examining such passages as 'To cut open the human body, to reach in and pluck out the offending part, the part that would destroy the whole, and then to stitch the body up – it has a beautiful simplicity that the rest of medicine does not own', Anderson discusses a number of conceptual metaphors which he argues have 'enormous implications'.[23] Philip R. Reilly has presented a legal-based medical account of Progressive Era America's 'surgical solution' (i.e., involuntary surgical sterilization) as the preferred method to alleviate the growing numbers of mental and social 'defectives'.[24]

Conceptualizing the 'Surgical Body'

In our visually oriented society, scholarship about the human body has reached an unprecedented level. No disciplinary boundaries delimit those recognized as authorities on the body. Anthropologists and literary critics, together with art and medical historians, have begun to re-examine, reinterpret, and revise representations of the human form. In the maelstrom of postmodernism, the most popular view of the human form is that of a deconstructed body. Some scholars claim that we have culturally deconstructed the body into components which can no longer be reassembled. Have we completely lost our assembly instructions? Who were the 'body snatchers'? If we, as fellow human beings, can no longer agree upon what was once envisioned as the body, have we lost part of what it means to be human?

The extent to which the body expresses an individual's identity or, more symbolically, a collective cultural identity remains a crucial question.[25] Humans adorn their outer surfaces with various markings and coverings that reflect images of their inner selves. However, markings such as tattoos, piercings, and mutilations may, in certain instances, represent cultural mores. Frances E. Mascia-Lees and Patricia Sharpe have argued that these markings and other adornments indicate that the body is regularly used as a canvas upon which a culture's truths and anxieties materialize.[26] However, marking the body also paradoxically obscures its presence.

Given this cultural preoccupation with the body, it may at first be difficult to see why so much scholarship has been directed to what academics have termed 'the disappearance of the body'. Works have emerged under the titles *Denaturalization of the Body, The Body's Recollection of Being, Posthuman Bodies,* and *The Absent Body.*[27] How can the body at once be so visibly enshrined by our culture and also have physically, or at least figuratively, disappeared?

Part of this cultural dilemma may be clarified by conceptualizing a surgical view of the body, in short, a surgical body. Before the growth of Renaissance anatomy, surgeons and their patients viewed the body in an holistic sense.[28] Disseminating the knowledge gained from dissections resulted in a paradigm shift of the surgical body. The 'modern' surgical body gradually became viewed as a mechanical machine composed of discrete parts.[29] By the Enlightenment, surgical craftsmen were mechanically reconstructing and replacing damaged and lost bodily parts.[30] Similar to an artist's ability to pick and choose distinct images as represented in William Hogarth's 1753 *Analysis of Beauty*, surgeons could supply deficient, defective or desired bodily parts *à la carte.*[31] The surgical art became more limb-oriented than body-oriented. Restoring use to limbs held particular socio-economic importance as such procedures allowed soldiers and sailors to continue defending their nation and civilians to return to their normal means of employment.

In order to conceptualize a more precise form of the surgical body, specific surgeons' and patients' views are needed. Biographical accounts of surgeons and their patients can help provide this required information.

Biography as History

Biography remains one of the most enduring genres of writing. Richard Holmes, the best-selling biographer of Samuel Taylor Coleridge, Percy Bysshe Shelley and other romantics argued that the

> great appeal of biography seems to lie, in part, in its claim to a coherent and integral view of human affairs. It is based on the profoundly hopeful assumption that people really are responsible for their actions, and that there is a moral continuity between the inner and the outer man.[32]

Some authors discount biography as history, claiming that the chosen subjects are typically 'literary rather than historical', or that the authors 'opt for narrative rather than analysis'.[33] Ian Hamilton, in reviewing how biographers and their subjects collaboratively create reputations and legacies, claimed that the process of biographical writing has often been construed much like 'arguing about abortion or capital punishment: minds tend to be made up before you start'.[34] Others query whether biography is 'merely a higher form of literary gossip'.[35]

I contend that all biography is, by definition, history – life history. Still, the level of historical accuracy and historiographical input is wide ranging. *Biography*, the gossipy American Arts & Entertainment television channel magazine, presents quite a different view of its subjects than does *Biography*, the scholarly quarterly published by the renowned Center for Biographical Research in Hawaii.

Science and medicine have long been popularized through biography.[36] 'Veritable industries' have been created in attempts to chronicle and explain the lives of individuals including Christopher Columbus, William Harvey, Isaac Newton, Charles Darwin, Florence Nightingale, Louis Pasteur, Joseph Lister, Marie Curie, Albert Einstein, and Sigmund Freud; individuals who, biographers claim, have significantly altered the course of science or medicine.[37] Of late, however, biographers have also begun to explore the lives of less well-known individuals. This change in focus, as Thomas Hankins has shown, is consistent with the general historiographical movement away from Whiggish heroic accounts towards writing history from the view of the common individual (i.e., history 'from below').[38] From another viewpoint, this shift away from a 'Great Doctors' male-oriented history appears to have resulted from recent reassessment of what females have contributed to science and medicine.[39] Well known among these recent revisionist accounts are Regina Morantz-Sanchez's and Londa Schiebinger's biographical sketches of the women they recognize as notable physicians and scientists, respectively.[40]

Attempts to redress earlier heroic accounts of surgeons by mapping them on 'a wider ... social canvas' are slow in coming.[41] This process has been hampered, in part, by the difficulty of discerning the extent to which a surgeon's practice was distinguishable from related occupations.[42] According to the historical model of 'marketplace practice', the practices of physicians, surgeons, apothecaries, and barbers were separated by quite fluid boundaries. Furthermore, generalizing about the type of surgical care most people received is, as Margaret Pelling and Charles Webster have convincingly argued, quite a complicated task when considering that unlicensed or unauthorized healers appear to have dominated the field.[43]

Among the most elaborate attempts at extrapolating a surgeon's writing to describe contemporary society is Marie-Christine Pouchelle's biographical account of the fourteenth-century surgeon, Henri de Mondeville. Beyond describing this surgeon's 'profession', Pouchelle used de Mondeville's *Chirurgerie* to develop a broad account of medieval attitudes toward the body.[44] Robert Jutte, Joan Lane, and Aloys Henning have developed more conventional models of the social history of surgery through their use of biography.[45] Anne Digby has literally mapped the geographical range of two late eighteenth-century surgeon's practices.[46]

It has been said of Turner's contemporary John Woodward that, although 'not a great man', he was a man of 'near greatness, ... who left his mark upon his own time, and ... for a long time afterward, but who slipped ... gradually ... into oblivion'. By examining Woodward's 'many-sided' characteristics, his 'sundry interests' and his 'several careers', Joseph Levine has vastly expanded our understanding, not only of Woodward, but more significantly of the contemporary meaning of the 'ancient–modern' dispute in which Woodward so ardently participated.[47] With similar skill, Roy Porter has taken the life of Thomas Beddoes, a physician whose reputation after his death in 1808 'soon became just a historical footnote', and reconstructed an historical account of the meaning of health and medicine, the 'oral culture' of sickness, and a physician's confrontations with the 'Enlightened classes'.[48] Most recently, Harold Cook, in a prize-winning effort, has effectively integrated the story of an individual practitioner, Joannes Groenevelt, a Dutch physician in London, into an elaborate account of Early Modern English and Dutch societies.[49]

This book provides an account of the career and writings of the currently little-known surgeon and physician, Daniel Turner (1667-1741).[50] Turner's prolific writings provide valuable insight into the surgical practice of a commonplace Enlightenment surgeon. Examining Turner's personal, 'professional' and genteel achievements enhances our understanding of the strength of the boundary between surgeons and physicians in Enlightenment 'marketplace' practice. In addition to reconstructing some of the social context within which Turner worked, I also identify key intellectual motivations underlying the personal choices that Turner made throughout his career. Indeed, his life history offers a remarkable example of the struggles, successes, and failures of one individual's attempts to move upward in Enlightenment London. This account is neither psychobiography nor 'micro-history'. Rather, by using Turner's life solely as a lens to examine contemporary society, I concentrate more upon biography in order to offer a 'respectable fragment' of some of the highlights of one individual's life work which specifically illuminate certain aspects of Enlightenment surgical practice.[51] Overall, this analysis of both Turner's writings and life activities corroborates Richard Holmes' declaration about biography, that the 'public and the private life do, in the end, make sense of each other; and the one is meaningless without the other'.[52]

Notes

1 Perhaps Sir D'Arcy Power's historical writings best exemplify this approach. Many of his works are found, together with a complete bibliography in his *Selected Writings 1877-1930* (Oxford: Clarendon Press, 1931). Jessie Dobson's insightful account into 'The Training of a Surgeon', *Annals of the Royal College of Surgeons of England*, xxxiv (1964), 1-36 is weighted toward early practice, as is T. C. Allbutt's *The Historical Relation of Medicine and Surgery to the End of the Sixteenth Century* (London: Macmillan, 1905). R. Theodore Beck's *The Cutting Edge: Early History of the Surgeons of London* (London: Lund Humphries, 1974) traces surgical history from *The Leechbook* (circa 970) through Thomas Vicary and his contemporaries of the mid-sixteenth century. Surgery is also presented as a succession of advancements in Gert Brieger's 'The Development of Surgery: Historical Aspects Important in the Origin and Development of Modern Surgical Science' in D. C. Sabiston (ed.), *Christopher's Textbook of Surgery*, 10th edn (Philadelphia: W. B. Saunders Co., 1972), 1-25, and in Owen H. Wangensteen and Sarah D. Wangensteen, *The Rise of Surgery: From Empiric Craft to Scientific Discipline* (Folkestone, Kent: William Dawson & Sons, 1978). For a review of Richard Wiseman, see Alan DeForest Smith, 'Richard Wiseman: His Contributions to English Surgery', *Bulletin of the New York Academy of Medicine*, xlvi (1970), 167-182, and John Kirkup's introduction in the reprint of Wiseman's *Of Wounds, Of Gun-shot*

Wounds, Of Fractures and Luxations (Bath: Kingmead, 1977), xi-xxi. Key works on John Hunter include L.S. Jacyna's 'Images of John Hunter in the Nineteenth Century', *History of Science*, xxi (1983), 85-108, and Elizabeth Allen, J.L. Turk, and Sir Reginald Murley (eds), *The Case Books of John Hunter, FRS* (London: Royal Society of Medicine Services, Ltd., 1993).

2 Fenwick Beekman, 'The Rise of British Surgery in the Eighteenth Century', *Annals of Medical History*, n.s., ix (1937), 549-66. See also Sir Clifford Naunton Morgan, 'Surgery and Surgeons in 18th-Century London', *Annals of the Royal College of Surgeons of England*, xxxxii (1968), 1-37. Samuel Sharp provided one of the earliest accounts of eighteenth-century surgery in *A Critical Enquiry into the Present State of Surgery* (London: J & R Tonson, 1750). See also Benjamin Gooch, *Practical Treatise of Wounds and other Chirurgical Subjects to which is Prefixed a Short Historical Account of the Rise and Progress of Surgery and Anatomy* (Norwich: published by the author, 1767), and George Parker, *The Early History of Surgery in Great Britain, its Organization and Development* (London: A & C Beach, 1920). The eighteenth-century coverage in each of these works focused on the latter half of the century. Ghislane Lawrence also skipped over the early eighteenth century in her account of 'Traditional' Surgery in W.F. Bynum and Roy Porter (eds), *Companion Encyclopedia of the History of Medicine* (London: Routledge, 1993), vol. 2, 961-83. 'Modern' surgery has been described as either that in the post-anesthetic era as in Frederick F. Cartwright's *The Development of Modern Surgery* (London: Arthur Baker, Ltd, 1967) or in the post-antiseptic/aseptic era as in Ulrich Trohler's overview of 'Modern' surgery in W.F. Bynum and Roy Porter (eds), *Companion Encyclopedia of the History of Medicine* (London: Routledge, 1993), vol. 2, 984-1029.

3 Susan C. Lawrence, *Charitable Knowledge: Hospital Pupils and Practitioners in Eighteenth-Century London* (Cambridge, Massachusetts: Cambridge University Press, 1996). The same period is central to Ulrich Tröhler's 'Quantification in British Medicine and Surgery, 1750-1830: With special reference to its introduction into therapeutics' (Ph.D. thesis, University of London, 1978), whereas Eric Shelton-Jones also omitted study of the early eighteenth century in his 'The Barber-Surgeons Company of London and Medical Education 1540-1660' (M.Phil. thesis, University of London, 1981). One notable exception in Norris Saakwa-Mante's discussion of early eighteenth-century surgeon John Atkins, in a chapter of his Harvard thesis tentatively entitled 'Constructing Race for Georgian Navy

Surgeons: The Discourse of John Atkins'.

4 William R. Le Fanu, 'The Lost Half-Century in English Medicine, 1700-1750', *Bulletin of the History of Medicine,* xlvi (1972), 319-48.

5 Frederic W.-B. Deleyiannis described this 'disintegration' of the Company in 'The United Company of Barbers and Surgeons of London, 1540-1745: Union and Disintegration' (M.A. thesis, Cambridge University, 1990). Some pre-1745 records of the Barber-Surgeons' Company have also been lost, thereby preventing a complete account of these years from an institutional view. Sidney Young claimed, in 1890, that the Barber-Surgeons' Company's Court of Assistants' Minutes Books from 1651 to 1689 were missing. See his *Annals of the Barber-Surgeons of London* (London: Blades, East & Blades, 1890), iv and 220. Jessie Dobson and R. Milnes Walker state that additional records were lost during the Second World War when the Barber's Hall and the Clerk's offices were destroyed. See *Barbers and Barber-Surgeons of London* (Oxford: Blackwell Scientific Publications, 1979), xv.

6 I have compiled this list of surgical writings from the chronological catalogue of holdings at the Wellcome Institute for the History of Medicine (London), as well as consulting the collections of the British Library, the Royal Society, the Royal Colleges of Surgeons of England and Edinburgh, the Historical Library, Yale University School of Medicine (New Haven), the Clendening Medical Library (Kansas City), and the Short Title Catalogues of the National Library of Medicine (Bethesda). During this period, at least sixteen different domestic manuals also appeared, most of which included sections of surgical remedies in addition to 'domestic concerns' such as cookery and cosmetics. For a more thorough account of the surgical remedies in these manuals see Philip K. Wilson, 'Acquiring Surgical Know-How: Occupational and Lay Instruction in Early Eighteenth-Century London', in Roy Porter (ed.), *The Popularization of Medicine 1650-1850* (London: Routledge, 1992), esp. 45-50.

7 I previously discussed the surgical writings from this period which appeared in the English vernacular in 'Vernacularisation vs. Vulgarisation of Early Eighteenth-Century English Surgical Writings', *Transactions of the Eighth International Congress on the Enlightenment* (Oxford: Voltaire Foundation, 1993), v.7. Science et technologie, 1169-72.

8 See 'A London Surgeon's Career: Joseph Binns', chapter 3 in Lucinda McCray Beier's *Sufferers & Healers: The Experience of Illness in Seventeenth-Century England* (London: Routledge & Kegan Paul, 1987), 51-96, and the revised version, 'Seventeenth-Century English

Surgery: The Casebook of Joseph Binns', in Christopher Lawrence (ed.), *Surgical Theory, Medical Practice: Studies in the History of Surgery* (London: Routledge, 1992), 48-84.

9 Margaret Pelling 'Appearance and Reality: Barber-Surgeons, the Body and Disease', in A.L. Beier and Roger Finlay (eds), *London 1500-1700: The Making of the Metropolis* (London: Longman, 1986), 82-112.

10 Christopher Lawrence, 'Democratic, Divine and Heroic: the History and Historiography of Surgery', in C. Lawrence (ed.), *Surgical Theory, Medical Practice*, 1-47. For a modern self-reflection into the surgical decision-making process, see Charles M. Abernathy and Robert M. Hamm, *Surgical Intuition: What It Is and How To Get It* (Philadelphia: Hanley & Belfus, Inc., 1995).

11 Owsei Temkin, 'The Role of Surgery in the Rise of Modern Medical Thought', *Bulletin of the History of Medicine*, xxv (1951), 248-259.

12 Vivian Nutton, 'Humanist Surgery' in A. Wear, R.K. French, and I.M. Lonie (eds), *The Medical Renaissance of the Sixteenth Century* (Cambridge: Cambridge University Press, 1985), 75-99.

13 Andrew Cunningham, *The Anatomical Renaissance. The Resurrection of the Anatomical Projects of the Ancients* (Aldershot, Hampshire: Scolar Press, 1997), 7.

14 Katherine Park, 'Healing the Poor: Hospitals and Medical Assistance in Renaissance Florence', in Jonathan Barry and Colin Jones (eds), *Medicine and Charity Before the Welfare State* (London: Routledge, 1991), esp. 30-9. Covering a similar period, Nancy Siraisi addressed a series of concerns about 'Surgeons and Surgery' in her *Medieval and Early Renaissance Medicine: An Introduction to Knowledge and Practice* (Chicago: University of Chicago Press, 1990), 153-86, with such clarity and insight that this work serves as a pertinent starting point for historians discussing surgery of any period.

15 Toby Gelfand, *Professionalizing Modern Medicine: Paris Surgeons and Medical Science and Institutions in the Eighteenth Century* (Westport, Connecticut: Greenwood Press, 1980).

16 Roger Cooter, *Surgery and Society in Peace and War: Orthopaedics and the Organization of Modern Medicine* (Houndmills, Basingstoke, Hampshire: Macmillan Press Ltd, 1993).

17 Jean Donnison, *Midwives and Medical Men: A History of the Struggle for the Control of Childbirth*, 2nd edn. (New Barnet, Hertfordshire: Historical Publications, Ltd., 1988).

18 Ornella Moscucci, *The Science of Woman: Gynaecology and Gender in England, 1800-1920* (Cambridge: Cambridge University Press, 1990). See also Jane Eliot Sewell, 'Bountiful Bodies: Spencer Wells,

Lawson Tait, and the Birth of British Gynaecology' (Ph.D. thesis, Johns Hopkins University, 1991).

19 Ludmilla Jordanova, *Sexual Visions: Images of Gender in Science and Medicine Between the Eighteenth and Twentieth Centuries* (Madison: University of Wisconsin Press, 1989), esp. 150-3.

20 Ann Dally described women's ordeals with surgeons and surgery based on nineteenth- and twentieth-century sources in *Women Under the Knife: A History of Surgery* (London: Hutchinson Radius, 1991).

21 Ann Dally, *Fantasy Surgery; 1880-1930: With Special Reference to Sir William Arbuthnot Lane* (Amsterdam: Rodopi, 1996). For an insightful perspective on American surgery from this period see Dale C. Smith, 'Appendicitis, Appendectomy, and the Surgeon', *Bulletin of the History of Medicine*, lxx (1996), 414-41.

22 Stefan Hirschauer, 'The Manufacture of Bodies in Surgery', *Social Studies of Science*, xxi (1991), 279.

23 Charles M. Anderson, *Richard Seltzer and the Rhetoric of Surgery* (Carbondale: Southern Illinois University Press, 1989), 10.

24 Philip R. Reilly, *The Surgical Solution. A History of Involuntary Sterilization in the United States* (Baltimore: Johns Hopkins University Press, 1991).

25 This current of thought permeates much of the voluminous research on the body. Key works which have addressed the Enlightenment body are Barbara Marie Stafford, *Body Criticism: Imaging the Unseen in Enlightenment Art and Medicine* (Cambridge, Massachusetts: The MIT Press, 1991); Roy Porter, 'Bodies of Thought: Thoughts about the Body in Eighteenth-Century England' in Joan H. Pittock and Andrew Wear (eds), *Interpretation and Cultural History* (New York: St. Martin's, 1991), 82-108, Lynn Hunt (ed.), *Eroticism and the Body Politic* (Baltimore: Johns Hopkins University Press, 1991), Estelle Cohen, 'The Body as a Historical Category: Science and Imagination, 1660-1760', in Mary G. Winkler and Letha B. Cole (eds), *The Good Body. Asceticism in Contemporary Culture* (New Haven: Yale University Press, 1994), 67-90; and Mary Fissell, 'Gender and Generation: Representing Reproduction in Early Modern England', *Gender & History*, vii (1995), 432-56. Two exceptional works of related interest are Carol Houlihan Flynn, *The Body in Swift and Defoe* (Cambridge: Cambridge University Press, 1990), and Aileen Douglas, *Uneasy Sensations. Smollett and the Body* (Chicago: University of Chicago Press, 1995).

26 Frances E. Mascia-Lees and Patricia Sharpe, 'The Marked and the Un(re)Marked: Tattoo and Gender in Theory and Narrative', in Frances E. Mascia-Lees and Patricia Sharpe (eds), *Tattoo, Torture,*

Mutilation and Adornment. The Denaturalization of the Body in Culture and Text (Albany: State University of New York Press, 1992), 164.

27 Frances E. Mascia-Lees and Patricia Sharpe, *Tattoo, Torture, Mutilation and Adornment. The Denaturalization of the Body* (Albany: State University of New York Press, 1992); David Michael Levin, *The Body's Recollection of Being: Phenomenological Psychology and the Deconstruction of Nihilism* (London: Routledge and Kegan Paul, 1985); Judith Halberstam and Ira Livingston (eds), *Posthuman Bodies* (Bloomington: Indiana University Press, 1995); and Drew Leder, *The Absent Body* (Chicago: University of Chicago Press, 1990).

28 Tony Hunt provides a literal interpretation of the iconography in the 13th-century manuscript prepared by Roger Frudard of Parma's students in *The Medieval Surgeon* (Woodbridge: The Boydell Press, 1992). For an excellent discussion of the cultural perspective of Renaissance dissection see Jonathan Sawday, *The Body Emblazoned. Dissection and the Human Body in Renaissance Culture* (London: Routledge, 1995). See also Caroline Walker Bynum, *The Resurrection of the Body in Western Christianity* (New York: Columbia University Press, 1995).

29 David F. Channell lucidly traces the intellectual shifts into the mechanical and organic worldviews in *The Vital Machine: A Study of Technology and Organic Life* (Oxford: Oxford University Press, 1991).

30 Similar procedures had, however, been performed for centuries, although on a limited basis. Enlightenment practitioner Richard Boulton described the 'ancient' four-fold art of surgery as consisting of 1) synthesis – 'to join together Parts unnaturally separated', 2) diaresis – 'to separate Parts which preternaturally happen to be joined together', 3) exaeresis – 'to take away what is superfluous', and 4) anaplerosis – 'to add what is wanting' (*A System of Rational and Practical Chirurgery* (London: W. Taylor & W. Innys, 1713), 6). Benjamin Gooch added two additional activities, 1) prosthesis – 'supplying deficiency', and 2) diorthosis – 'restoring parts to their proper places' in his *Practical Treatise of Wounds and other Chirurgical Subjects to which is Prefixed a Short Historical Account of the Rise and Progress of Surgery and Anatomy* (Norwich: The Author, 1767), vol. 1, 6.

31 Fiona Haslam more thoroughly analyses the medical content of Hogarth's popular works in her *From Hogarth to Rowlandson: Medicine in Art in Eighteenth Century Britain* (Liverpool: Liverpool University Press, 1996). Although surgeons still do not have the flexibility of Hogarth, Joseph Vacanti, a Boston Children's Hospital

surgeon, recently claimed that it is only a matter of time before 'we'll learn to generate living prosthetics for every organ system in the body'. (Geoffrey Cowley, 'Replacement Parts', *Newsweek*, cxxix (27 January 1997), 66). In this sense, art forms of the body may replace natural forms.

32 Richard Holmes, *Footsteps. Adventures of a Romantic Biographer* (New York, Penguin, 1985), 175.

33 Raphael Samuel, *Theatres of Memory. Volume 1: Past and Present in Contemporary Culture* (London: Verso, 1994), 4.

34 Ian Hamilton, *Keepers of the Flame: Literary Estates and the Rise of Biography* (London: Pimlico, 1993), vii.

35 *Biography, Granta 41* (New York: Penguin, 1992), back cover notes.

36 David Novarr has provided a most useful anthology of various approaches to the art and theory of biography in *The Lines of Life: Theories of Biography, 1880-1970* (West Lafayette, Indiana: Purdue University Press, 1986). See also Ulick O'Connor, *Biographers and the Art of Biography* (Dublin: Wolfhound Press, 1991).

37 Susan Sheets-Pyenson used this term in her helpful 'New Directions for Scientific Biography: The Case of Sir William Dawson', *History of Science*, xxviii (1990), 399-410.

38 Thomas L. Hankins, 'In Defence of Biography: The Use of Biography in the History of Science', *History of Science,* xvii (1979), 1-16. Michael Shortland and Richard Yeo have enhanced this field with their edited collection, *Telling Lives in Science: Essays on Scientific Biography* (Cambridge: Cambridge University Press, 1996), the first thorough attempt to examine the development of scientific biography.

39 Lois Magner has attempted to realign the balance of biographical focus by including many women in her edited *Doctors, Nurses, and Medical Practitioners: A Bio-Bibliographical Sourcebook* (Westport, Connecticut: Greenwood Press, 1997). Still, some recent authors like Sherwin Nuland perceive a demand for the more traditional 'Great Doctors' approach with writings like his *Doctors: The Biography of Medicine* (New York: Random House, 1995), albeit Nuland devotes a chapter to 'Helen Taussig and the Blue-Baby Operation'.

40 Regina Markell Morantz-Sanchez, *Sympathy and Science: Women Physicians in American Medicine* (New York: Oxford University Press, 1985), and Londa Schiebinger, *The Mind Has No Sex?: Women in the Origins of Modern Science* (Cambridge, Massachusetts: Harvard University Press, 1989). For a detailed account of a woman's successful crusade as a surgeon in the nineteenth century, see Regina Morantz-Sanchez's 'Making It in a Man's World: The Late-

Nineteenth-Century Surgical Career of Mary Amanda Dixon Jones', *Bulletin of the History of Medicine*, lxix (1995), 542-68. One considerably earlier example is Kate Campbell Hurd Mead's *History of Women in Medicine from the Earliest Times to the Beginning of the Nineteenth Century* (1938). For further discussion of American women as practitioners and patients see Rima D. Apple (ed.), *Women, Health, and Medicine in America* (New York: Garland Publishing, Inc., 1990).

41 C. Lawrence, 'Democratic, Divine and Heroic', 13.

42 Roy Porter, Harold Cook, and Lucinda Beier among others have described medical 'services' of the seventeenth and eighteenth centuries as being provided through a 'marketplace' of practice.

43 Margaret Pelling and Charles Webster, 'Medical Practitioners', in Charles Webster (ed.), *Health, Medicine and Mortality in the Sixteenth Century* (Cambridge: Cambridge University Press, 1979), esp. 182.

44 Marie-Christine Pouchelle, *The Body & Surgery in the Middle Ages*, translated by Rosemary Morris (Cambridge: Polity Press, 1990).

45 See Aloys Henning's *Die Affäre Hillmer: Ein Okulist aus Berlin in Petersburg 1751* (Frankfurt am Main: Peter Lang, 1987) and an abbreviated English translation as 'A German oculist in Russia', *Documenta Ophthalmologica*, lxxvii (1991), 277-93. Robert Jütte's 'A Seventeenth-Century German Barber-Surgeon and his Patients', *Medical History*, xxxiii (1989),184-98, together with Joan Lane's 'Eighteenth-Century Medical Practice: A Case Study of Bradford Wilmer, Surgeon of Coventry', *Social History of Medicine*, iii (1990), 369-386, and Joan Lane and Anne Tarver's 'Henry Fogg (1707-1750) and his Patients: The Practice of an Eighteenth-Century Staffordshire Apothecary', *Medical History*, xxxvii (1993), 187-196 provide exemplary, brief biographical accounts which contextualize the practices of ordinary practitioners.

46 Anne Digby diagrammed the geographical range of William Goodwin's and William Elmhirst's general surgical practices in *Making A Medical Living: Doctors and Patients in the English Market for Medicine, 1720-1911* (Cambridge, Massachusetts: Cambridge University Press, 1994), 112-116.

47 Joseph M. Levine, *Dr. Woodward's Shield: History, Science and Satire in Augustan England* (Berkeley: University of California Press, 1977), 3-4.

48 Roy Porter's biography, *Doctor of Society: Thomas Beddoes and the Sick Trade in Late-Enlightenment England* (London: Routledge, 1992), probably fulfils many historians' expectations of integrating

the story of an individual with a story of society.

49 Harold J. Cook's *Trials of an Ordinary Doctor: Joannes Groenevelt in Seventeenth-Century London* (Baltimore: Johns Hopkins University Press, 1994) won the William H. Welch medal from the American Association for the History of Medicine in 1997. For a more synoptical account of Groenevelt, see Cook's 'Medical Innovation or Medical Malpractice? Or, A Dutch Physician in London: Joannes Groenevelt, 1694-1700', *Tractrix*, ii (1990), 63-91.

50 Turner is mentioned in most standard biographical compilations of surgeons and physicians. But beyond a few brief biographical articles, mostly in dermatological periodicals, Turner's writings are little known even among medical historians. Writings which discuss Turner include John E. Lane, 'Daniel Turner and the First Degree of Doctor of Medicine Conferred in the English Colonies of North America by Yale College in 1723', *Annals of Medical History*, 2nd series, ii (1919), 367-80; L.J.A. Lowenthal, 'Daniel Turner and "De Morbis Cutaneis"', *Archives of Dermatology*, lxxxv (1962), 517-23; P.J. Hare, *Our Credulous Countryman* (Edinburgh: Constable Publication, 1968); Ruth J. Mann, 'Daniel Turner, the First British Dermatologist', *Mayo Clinic Proceedings*, li (1976), 62-66. Alan Lyell, 'Daniel Turner (1667-740) LRCP London (1711) M.D. Honorary, Yale (1723) Surgeon, Physician and Pioneer Dermatologist: The Man Seen in the Pages of His Book on the Skin', *International Journal of Dermatology*, xxi (1982), 162-170; Idem, 'Daniel Turner, and the First Controlled Therapeutic Trial in Dermatology', *Clinical and Experimental Dermatology*, xi (1986),191-194.

51 I borrow D.A. Stauffer's term as cited by Donald J. Winslow in 'Glossary of Terms in Life Writing Part I', *Biography*, i (1978), 66.

52 Holmes, *Footsteps*, 175.

2

Entering the Surgical Trade

Conceived in the year of London's great fire, Daniel Turner was born on 18 September 1667, the third son of John and Rebecca Turner.[1] Standard biographical sources claim Daniel Turner was born in London, however surviving parish records offer no conclusive evidence of his birthplace. Turner spent his early years in Holborn, near 'Gray's-Inn-Gate'.[2] Later, his family moved to the St Andrew, Holborn parish.[3]

In contrast to the vivid accounts Turner later provided about his surgical training, he revealed no clues about his early education. Such withholding of information suggests that Turner viewed his background as commonplace or perhaps somewhat degrading. Extant London grammar school records fail to provide evidence as to the whereabouts of his earliest education.[4] As a student, he probably gained a rudimentary knowledge of Latin and Greek.[5] His frequent use of these foreign tongues in later writings suggests a familiarity with both languages. However, one critic claimed Turner communicated through no more than a 'poor, low, paultry school-boy's Latin'.[6] Turner likely received a strict moral Anglican upbringing. His public writings and private devotional suggest that he revered the Bible as his ethical guide throughout life.[7]

Becoming a Surgeon through Apprenticeship

By traditional standards, London apprenticeships entailed seven years of servitude under a master of a particular guild or company. Since 1540, London surgeons and barbers were combined into the single company of Barber-Surgeons (Figure 2.1). However, no one actually practised as a 'barber-surgeon' in London. Barbers did bleed patients as part of their regular practice, but this was the only surgical-like procedure that the surgeons officially sanctioned.[8]

A few lists of late seventeenth-century Barber-Surgeon apprenticeships survive.[9] It remains difficult, however, to ascertain precisely what apprentices accomplished during their servitudes. Few diaries have survived if, indeed, many ever existed.[10] Legal documents typically indicate instances of malevolent masters and recalcitrant apprentices, yet mention little if any of the training that apprentices received.[11]

Records of the Barber-Surgeons' Company of London provide some information about Turner's surgical training. He first applied himself as an apprentice to the surgeon Charles Bateman, probably in 1684 (Figure 2.2).[12] Bateman descended from a prominent lineage of surgeons that continued into eighteenth-century London. When Turner became an apprentice, Bateman had at least three other apprentices: Jeremiah Merry, Catton Chamberlaine, and Samuel Faulkner.[13] After only two years of servitude to Bateman, Turner was 'turned over' to another master, the London surgeon Thomas Lichfield on 4 February 1686.[14] Both Lichfield and Bateman were 'freemen' of London's Barber-Surgeons' Company, meaning they were granted the 'freedom' to practise their trade within the city.

By the late seventeenth century, the Barber-Surgeons' Company, one of the capital's 63 'minor' companies, had become one of the largest.[15] Company historian, Sidney Young estimated that there were, in any year between 1670 and 1745, 75 practising freemen of this Company.[16] Figure 2.3 indicates that between 1690 and 1715, the years Turner was involved with the Company, barbers comprised between one-half and two-thirds of the freemen of this company.[17] The 'others' identified in this figure represent freemen including the

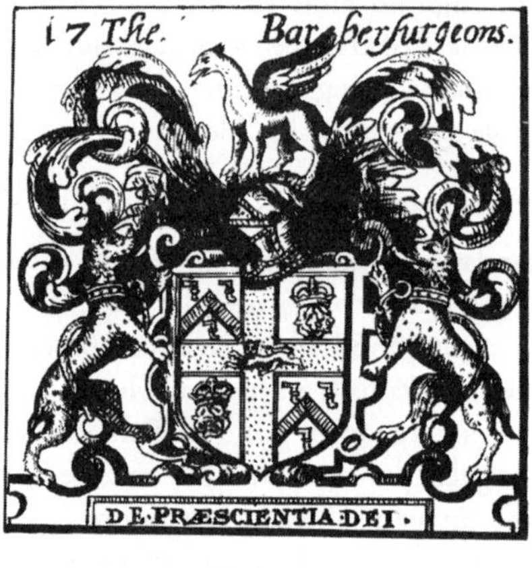

Figure 2.1
Crest of the Barber-Surgeons' Company of London (Wellcome Institute Library, London)

razor and instrument makers, perfumers, haberdashers, distillers, cutlers, taylors, patten makers, leather trimmers, book binders, painters, blacksmiths, weavers, drapers, and other trade workers whose talents allowed the company to operate self-sufficiently.

The Barber-Surgeons' Company was governed by a master, three wardens, and a twenty-member Court of Assistants.[18] During Turner's servitude, his master, Thomas Lichfield was a member of the Court. The surgical half of this governing body examined entering surgical apprentices in their 'ability in reading and understanding the Latin Tongue'.[19] Once apprentices completed their seven-year servitudes, elected Company examiners assessed their

> Skill, Experience, and Knowledge ... not only in the External and Actuall Practice [of Surgery,] But also in their Internal Speculation of the Natural Causes and Remedies of all ... Infirmities or Diseases Incident to their ... Profession.[20]

Approved candidates received a diploma permitting them to practise surgery in London or within its 7-mile perimeter in a manner conforming with the Company's 'Rules of Practice'. Company wardens were called upon to judge any surgeon who was claimed to have 'Ignorantly unskillfully or willfully' administered remedies

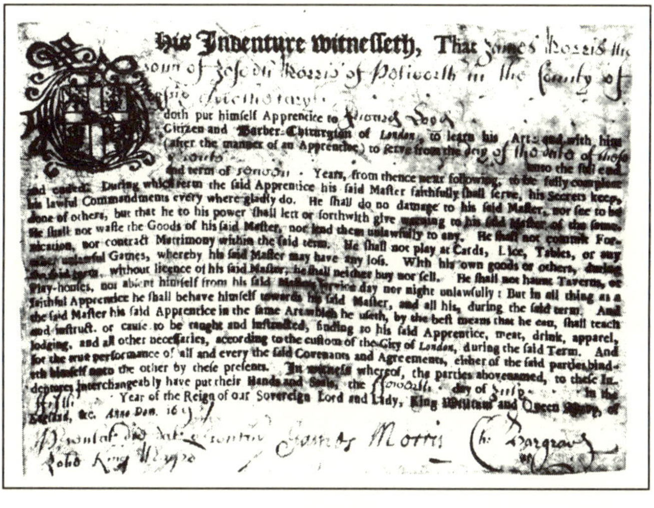

This Indenture witnesseth, That James Morris the sonn of Joseph Morris of Policorth in the County of [illegible]

doth put himself Apprentice to [illegible]
Citizen and Barber-Chirurgion of *London*, to learn his Art; and with him (after the manner of an Apprentice) to serve from the day of the date of these [illegible] unto the full end and term of seven Years, from thence next following, to be fully compleat and ended. During which term the said Apprentice his said Master faithfully shall serve, his Secrets keep, his lawful Commandments every where gladly do. He shall do no damage to his said Master, nor see to be done of others, but that he to his power shall lett or forthwith give warning to his said Master of the same. He shall not waste the Goods of his said Master, nor lend them unlawfully to any. He shall not commit Fornication, nor contract Matrimony within the said term. He shall not play at Cards, Dice, Tables, or any other unlawful Games, whereby his said Master may have any loss. With his own goods or others, during the said term, without licence of his said Master, he shall neither buy nor sell. He shall not haunt Taverns, or Play-houses, nor absent himself from his said Masters service day nor night unlawfully: But in all thing as a faithful Apprentice he shall behave himself towards his said Master, and all his, during the said term. And the said Master his said Apprentice in the same Art which he useth, by the best means that he can, shall teach and instruct, or cause to be taught and instructed, finding to his said Apprentice, meat, drink, apparel, lodging, and all other necessaries, according to the custom of the City of *London*, during the said Term. And for the true performance of all and every the said Covenants and Agreements, either of the said parties bindeth himself unto the other by these presents. In witness whereof, the parties abovenamed, to these Indentures interchangeably have put their Hands and Seals, the [illegible] day of [illegible] In the [illegible] Year of the Reign of our Sovereign Lord and Lady, King William and Queen Mary, of England, &c. *Anno Dom.* 16[illegible]

James Morris

Figure 2.2

One of the few surviving contemporary indentures into seven years of servitude as a Barber-Surgeons' apprentice

(Wellcome Institute Library, London)

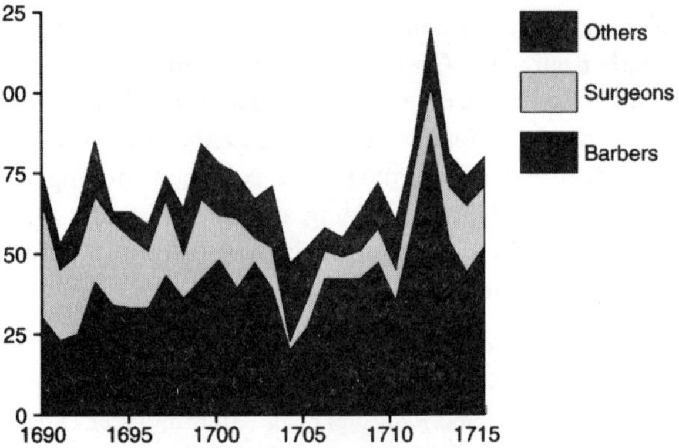

Figure 2.3
Freeman Admissions into the Barber-Surgeons' Company of London
(Compiled from Guildhall Library MS 5265)

'Contrary Repugnant or Incongruent' to the 'true Indications of Surgery'.[21] Additionally, they apportioned necessary corrective and punitive measures as stipulated in their Company's by-laws.

During Turner's servitude, Lichfield oversaw the training of three other apprentices: his son, John Lichfield, Roger Fenwick, and Hy Watson.[22] As was common in this period, Turner and the other apprentices most likely resided in Lichfield's home, in the St Botolph without Bishopsgate parish, throughout their servitude.

Turner remained in Lichfield's servitude through 1691. On 2 February of that year, Turner was admitted into the freedom of the Barber-Surgeons' Company.[23] Eight years passed, however, before Turner was 'sent for' by the Company to take his examination on 23 March 1699/1700.[24] Turner's master, Thomas Lichfield, was Master of the Barber-Surgeons' Company in 1699, and most likely sponsored Turner's candidacy for examination. At the Examination Committee meeting on 12 June 1700, Turner was presented before the Company's examiners, including Company Wardens John Pinke, James Wall, and Bartholomew King, as well as liverymen including William Oades, William Layfield, Henry Rossington, Zachariah Gibson, Mr Babington, and Sergeant-Surgeon Thomas Gardiner.[25] The examiners approved of Turner's answers and affixed the Company's seal upon his 'letter testimoniall'.[26] Turner was charged a fee for this 'privilege', and according to tradition, would have presented each of his examiners with a pair of gloves.[27] The following 15 October, Turner was admitted into the 'livery' or clothing of the Company.[28] More money would have been paid for this privilege, as well as for the robe and regalia of a liveryman.

Alternatives to Apprenticeship

Turner later advocated apprenticeship as the ideal form of surgical training. However, during his own apprenticeship, the Company of Barber-Surgeons experienced much of the city-wide general breakdown of guild control.[29] The time-honoured method of apprenticeship as the sole mode of entry into the practice of surgery had begun to erode. Specifically, the number of apprentices trained under surgeons who were recognized as freemen of the Company was declining. Figure 2.4 is a graph of the proportional distribution of barbers and surgeons who were registered as apprentices each year between 1680 and 1715.[30] As this Figure suggests, the number of surgeon apprentices who registered with the Company (i.e., the slashed line segment) began to decrease (i.e., narrow) after 1680, and more markedly declined after 1700. The diminishing numbers of surgeons trained by servitude more distinctly shown on Figure 2.5.[31]

Alternative entrées into surgical practice which circumvented lengthy servitudes began to gain favour. For example, the surgeons at St Bartholomew's and St Thomas' hospitals frequently kept pupils or 'cubbs' in addition to apprentices. By the mid-1690s, many cubbs

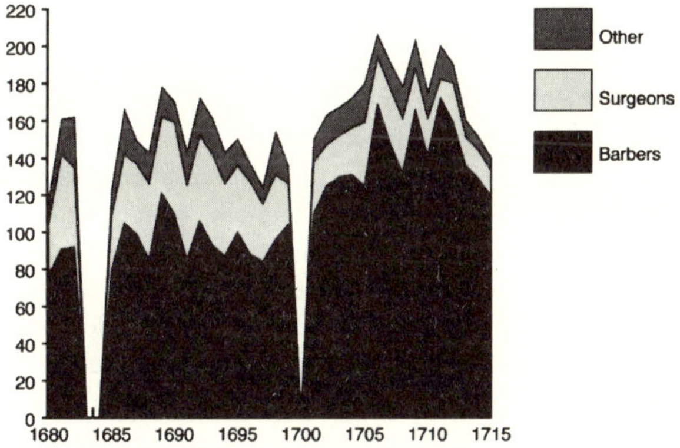

Figure 2.4
Apprentices registered at the Barber-Surgeons' Company of London
(Compiled from Guildhall Library MS 5266)

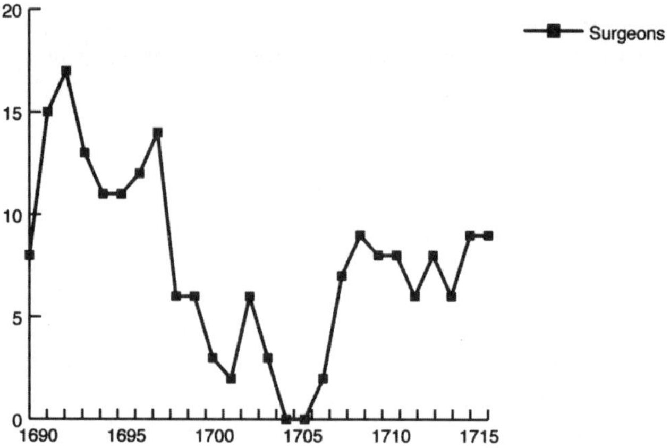

Figure 2.5
Surgeons trained by servitude who were admitted into the Barber-Surgeons' Company of London (Compiled from Guildhall Library MS 5265)

had established themselves as surgical practitioners elsewhere in the city after reputedly gaining only six months' to a year's hospital experience. This reduced training period fuelled many arguments from Barber-Surgeons' Company freemen who denounced hospitals as 'breeding ... many Illiterate and unskillful pretenders to chyrurgery'.[32] Since few records remain of this type of hospital training, historical enquiry into cubb training and practice remains difficult. However, accounts from surgical reformers like Turner suggest that the number of London cubb-trained surgeons continued to increase throughout the early eighteenth century.[33]

Military and navy service also provided an abbreviated training period for many London surgeons. Maintaining seamen's health was central to the growth of British commerce during this period.[34] The high prevalence of disease at sea, spread through close contact, inadequate food, and poor ventilation, created a great demand for sea surgeons.[35] This demand was considerably increased during times of war. For instance, 113 London surgeons and surgeon's mates were licensed into practice during a three-month siege of the war of the League of Augsburg (1692/93).[36]

Examiners from the Barber-Surgeons' Company held an official responsibility to recommend surgeons and surgeon's mates for particular classes of ships in the Royal Navy. By 1709, the Barber-

Surgeons' Company claimed to annually certify five hundred sea surgeons and their mates.[37] However, searches among the extant records of the Barber-Surgeons' Company corroborate R. R. James' claim that fewer than this number of sea surgeons and their mates were actually certified each year.[38] But even a hundred or more sea surgeons presented the Company a formidable examination task.

Throughout the early Enlightenment, sea-surgeons made up the greatest proportional representation of surgeons qualified before Barber-Surgeons' Company examiners (see Figure 2.6). Cromwell's 1654 ordinance remained in effect, whereby ex-military and naval surgeons, in recognition of their service to the Commonwealth, could take up their trade as civilians and remain free from the Barber-Surgeons' jurisdiction once their military duty had ended (i.e., for many, once a war was settled).[39] The increase in naval surgeons during wartime opened pathways for upward social mobility once the battles had ceased.[40]

Although most sea-surgeons received official certification from Barber-Surgeon examiners before entering into service, some embarked upon sea surgery having only purchased a licence from the Bishop of London or the Archbishop of Canterbury. This method of licensing, an episcopal 'right' since 1534, was claimed to be 'so very easy, that [anyone with] ... a small summ [sic] of money, has seldom despair'd of that kind of protection'.[41] Upon tabulating the sixty-eight episcopal licences which one source claimed were granted to surgeons and 'barber-surgeons' between 1680 and 1725, it seems that 34.5% of these

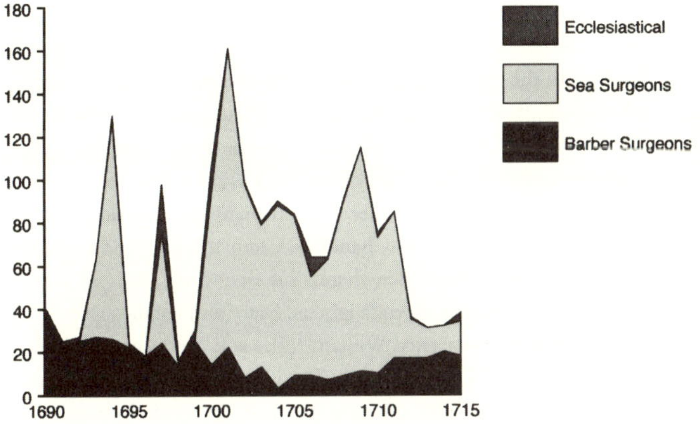

Figure 2.6
Surgeons Qualified by the Barber-Surgeons' Company of London

licences were presented in 1697. It is most likely that these individuals were returning to civilian practice after the Treaty of Ryswick was signed that year, ending the war between Anglo-Dutch allies and the French.[42]

The proportion of ecclesiastically licensed surgeons to those trained by servitude or as sea surgeons was minimal (refer back to Figure 2.6). However, their presence created much apprehension among many freemen of the Barber-Surgeons' Company. Surgical reformers, like Turner, regarded this method of qualification as a 'gross perversion' because 'his Lordship [was] ... no judge ... [of] surgery'.[43] The Barber-Surgeons' Company 'humbly begg[ed]' the ecclesiastical authorities 'not to license any person ... who hath not first obtained a Testimoniall under the Seale of the Company certifying the [prior] examination of such person['s] ... Skill & Ability for ... exercis[ing]' the surgical art.[44] However, it was only after issuing a series of such petitions that the Bishop of London complied with their request. His decision was not proclaimed until May 1713, one month after the Treaty of Utrecht was signed. This treaty itself procured a stretch of relatively peaceful times for England during which few if any new surgeons were immediately needed for tending wartime wounds.

Notes

1 Throughout this book, I have retained Old Style dating. Thus, 1666 remained recognized on the Julian calendar through March 1666/67. Additionally, I have retained the original eighteenth-century spelling and grammar in my quoted passages. Daniel Turner recorded his birth date in 'Religio Medici Reformata: or, Private Devotion, in 2 parts. conteining [sic] certain Forms of Prayer, Thanksgiving &c. To be used in the times of Health & Sickness. suited to the Authours Occasions', British Library, Additional Manuscripts, MS 14404, f.23. Turner also noted his baptism as 17 October of the same year (f.24). I am grateful to Richard Palmer and W.F. Bynum for directing me to this manuscript. Daniel's father, John Turner, was a London citizen and freeman of the Tallow-Chandlers' Company. His oldest son, John, followed in this trade, whereas his second son, Samuel, entered the Taylor's Company. Two daughters, Mary and Sarah, survived infancy, and Mary married William Miles and Sarah married John Cleeve. Guildhall Library, Tallow Chandlers Company, Register of Apprenticeship Bindings, manuscript 6158 (3), f.110, indicates that John Turner became apprenticed to his father for seven years on 29 March 1677. Samuel Turner later in life was a merchant taylor but appears to have apprenticed as a haberdasher (Land Lease

Hertfordshire Record Office MSS D/EAS 3131 and D/EAS 1610-1).

2 Daniel Turner, *The Ancient Physician's Legacy Impartially Survey'd* (London: John Clarke, 1733), 135, and *idem*, *The Drop and Pill of Mr. Ward Consider'd* (London: John Clarke, 1735), 6.

3 John Turner's probated will, Public Record Office, Chancery Lane, Prob. 11/440.

4 Although several of the London Companies sponsored particular grammar schools, W. K. L. Prosser, Clerk of the Tallow Chandlers Company claimed this Company held no such connections (personal communication).

5 George C. Brauer claimed that by the time of Turner's schooling, Greek was no longer deemed as 'essential' as Latin. See his *The Education of a Gentleman: Theories of Gentlemanly Education in England: 1660-1775* (New York: Bookman Associates, 1959), 83.

6 John Douglas, *A Dissertation on the Venereal Disease*, part III (London: for the Author, 1739), 156.

7 Catechisms as well as teachings of morals and manners were, according to Foster Watson's *The English Grammar Schools to 1660: Their Curriculum and Practice* (Cambridge: Cambridge University Press, 1908), part of most young school-boys' education (see esp. 69-85, 98-136).

8 R. Campbell, in his 1747 *The London Tradesman*, claimed that letting blood and drawing teeth comprised 'the only Part of Surgery' that barbers 'ever pretended to practice' (London: David & Charles, 1969, 1st edn 1747), 204.

9 R. Rutson James, 'Apprentice books at Barber-Surgeons' Hall', *British Medical Journal*, ii (1944), 288 mentions the whereabouts of records listing London barber-surgeon apprentices back to 1603. Provincial apprentice lists have been consulted in Margaret C. Barnet's 'The Barber-Surgeons of York', *Medical History*, xii (1968), 19-30; Margaret Pelling's 'Occupational Diversity: Barber-Surgeons and the Trades of Norwich, 1550-1640', *Bulletin of the History of Medicine*, lvi (1982), 484-511; and James H. Thomas' 'Hampshire and the Company of Barber-Surgeons, 1658-1720', *Hampshire Family Historian*, x (1983), 15-18.

10 Joan Lane has gleaned several important clues about apothecary-surgeons' apprenticeships from a few diaries in her thorough distillation of 'The Role of Apprenticeship in Eighteenth-Century Medical Education in England', in W.F. Bynum and Roy Porter (eds), *William Hunter and the Eighteenth-Century Medical World* (Cambridge: Cambridge University Press, 1985), 57-103.

11 Thomas R. Forbes, 'Apprentices in Trouble: Some Problems in the

Training of Surgeons and Apothecaries in Seventeenth-Century London', *Yale Journal of Biology and Medicine,* lii (1979), 227-37. The mischievous side of apprenticeship is also revealed in the sixty-two short entries from Barber-Surgeons' Company records Sidney Young selected for his *Annals*, 261-70.

12 The precise date Turner began his apprenticeship is unknown since the Register of Apprenticeship Bindings of the Barber Surgeons' Company, Guildhall Library manuscript 5266, vol. 2 (1672-1707) is missing its records between 26 July 1683 and 1 May 1685. However, Turner later claimed having served a traditional seven-year apprenticeship which was completed in 1691. See his *Present State of Chyrurgery, with some Short Remarks on the Abuses Committed under a Pretence to the Practice. And Reasons offer'd for Regulating the Same* (London: R. Tookey, 1703), 8.

13 Apprenticeship Bindings, Barber-Surgeons' Company, Guildhall Library manuscript 5266, vol. 2. On 19 August 1698, the Company's Court of Assistants prohibited any Freeman from taking more than two apprentices 'at one time without the[ir] consent'.

14 Barber-Surgeons' Company Apprenticeship Books, Royal College of Surgeons of England Library, transcript by R.R. James, Book VI (3 July 1683 – 6 August 1689). The reason for this turn-over remains unknown.

15 J.R. Kellett compared the sizes of various London companies, including the Barber-Surgeons' Company, in his 'The Breakdown of Gild and Corporation Control Over the Handicraft and Retail Trade in London', *Economic Historical Review,* x (1958), 388-94.

16 S. Young, *Annals*, 259. Historians frequently cite this figure as accurate. I use it with much more reservation since Young has not provided any clues or left any notes as to how he arrived at this 'average'. For a slightly later period, David Wright's 'An Index of London Surgical Practitioners, 1736-1811, compiled from the Trades Directories' in the Guildhall Library, London (SL 47 oversize), is most helpful.

17 Volumes 2 and 3 of the Register of Freedom Admissions, Guildhall MS 5265 divide between April and May 1704. Thus, the 1704 dip in Figure 2.3 may reflect an insufficient recording (loss?) of freeman admissions at this time. The artificiality of this dip must not, however, be over-emphasized, for the 1705 records which indicate a comparatively diminished number of freeman admissions appear to be complete.

18 Half of the Court was composed of barbers, half of surgeons. Barbers and surgeons annually rotated the Company's mastership. A

dispute arose in 1700 when more surgeons than barbers made up the Company's four Governors (the master plus the three wardens). On 9 July 1700, equal representation between barbers and surgeons was re-established. See the Company's Court Minutes, MS 5257(6).

19 'The Rules, Orders and Ordinances of the Mistery and Commonally [sic] of Barbers and Surgeons of London', 13 January 1708, Barber-Surgeons' Company MS A/2/1, 36.

20 *Ibid.*, 29.

21 *Ibid.*, 34.

22 Apprenticeship Bindings, Guildhall MS 5266, vol. 2.

23 Court Minutes, MS 5257(6).

24 I cannot explain this eight-year gap except to say that it appears to have been uncommon for surgeons to wait many years to be officially examined after having been taken into the freedom.

25 Court Minutes, MS 5257(6).

26 *Ibid.* Richard Lee, Joseph Bateman (son of Turner's first master, Charles Bateman), John C(?)ooke, Jeremy Wright, and William Petty (with whom Turner later regularly consulted) also passed their surgeons' examinations on 12 June 1700.

27 By 1721, the examiners asked their successful candidates to remember them with a gift of money, reputedly to buy the gloves themselves, rather than offering them a new pair of gloves directly. J. Dobson and R. M. Walker also noted that freemen, upon admission to the Company, were expected to present the Company a silver spoon upon which their name had been engraved. See *Barbers and Barber-Surgeons of London*, 46.

28 Court Minutes, MS 5257(6).

29 J. R. Kellett claimed the erosion of guild and corporation control was precipitated by the population's expansion into the conurbation of London forming beyond the confines of the City wall. See 'Breakdown of Gild Control', 381-94. Early indication of this suburban growth was seen after the 1665 plague and great fire of the following year. Other London tradesmen were, according to Kellett, driven into the suburbs in the 1680s and 1690s when the City faced severe financial indebtedness (382). The rise of 'unfree' trade and manufacturing in the suburbs further devaluated apprenticeship. This new trade established a great suburban wealth which, when coupled with the debts of war, precipitated further financial decline within the municipality. D.W. Jones provides a further analysis in his 'London Merchants and the Crisis of the 1690's' in P. Clark and P. Slack (eds), *Crisis and Order in English Towns, 1500-1700* (London: Routledge & Kegan Paul, 1972), esp. 311-12. Ulrich Im Hof also

claimed that by the 18th century, 'The time was past when the guilds had set the tone and represented the progressive element'. Rather, they had become 'social clubs whose members were anxious to preserve their ancient privileges', *The Enlightenment* (Oxford: Blackwell Publishers, 1997), 58.

30 Compiled from data extracted from Apprenticeship Bindings, Guildhall MS 5266. Records for 1683, 1684, and 1700 are partially incomplete, therefore my graph slightly under-represents (probably only slightly) the number of apprentices registered during these years. The 'Other' in Figure 2.4 once again represents the trade workers whose various skills were utilized within the Barber-Surgeons' Company.

31 Graphed according to data compiled from Freedom Admissions, Guildhall MS 5265.

32 J. F. South, *Memorial of the Craft of Surgery*, 246-7.

33 For example, see [Robert Poole], *Physical Vade Mecum: or, Fifth Gift of Theophilus Philanthropos* (London: E. Duncomb, 1741), Dedication, and the accounting of St Thomas' hospital surgeon assistants in the 'Register of Pupils and Dressers', The Medical Library, St Thomas' Campus, United Medical Schools of Guy's and St Thomas' Hospitals, MS 31.d.2, a listing which began on 11 January 1723.

34 On the Navy and commerce, see John Brewer, *Sinews of Power: War Money and the English State, 1688-1783* (London: Unwin Hyman, 1989), 29-63, 167-90. See also Richard Harding, *The Evolution of the Sailing Navy, 1509-1815* (London: Macmillan Press, 1995).

35 Arnold Zuckerman discussed many of the conditions of navy life in his 'Disease and Ventilation in the Royal Navy: The Woodenship Years', *Eighteenth-Century Life*, n.s. 3, xi (1987): 77-89. For a more comprehensive account, see N.A.M. Rodger, *The Wooden World: An Anatomy of the Georgian Navy* (Glasgow: William Collins Sons & Co., 1986).

36 J. J. Keevil, *Medicine and the Navy 1200-1900, Vol. 2: 1649-1714* (Edinburgh: E & S Livingstone, 1958), 257. For specific details and tabulations of the number of ships annually called to war see E. H. H. Archibald, *The Fighting Ship in the Royal Navy A.D. 897-1984* (Dorset: Blandford Press, 1984).

37 Keevil, *Medicine and the Navy*, Vol. 2, 263.

38 R. R. James, [Admiralty], Surgeon's Passing Certificates, Royal College of Surgeons of England Library, MS 129A f.12-13.

39 This special privilege of military surgeons has been cited in works throughout the past three centuries. See, for example, Lloyd G.

Stevenson, 'A Note on the Relation of Military Service to Licensing in the History of British Surgery', *Bulletin of the History of Medicine,* xxvii (1953), 422. Two cases arguing for this privilege of practice appear in the Court Minutes for 15 April and 6 September 1709. Geoffrey Holmes provides an alternative explanation that ambitious youngsters selected military and naval service as a way to gain more extensive training than that offered by apprenticeship. See his *Augustan England: Professions, State and Society 1680-1730* (London: Allen & Unwin, 1982) as cited by R. Porter and D. Porter in *Patient's Progress,* 20-21. Although this may have been the case in some instances, those ambitious individuals who rose to high ranks within the Barber-Surgeons' Company had exclusively served full apprenticeships.

40 Lawrence Stone, 'Social Mobility in England, 1500-1700', *Past and Present,* xxxiii (1966), esp. 25.

41 D. Turner, *Present State,* 15. John R. Guy thoroughly reviewed the statutes providing for episcopal licensing in his 'The Episcopal Licensing of Physicians, Surgeons, and Midwives', *Bulletin of the History of Medicine,* lvi (1982), 528-42.

42 Data for this graph were gathered from J. H. Bloom and R. R. James, *Medical Practitioners in the Diocese of London, Licensed under the Act of 3 Henry VIII, c.II. An Annotated List 1529-1725* (Cambridge: Cambridge University Press, 1935). The 'other' category denotes individuals identified as physicians or apothecaries, without any mention of surgical expertise.

43 D. Turner, *Present State,* 15.

44 'The humble petition of the Masters or Governors, Assistants, Livery & Freeman of the Mystery & Commonality of Barbers & Surgeons of London', 1 June 1710 as transcribed in S. Young, *Annals,* 348.

3

The Surgical Art

Perhaps there never was a Period of Time in which any Art was more cultivated than Surgery has been for these last thirty Years.
Samuel Sharpe (1750)[1]

Before examining the particular surgical view of the body or Daniel Turner's attempts to reform surgery, we need some insight into a typical surgical practice. Turner's detailed case histories provide such insight. Each case, or in Turner's words, 'History by way of Example', exemplified the practical aspect of treating a disorder which London surgeons were likely to encounter.[2] These histories also provide a superb source from which to 'uncover the human condition as it was experienced', a factor missing from most historical accounts of surgery.[3]

Turner's *Art of Surgery*

In 1722, Daniel Turner's *Art of Surgery* first became available through booksellers Charles Rivington, James Lacy and John Clarke[4] (see Figure 3.1). This work joined the multiple editions of twenty-seven other surgical writings which had been published in the English vernacular since 1685.[5] Unlike the concise, often pocket-sized manuals of surgical practice such as Hugh Ryder's *Practical Chirurgery* (1689), John Moyle's *The Experienced Chirurgion* (1703), or James Handley's *Colloquim Chyrurgica* (1710, 2nd ed), Turner's two-volume publication represented a massive text of the 'Art' more comparable, in length, to William Salmon's *Ars Chirurgica* (1698) or Richard Wiseman's *Eight Chirurgical Treatises* (1705, 5th ed). Turner designed his work to aid readers who, through apprenticeship, were already 'tolerably grounded' in surgery rather than to 'instruct the finish'd Surgeon' or 'initiate mere Tyros'. In principle, this work offered readers 'Hints', so Turner claimed, about the 'general Idea' of surgery.[6]

Turner's general description of the surgical art was consistent with most contemporary accounts. He divided this work into the categories of Tumours, Wounds, Ulcers, and Fractures. Although holding to these conventional categories, he appeared rather indifferent as to the precise arrangement of his text: 'Whether or no ... [the] Discourse [On Ulcers] should not have preceeded the ...

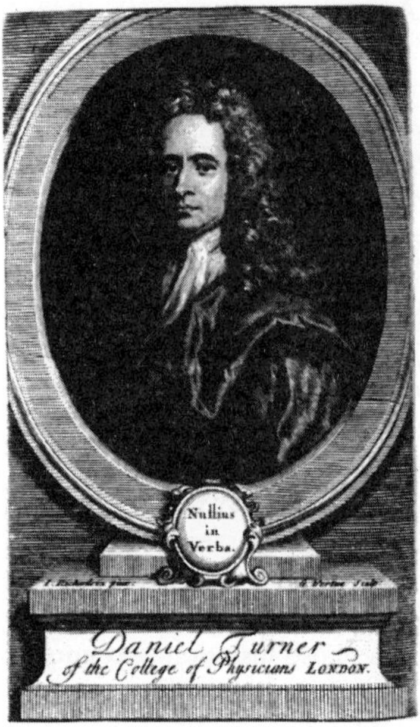

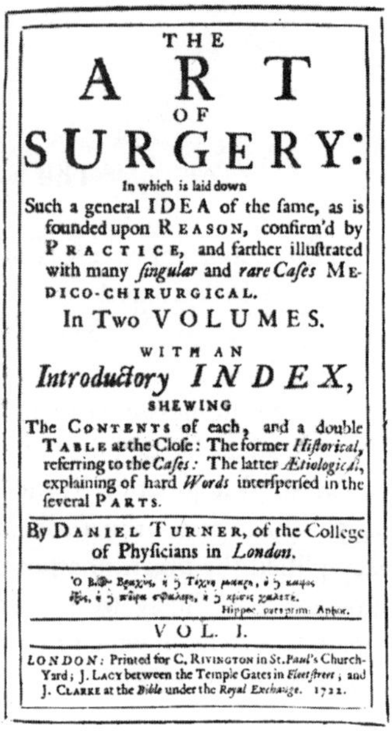

THE
ART
OF
SURGERY:
In which is laid down
Such a general IDEA of the same, as is founded upon REASON, confirm'd by PRACTICE, and farther illustrated with many *singular* and *rare Cases* MEDICO-CHIRURGICAL.
In Two VOLUMES.
WITH AN
Introductory *INDEX*,
SHEWING
The CONTENTS of each, and a double TABLE at the Close: The former *Historical*, referring to the *Cases*: The latter *Ætiological*, explaining of hard *Words* interspersed in the several PARTS.

By DANIEL TURNER, of the College of Physicians in *London*.

Ὁ βίος βραχὺς, ἡ δὲ τέχνη μακρὴ, ὁ δὲ καιρὸς ὀξὺς, ἡ δὲ πεῖρα σφαλερὴ, ἡ δὲ κρίσις χαλεπή.
Hippoc. Aphor.

VOL. I.

LONDON: Printed for C. RIVINGTON in *St. Paul's* Church-Yard; J. LACY between the Temple Gates in *Fleetstreet*; and J. CLARKE at the *Bible* under the *Royal Exchange*. 1722.

Figure 3.1

Daniel Turner, engraved by G. Vertue after J. Richardson, *c.*1712-14.
The title page of Turner's *Art of Surgery* (author's personal collection).

former [On Wounds] according to the Method of some Writers, may be disputed'. For Turner, the importance of the work lay not in its arrangement, but rather in conveying the necessary instructions for surgical readers within each division.

In addition to the above-mentioned divisions, Turner included a fifth section on Diseases Peculiar to Women. This concentration upon women's diseases sharply distinguished Turner from his English contemporaries. Such diseases were more typically described in English midwifery writings.[7] However, as his case studies illustrate, female midwives often turned to surgeons to treat women when their own attempts had failed. Therefore, Turner proceeded to instruct surgeons about the specific part of midwifery which he and several surgical colleagues had frequently been called to attend.

In Turner's *Art of Surgery*, he described the surgical conditions of 110 different individuals whose treatments he had personally attended or supervised. This work, however, is not a complete sequential record of his cases, like those of seventeenth-century London surgeons Joseph Binns or W. Wood, or Plymouth surgeon

James Yonge. One, therefore, is unable to identify Turner's patient load at any given time, the date he treated specific patients, the precise length of treatment, or the patients' regard for Turner as a practitioner.[8] Nevertheless, his work is instructive in providing a typical surgeon's viewpoint of his practice and patients as it elaborately describes many of the conditions for which ordinary city civilians sought surgical care during a particular period.

Turner's Surgical Patients

Turner treated patients from all social classes. Seventeen of the patients were identified as either Gentlemen or Gentlewomen.[9] Tradesmen and artisans, like the tallow chandler's family into which Turner was born, appear to have comprised most of his patient load. Among these tradesmen, Turner treated the barber, Mr Marks, the bookseller, Mr Jay, as well as 2 butchers, an apothecary, a distiller, an artificer, a shoemaker, a weaver, a victualler, a wire-drawer, a corn chandler, a carpenter, a linen draper, a shop keeper, a brazier, a baker, an ostler, and a thread seller. All of these patients were men. Turner also attended the wife of a butcher and five children of tradesmen. Seven servants, and four sea or military men were treated, including

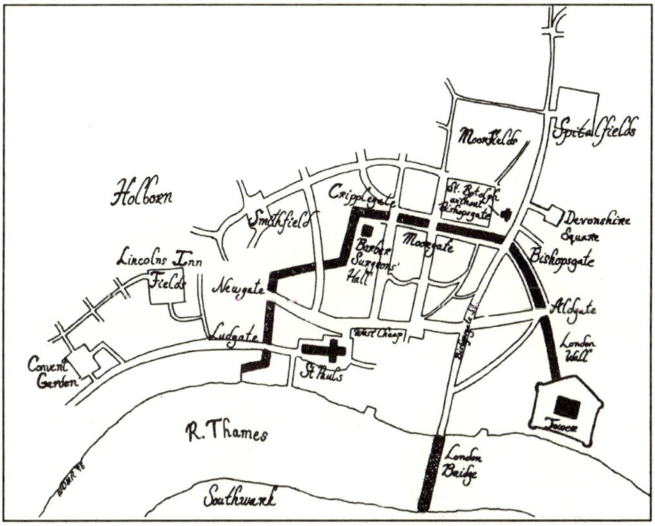

Figure 3.2
Turner lived and worked within this geographical boundary of London
(Original drawing by Warren D.M. Reed)

Captain H—-y of the Guard, as were nine 'poor' or 'charity' patients.

Turner's case reports suggest that he conformed to practising within the seven-mile boundary proscribed by the Barber-Surgeons' Company. Of the 44 patients whom Turner identified by residence, most lived either around St Botolph without Bishopsgate (Turner's home parish) or in the north central parishes within the London wall. Seventeen lived along or near Bishopsgate Street, three of these residing in local Inns, whereas eight lived in Turner's neighbourhood. Six patients lived to the immediate north in Shoreditch and Spitalfields, three to the immediate west in Moorfields, and eight within the City wall along Cornhill, Poultry, or Wood Streets. Only five patients were identified as living 'remote' from Turner; a few of these came 'from the Country', and one travelled fifty miles to reach London. Figure 3.2 provides a geographical synopsis of the neighbourhoods in which Turner practised.

Accidents were the chief cause of the disorders Turner treated. Fractures were among the most common accidents for which patients called upon surgeons, and Turner claimed that in 'more than 20 Years' of surgical practice, he 'seldom had fewer than four or five [patients with fractures] of one kind or other, at once under my Inspection'.[10] These cases from private practice conform with contemporary hospital accounts which describe fractures as among the most common surgical disorders.[11]

The accidents from which Turner's patients suffered varied widely, from the man who sliced his finger while cutting cheese to a child who suffered a fractured skull having been struck in the head by a misguided catstick thrown during a cockfight in Southwark (see Figure 3.3). Many accidents owed their origin to sport. For example, Mr Jay, the bookseller, was hit in the eye by a ball 'struck from the Racket' at Five-Courts in Moor-fields, whereas a young boy accidentally 'pierc'd' the corner of his eye when the point of the needle 'suddenly slipt' while he was stitching up the leather seams of a football. A few accidents were occupational. A porter attributed the growth on his shoulder to carrying heavy bags. One coachman was attacked while sitting on his coach box, whereas another broke his arm from the kick of his horse. I believe it may also have been occupationally related that a servant employed to draw drinks for a victualler developed ascites from his 'tippling' habit. Horses also caused a number of accidents. One man was bruised from the saddle of a horse, another man was kicked in the leg by the horse he was 'trying to break', whereas an ostler (i.e., a horse stableman) was thrown from the horse he was tending. Pedestrian accidents and violence were

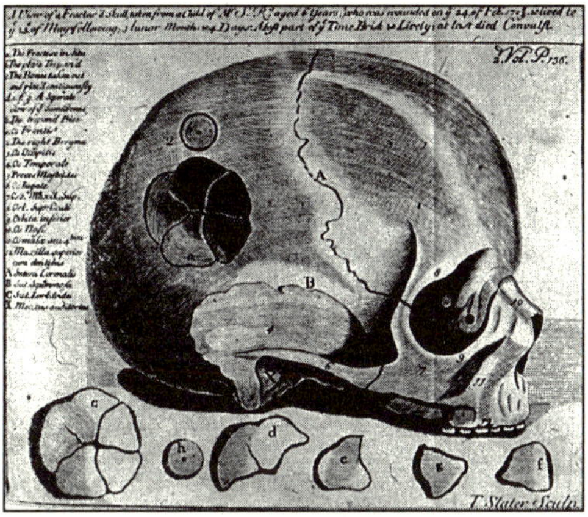

Figure 3.3

Detailed view of the fractured skull and trepanning site of the boy Daniel Turner treated in 1709 (D. Turner, *Art of Surgery*, 1732; Wellcome Institute Library, London)

also common on London streets. One gentlewoman slipped on a 'Peas-cod-shell', falling upon the marble-pavement, fracturing her 'Crupper-bone' (i.e. tailbone or coccyx). Another woman was thrown from her chaise, and still another severed her tongue as the result of an epileptic seizure. Eight patients' wounds were due to fights or scuffles with swords, knives, and fists, whereas an additional four patients' disorders were self-inflicted. Finally, some accidents occurred at home. One elderly gentleman while asleep in his chair 'after a large evening's draught', fell out of the chair and dislocated his humerus. Another patient dislocated her jaw at home 'merely by the force of yawning'. (Table 3.1 provides a brief surgical description of all the patients' disorders Turner discussed in his *Art of Surgery*).

Most of the accident victims were brought either directly to Turner, to a nearby inn, domestic residence, or to the patient's settlement whence a messenger was sent requesting Turner's attendance. For many, Turner was apparently the closest surgeon available. In one situation, he just happened to be passing by, and was recognized by 'one in the Crowd' who 'earnestly begged' his assistance for 'a poor man bleeding to Death'.[12] In another case, a patient was referred to Turner by a midwife who knew of his success in treating previous cases 'of the like kind'.[13]

The length of time his patients endured their disorder before seeking surgical assistance varied widely. Accident victims received

Disorder	Frequency	Bodily Region (when specified)
	Tumours	
Hernia	11	6-Testicular, 3-Intestinal
Ascites/Hydrops	5	4-Scrotal, 1-Legs & 'Cod'
Inflammation	4	Arm, Tonsil & Tongue, Joint, Leg
Sarcoma	4	Shoulder, Upper Back, Testis
Hydrocephalus	3	Head
Phlegmon	2	Knee, Ankle
Scirrhous	2	Breast
Cancer	2	Anus, Lip
Scrofula	2	Neck; Glands
Ganglionide	2	Shoulder
Multiple	2	Scalp
Erysipelas	2	Face
Oedematous	1	Leg & Foot
Bubo	1	Groin
Bronchocele	1	Lung
Polyp	1	Nose
Rupture	1	Inguinal
Flatulent	1	Knee
Stones	1	Bladder
	Wounds	
Wound	7	Shoulder, Leg, Neck, Temporal Muscle, 2-Eyes, Head
Cut/Slash	6	Face, Arm, 2-Wrist, Neck, Finger
Severed	4	3-Throat, 1-Tongue
Stab	2	Chest, Belly
Laceration	1	Biceps Tendon
Fracture	1	Skull
	Ulcers	
Ulcer	5	4-Leg, 1-Arm, 1-Back
With Tumour	3	2-Buttocks, 1-Ribs
Excoriation	1	Leg
	Fractures	
Broken	10	4-Skull, Humerus, Thigh, Leg, Coccyx, Patella, Jaw
Dislocation	7	4-Humeri, Femur, Ankle, Jaw
Depression	1	Skull
Ossified Callus	1	Leg
	Women's Disorders	
Prolapse	9	6-Uterine; 2-Vaginal; 1-Anal
Bubo/Tumour	3	Groin
Milk Tumour	2	Breast

Table 3.1

Patients' disorders detailed in Turner's *Art of Surgery*

immediate care. Others, like three-quarters of those suffering diseases 'peculiar to women', were brought to Turner's attention a few days post partum. Many others, however, suffered from more chronic conditions by the time they reached a surgeon. Patients afflicted with tumours, for example, delayed seeking care. Five patients waited 'some days'; two, 'some weeks'; four, 'some months'; five, 'a long time'; and eleven waited 'several' or 'many' years. One man watched his tumour 'filling leisurely for seven years' before seeking Turner's assistance.[14] These cases corroborated the historical generalization that 'surgical conditions' were often 'long-term' disorders.[15] Except for accident victims, these cases suggest that patients retained a right to wait for considerable periods of time before relinquishing the care of their bodies to the hands of surgeons.

Turner's Surgical Treatments

Historians have described bloodletting as the 'commonest of all treatments for any kind of illness' and the 'epitome' of surgical practice.[16] Bleeding basins, also known as 'barber's bowls' or bloodporringers, which were displayed on the sign boards and in shop fronts, were publicly recognized as the symbol of the surgical trade. Turner, too, regarded the letting of blood as a primary part of the surgical art (see Figure 3.4). There were a number of occasions, however, when he purposely avoided the procedure.[17] For instance, some patients had bled so profusely from gaping wounds and fractures that their constitution was, so he deemed, too weak to endure the letting of more blood. When treating one woman who had cut her carotid artery, Turner claimed he 'would have bled her in the Contrary arm, but in consideration of the great Loss ... she had just before sustain'd by her Wound', he omitted venesection.[18] In other cases, accident victims had been bled by a barber, apothecary or surgeon who had arrived at the scene before Turner. In these situations, Turner deemed further bloodletting unnecessary. Table 3.2 identifies specific methods and medications Turner used to treat his patients. This table shows that bloodletting was not performed on every surgical patient.

Indeed, Turner warned against bleeding all patients. This caution stemmed, in part, from the hazardous consequences he claimed this procedure often produced. Several of Turner's cases exemplify that letting blood through venesection, scarification, and leeching at times posed hazards. For example, disastrous consequences could arise from letting blood without due consideration of the patient's 'Age, Strength, Habit, and Way of Living'. In one instance, Turner

	Tumour	Wound	Ulcer	Fracture	Women's Diseases
Number of patients for whom treatment is known	37	18	10	14	14
Purging	21	8	6	3	4
Bleeding	8	7	9	4	6
Pledgit, Bolster, Dossil	9	11	7	3	5
Bandages	4	2	4	8	6
Plaister, Poultice	7	2	2	3	4
Cataplasm	9	3	6	4	4
Fomentation	9	2	2	2	10
Embrocation	3	7	0	2	2
Anodyne	5	4	3	2	3
Caustic	6	0	4	2	3
Digestive	13	4	8	1	4
Defensitive	1	0	1	3	0
Vesicatory, Blister	2	3	1	1	1
Styptic	2	2	0	0	3
Tonic	7	3	2	1	3
Wash	2	2	1	3	2
Turner's Cerate*	5	3	4	1	1
Other**	8	0	0	1	4

* Turner's cerate is further discussed in Chapter Four.

** anti-strumatics, emetics, salivation, alexipharmics, deobstruents, discutients, restringents

Table 3.2

Treatments that Turner's Patients Received
(Physical Methods and Medications)

was called upon to consult with another surgeon regarding a patient's severely inflamed arm due to the surgeon's venesection. After viewing the disorder, Turner proclaimed to the patient that the surgeon had been in 'no other way instrumental to [this] Accident, than in, ... bleeding her before her Body had been prepared by some lenient purgation'. The patient, however, retained her 'unalterable belief' that the surgeon rather than the state of her humours had caused her 'severe indisposition'. Turner accepted the further responsibility of this patient, but had much difficulty persuading her to undergo another venesection. Moreover, he found it equally difficult to 'reconcile her' to allow the surgeon 'who had bled her to give [him] Attendance'. She only consented to this upon the 'Terms' of Turner's 'Promise of standing by, at the Times of Dressing'.[19] Turner and the assisting surgeon succeeded in healing this patient in six weeks. For these weeks of effort, however, the surgeon assisting Turner received only half the crown he was owed for the initial venesection he performed.[20] This case illustrates how neglecting a proper surgical protocol readily brought surgeons public 'censure'.[21]

Purging was also a standard treatment for most surgical conditions,[22] but Turner argued that purges were not a mere 'Piece of Formality'.[23] Rather, he claimed their administration was often a necessary step to avoid fatalities. For example, he insisted that purgatives must be administered both pre- and post-operatively in order to avoid the symptomatic fever which often followed operations.

As a lenient purge, Turner most often recommended infusions or boluses of rhubarb or calomel.[24] Because their effect was not immediate, Turner administered them, whenever possible, three to four days in advance of an operation. As in bloodletting, he claimed that purgation was to be adjusted according to the age and constitution of the patient. In particular, infants were only to be purged as much as their 'tender Age could bear'.[25] Some patients, like those with fluid-filled swellings, were given daily doses of purgatives whereas Turner completely avoided 'throwing up' a clyster (i.e. an enema) in one patient suffering an abscess for 'fear' of 'checking' or 'divert[ing] the abscess' to a more 'advanc'd' or 'unsafe' stage.[26]

Turner also employed purgatives to counteract the adverse effects of other medications. He described their usefulness in promoting a 'good Temper as to [the] Stools' when anodynes were concurrently administered; otherwise the pain relievers, commonly containing opiates, would constipate the patients.[27] Conversely, he administered anodynes to patients with anal fistulae, 'not only to quiet the Pain, but to prevent [the patient from] suddenly going to stool'.[28]

Equally as important as Turner's use of venesection and purges was his concern for the patient's dietary regimen. In 40 of the 110 cases, Turner mentioned particulars about the patient's diet. He regularly prescribed a 'slender Diet' for 'some Days' both before and after an operation.[29] For oedema, he recommended a drying diet of easily digested meat, and for other 'hydropics', small broths, gruels, and panada (i.e., bread boiled in water) were recommended. A liquid diet was prescribed for a patient with erysipelas, and a similar diet was 'sucked ... through a spout' by a patient suffering from a fractured jaw bone. A 'spare' diet was given to a patient with a fractured patella, whereas guaiac diets were prepared for both a patient with a tumour on his buttocks and another with an excoriation on his leg. Turner also adjusted his patients' drinks according to their general habits. If one regularly 'tipl[ed] Strong Waters' and claimed he could not sleep without them, then Turner argued 'even in his Illness [the patient must] be allow'd daily half a Pint [of Claret] or a Dram or Two [of Distilled Spirits] at the surgeon's discretion'.[30] Although he noted that Hippocrates, for whom he held great reverence, refused his patients certain foods and drinks, Turner exclaimed: 'I fear some of our [patients] would think themselves undone, if they had not Flesh and Wine allow'd them'.[31]

Dietary abuse was a contributing factor to many surgical patients' disorders. One poor shoemaker's troubles were exacerbated, Turner argued, by a crude diet. An old Frenchwoman in Spitalfields was described as 'emaciated' and of a 'worn-out' habit. Excessive living brought about the 'full' and 'corpulent' habits Turner described of other patients. Additionally, some patients' sufferings were consequent to excessive drinking. It was only after 'drinking hard' that two men, Captain H—-y and Surgeon P——r drew swords which ultimately led to the former being 'prick'd in the belly'. The inability to cure one clergyman's hernia was in part due to his having 'too much indulged himself with strong liquors', and a victualler's servant's swollen state was attributed to his 'addict[ion] to tippling'.

The remedies Turner described were generally consistent with those recommended by contemporaries. The ointment he most often used was explicitly taken from Alexander Read's text, whereas many caustics, anodynes, and tonics were taken from Bates' *Dispensatory* or Fuller's *Pharmacopoeia*.[32] Occasionally, however, he promoted a new remedy he had found to be effective. For example, in contrast to contemporaries' remedies for treating scrofula, Turner suggested a remedy he considered equally effective but less costly and time

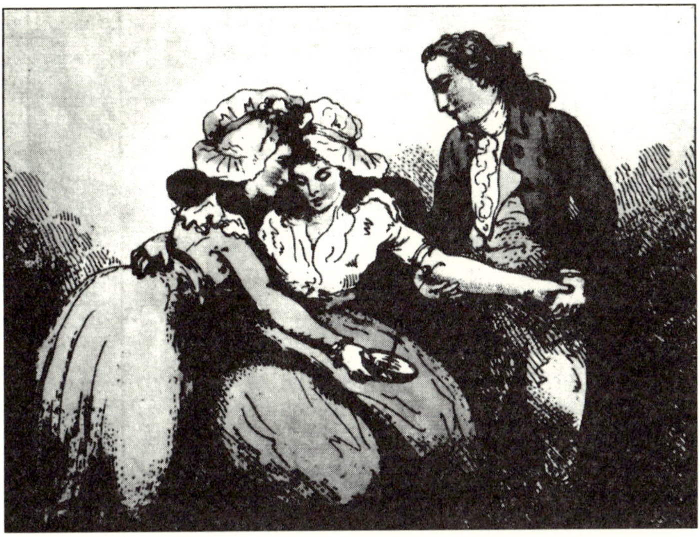

Figure 3.4
Surgeon bleeding the arm of a young woman who is being comforted by another woman (T. Rowlandson (?), 1784; Wellcome Institute Library, London)

consuming to prepare.[33] In other instances, he promoted the use of medications which he found through experience with his own patients to be 'less hazardous, [but] that will perform our Work'.[34] Perhaps the remedy which most distinguished Turner's medications from those promoted by contemporaries was his own special calamine-based cerate. 'Turner's Cerate' is more thoroughly discussed in Chapter Four.

Although Turner's medications were similar to those his contemporaries used, his case studies reveal some intriguing distinctions between the types of surgical compounds which different groups of patients received[35] (see Table 3.2). For instance, he administered medicines in the form of cataplasms (i.e., spread like a plaister in such a consistency as neither to adhere nor to run) to treat a number of his patients with ulcers and tumours. Over 70% of patients with women's diseases received warm fomentations applied to their tumours and prolapsed uteri. For one of these patients, Turner applied his commonly used Theriaca, 'spread on Cloth like a Pultis' as 'hot as she could suffer'.[36] Many of the patients with wounds received embrocations (i.e., fluid applications) of a more volatile nature. Patients with ulcers and wounds were frequently treated with digestives to promote the 'first stage' of healing.[37]

These data also suggest that ulcers, wounds, and tumours required more extensive use of the inward tenting of wounds with medicated dossils and plegits before bolstering them up. On the contrary, fractures and women's diseases demanded more externally applied bandages. As a precautionary measure, Turner noted that this procedure sometimes 'seem[s] a Paradox'. In the case of oedematous swellings, like that of King William's legs, bandaging clearly reduced the swelling. At other times, Turner warned that bandaging, particularly if inappropriate or performed by unskilled hands, actually produced such oedematous conditions.[38] Better precision in this procedure would, he argued, 'prevent many a bitter Groan of the Patient, as well as Heart-ach of the conscientious Practitioner'.[39]

Correlating Turner's use of cataplasms, fomentations, and other medicated applications with particular categories of disease distinguishes his surgical art from 'cure-all' remedies described in contemporary family self-help or domestic manuals. That is, Turner administered particular compounds for particular disorders rather than proffering panaceas like a quack, who typically claimed that plaisters were:

> good against all green wounds, old fistulas and ulcers, pains and aches in either head, limbs or bowels, contusions, tumours, or Queen's evil, sprains, fractures or dislocations, or any hurts whatsoever, receiv'd either by sword, cane or gunshot, knife, saw or hatchet, hammer, nail or tenterhook, fire, blast or gunpowder, &c. It will continue its virtues and be as useful seven years hence as at the present moment, so that you may lend it to your neighbours in the time of distress or affliction, and when it has perform'd forty cures 'twill be ne'er the worse, but still regain its integrity.[40]

Turner's surgical practice was quite time and labour intensive. Seventy percent of the wound patients required weeks of treatment. Fractures were generally treated for many months, as were three-quarters of his ulcer patients, half of those with women's diseases, and nearly half of those with tumours. At one extreme, Turner offered one tumour patient regular treatment for over a year. Typically, he tended patients' needs several times daily during the early course of treatment, but after a few weeks he saw them much less frequently. Four patients were sent to the hospital for extended care, and an additional two were recommended there, but refused to go. In contrast to the brief time physicians spent with their patients, the length of surgical treatment was considerably longer. In London, some physicians reputedly wrote their prescriptions while sitting in coffeehouses based upon a servant's or messenger's account of the disorder, and often never actually saw the patient they were treating.[41]

In general, Turner deviated from standard operative procedure only on an individual case basis. In one typical scenario, Turner found his wounded patient 'hot and restless' one morning after having suffered 'great Pain all Night'. Seeing the patient in this condition, Turner decided simply to take 'away some Blood, and contented [him]self for … the Time with only embrocating the … [area] above and below the Bandage' rather than completely redressing this patient's wound.[42] When Turner noticed that another patient's 'cough and hectic' still continued, he altered this patient's regimen.[43] Turner 'designedly omitted' fomenting one patient's wounded shoulder, whereas in another case, upon seeing 'no likelihood' of one poultice 'discussing' the humour of a different patient's tumour, Turner changed the poultice to one more likely to 'promote' the tumour's 'Maturation'.[44] Such improvisation upon the reaction or condition of the patient appeared to be part of the surgical art.

Turner's case histories reveal many particulars about surgical procedure. For example, Turner described that, when the situation allowed, patients were placed on a stool or table near a window so that the surgeon would have the best available light (see Figure 3.5). He also informed readers of the types and layout of instruments he planned to use. For example, the 'Pre-requisites' for reducing a fracture were placed 'in a large Dish, on a Stool or Table by the [patient's] Bed-side'. These items included a plaister compress, a defensative emplaster, a couple of bolsters of cloth, a roller, splints, tape, a basin of oxycrate, a pair of scissors, a penknife, and a pin-cushion with pins.[45] Additionally, wax candles were used for a variety of purposes. At times, they provided light under which the operator could see better. In other instances, their incandescence was useful for distinguishing fluid-filled from solid tumours, and their solid yet pliable consistency proved effective in probing various bodily cavities and wound sinuses.[46] To stop any excessive bleeding, Turner also had prepared cauteries in a chaffing dish of 'lighted Charcoal' to have 'just at Hand'.[47]

From his description, Turner appears to have had a large supply of surgical instruments available for use while operating in his home. When travelling to a patient's home or the site of an accident, he carried a much smaller variety of instruments loosely with him in his coat pockets; the more fine instruments were secured in his pocket

'Tweeser Case'. Among the instruments he carried were his lancet, probe, tweezers, scissors, various 'forcipes', several button cauteries, suture thread or silk, and 'Common Stitching' needles which, when needed, were held 'in the Fire till [they were] ... so temper'd as to Admit of bending'.[48] When particular medications were needed, the message was relayed to the local apothecary.

His overall operative procedure conformed with the recommendations of contemporary surgeons including Read and Wiseman. Only rarely did Turner distinguish his own mechanical operation from that of a recent surgical predecessor or colleague. For example, he sided with the 'frequently practis'd' method of using ligatures rather than styptics as a 'much easier way' to stop haemorrhaging.[49] Any deviation from earlier accounts was generally put forth as a cautionary suggestion. For instance, Turner suggested it was best to try to reduce a tumorous swelling before attempting to open it.[50] He also argued that lancets rather than caustics were more likely to 'Prevent' unsightly scars when treating facial wounds. Caustics, he claimed, which were laid on in the size of a 'Silver three-pence' will make 'an Eschar' as large as a six-pence within an hour.[51]

Turner's cases further illustrate that surgery was seldom a one-person job. Two, three, or more assistants were often relied upon to secure the patient or to hand Turner various instruments (see Figure 3.6). Some procedures required more manual assistance than others. To reduce one gentleman's dislocated humerus, for instance, Turner called upon the assistance of Mr Bentham, his neighbour in Devonshire Square. However, three 'strong fellows' were needed to hold and manoeuvre the dislocated femur of a more 'sprightly' young patient. 'Happening [to be] in his Neighbourhood', Turner also called for the assistance of surgeon Richard Bateman to help in this case. Since Bateman was away, his servant attended instead. Turner also recorded the help of various nurses, barbers, servants, and unnamed assistants. Turner was called in to assist other surgeons, too. Joseph Tanner, for example, called upon him to help reduce the dislocated humerus of a baker on Bishopsgate Street.

Turner consulted with a number of local surgeons and physicians, suggesting that urban surgical practice actually involved a wide interdependence or cooperative network of practitioners. Among the surgeons with whom he most frequently consulted were: Charles Bernard (12 cases), Richard Blundell (8 cases), William Petty (4 cases), and Richard Bateman and Edward Greene (3 cases each). On other occasions, Turner mentioned having worked with Anthony Herenden, William Layfield, William and Joseph

Babbington, Henry Boon, Joseph Tanner, Richard Harvey, Mr Cowling, and Mr Freemoult. He also consulted with physicians including Edward Tyson (4 cases), James Blondel (2 cases), and one case each with Richard Mead, Caleb Coatsworth, Charles Morton, Joannes Groenevelt, and Richard Blackburn.[52] Mr Boyce, the oculist, fit one of Turner's patients for a glass eye, Mr Johnson fit one for a truss, and 'his Instrument maker' fit another patient with a metal plate to protect the healthy skin surrounding the ulcer which Turner was treating.

Turner's cases indicate that he collaborated with many of London's surgical and medical elite. Bernard, for example, was one-time master of the Barber-Surgeons' Company, surgeon at St Bartholomew's Hospital, and Sergeant Surgeon to Queen Anne. Herenden, Layfield, Harvey, and Greene all served as master of the Barber-Surgeons' Company; Greene later served as surgeon to St Bartholomew's Hospital. Richard Blundell, according to economic historian Peter

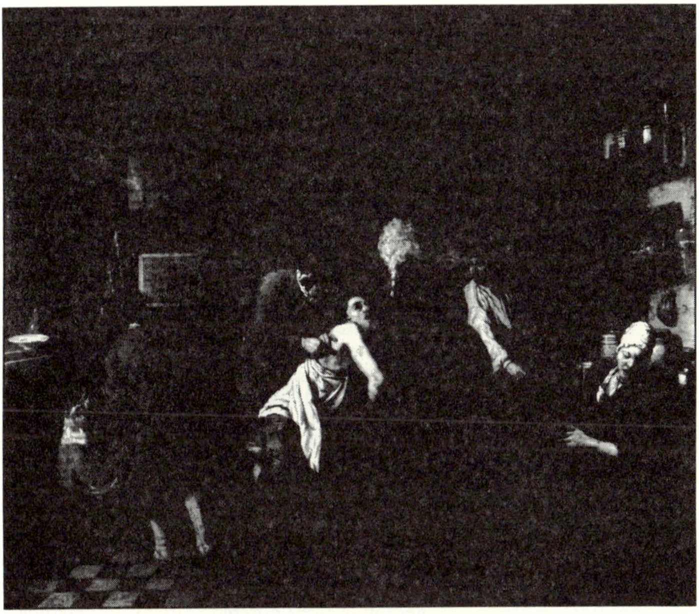

Figure 3.5
Surgeon Operating in his Surgery
(Jan Josef Horemans, the Elder, c.1722;
Wellcome Institute Library, London)

Earle, had established one of the most lucrative surgical practices in London.[53] Dr Tyson, among other capacities, served as anatomical curator to the Royal Society and promoted Turner's early work with anatomical dissections. Mead was pronounced the 'greatest physician of the Age' at the time of his death.[54] Coatesworth was one of the few individuals who, like Turner, practised surgery as a member of the Barber-Surgeons' Company before relinquishing that role in favour of medical practice. As to the characters of these men, Turner remarked that Blundell was a person 'thro' native temperament, more timerous ... than most others of so Sound a Judgement'.[55] James Ferne, a St Thomas' Hospital surgeon and master to William Cheselden was, according to Turner, 'a Gentleman of strict probity, good learning, and good Judgement'.[56] Turner esteemed William Petty as having 'all the Qualifications of an honest and able Artist'.[57]

Does Turner's collaboration with these elite practitioners imply that Turner, too, was among their ranks? Not necessarily, but it does

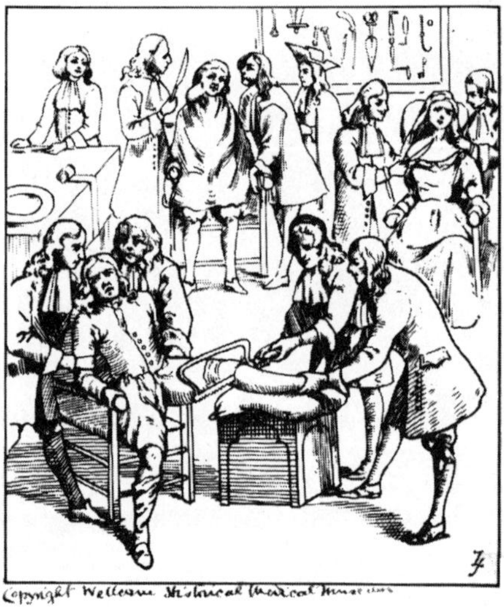

Figure 3.6
An operating room in a surgery with three different patients undergoing operations, all of whom are attended by more than one surgeon.
(Z.S., 1690; Wellcome Institute Library, London)

exemplify that Turner conformed to the by-laws of London's Barber-Surgeons' Company. Surgeons were, according to the 1708 by-laws, to 'Make Knowne' any 'Wounded, Hurt, or Diseased' patients found to be 'in Danger of any loss of Life or Maime of Limb' to 'one of the ... [Company's] Masters or Governors' who are 'skillfull and Expert in that Art'.[58] Supportive of these by-laws, Turner cautioned readers that in all difficult cases 'it will behove you, ... to consult with some ancient and learned master of your Art, that both your own Reputation, as well as your Patient's welfare, may be thereby secured'. He further argued this consultation should take place in a timely manner while the patient is still in a 'condition' to be cured.[59]

More significantly, Turner's case studies show precisely how these by-laws were put into practice. For example, after initially tending one young man's fractured skull, Turner called upon Mr Blundell for 'mature deliberation' over the course of therapy. Once they agreed the case warranted trephination, Anthony Herenden, a warden of the Barber-Surgeons' Company, examined the case and offered a more 'expert' opinion. In another situation, Turner sought advice from Sergeant Bernard on the second day of treating the potentially fatal wound of a patient who had been 'prick'd in the belly' during a sword fight. Elsewhere, William Layfield, master of the Barber-Surgeons' Company, was called upon to first consult with and then assist Turner in extirpating one woman's prolapsed and mortified uterus. For another patient, Turner met with Blundell, after which they offered their 'joint opinion' that this patient's foot should be amputated.[60]

From another perspective, Turner's repeated work with Edward Tyson and Charles Bernard, both proponents of an innovative experimental approach to practice, may indicate that Turner, too, adopted this agenda. Such positioning would have made him less popular with the 'old guard' of the Barber-Surgeons' Company, the Royal College of Physicians, and the Royal Society. The connection between Turner's association with Tyson and his claims for reforming surgical practice will be discussed in later chapters.

In some cases, the instigation for calling upon other surgeons came not from Turner, but from the patient. For example, when Turner was treating a ship captain's knee, the patient requested a consultation with Bernard. In another case, Turner recommended to a patient that if she 'and her Friends thought fit', he would 'cut out' the patient's breast tumours, whereupon the patient desired Bernard's opinion on the matter.[61] When Turner refused to interfere with the self-treatments one man had been applying to his ulcer 'for many years', the patient turned to surgeon Edward Greene for advice. This information substantiates sociologist N. D. Jewson's claim that eighteenth-century patients adjudicated a practitioner's competence and directly selected the therapy they deemed appropriate.[62] However, the patients Turner described were not all from the gentle class that Jewson discussed. Indeed, tradesmen and poor patients alike appear to have held this right of choosing whether to accept or refuse surgical therapy.

Many patients were attended by both surgeons and physicians concurrently. For instance, while Turner treated the tongue which one patient nearly severed in an epileptic fit, her physician, Edward Tyson, also treated her with an anti-epileptic concoction. Dr Tyson also stood by as Turner operated on the hydrocephalus of a young patient. Although Turner argued that these particular tumours generally 'fall under the Care of Physicians', complications from their treatment often led to ulceration, gangrene, and mortification. Without selectively ridiculing Tyson, Turner claimed that physicians' treatments of hydrocephalus patients typically 'make ... work for the Surgeon'.[63] On another occasion, in cooperation with Dr Mead, Turner administered lenient purges and frequently let blood while Mead provided internal remedies to aid one clergyman's hernia.[64]

Turner's patients, however, did not exclusively call upon orthodox practitioners. As he argued elsewhere, there was a 'natural Propensity in Humane [sic] kind, to attempt the speediest means of self-preservation'.[65] As many as eighteen of Turner's patients obtained treatments from some 'empiric' before seeking his care. Half of his patients suffering with ulcers were previously treated by such practitioners. One patient with a large ulcer on her arm had 'passed thro' several hands' before calling upon Turner,[66] whereas another young woman came to Turner directly 'out of the Hands of a Famous Empiric'.[67] Another individual, so Turner claimed, was 'almost ruined' by an empiric before Turner's care.[68]

For some patients, Turner appears to have been the last resort, but other patients' cases show that securing his help did not preclude them from returning to empirics. One fellow suffering from an inguinal rupture had acquired the surgical assistance of William Petty, who, in turn, called Turner in as a consultant. However, during their treatment a 'bold pretender' intervened, secured the patient's confidence, and steered him away from the surgeons. In another case, a pretender 'got into ... [the] good opinion' of a patient whom Turner was treating, and convinced him to quit Turner's care.[69] A different patient returned to Turner after her condition became worse following two months of treatment by an 'old woman'.[70] Thus, Turner's patients took much control in seeking out practitioners that they deemed most appropriate for particular conditions.

The surgical conditions and treatments of Turner's patients greatly affected their lives and the lives of those around them. Most drastically, 21 of the 110 patients died.[71] The highest mortality appears to have been among the tumour patients (28.9%). However, 54 of all the patients Turner discussed were eventually 'healed' or 'cured'. Many of these patients regained a 'better State of Health ... than [they had] enjoyed for months'.[72] Of all the treatments which Turner described, more complete 'cures' were obtained for patients suffering from woman's diseases (100%). This cure rate is, in part, due to the type of treatment they received. Half of the patients were simply treated by replacing or restraining prolapsed uteri. At the other extreme, only one-third of the patients with fractures were 'cured'. However, many more achieved at least partial usefulness of their limbs.

Most patients underwent months of therapy, being confined to bed and thereby away from their means of financial support. The victualler whom Turner treated for a lacerated bicep muscle was out of work for over six months, but upon returning to work found himself still able, with his 'lame Arm', to 'lift up a full Pot of Beer'.[73] A coachman, after being knocked from his coach box, was, after four months, also able to 'follow ... his old Employment'. Turner noted, however, that this patient never regained 'good Use' of one arm and his whole hand remained 'as they say, clumsey [sic]'.[74] Mr Prideaux's coachman was not capable of returning to his job because a callus never formed to cover and strengthen his broken arm. Instead, his master 'procur[ed] ... [him] a letter-carrier's place'. In like manner, Turner was unable to restore completely one gentlewoman's 'disjuncture' of her tailbone, and for years thereafter she was forced to use her finger to 'facilitate the exitus' of faeces. Of the patients treated with fractured limbs, several were left with crooked or shortened legs; one became 'bed-rid' as the result of her fractured thigh bone that 'never heal'd'; and several were forced to resort to walking with canes.

At times the results of Turner's treatments surprised him. One old man refused to allow Turner to amputate his leg after the bones had been 'shivered ... to pieces' when run over by a loaded cart. Despite Turner's persistent encouragement to amputate, the patient preferred to save his leg and opted for a lengthy course of treatment under Turner's care. Contrary to Turner's initial prognosis, the man recovered such remarkable use of his leg that, according to Turner, it gave him 'less trouble' than what 'in likelihood' would have 'attend[ed] a stump leg'.[75] By contrast, in another, admittedly more typical case a patient who refused the amputation of a mortified, dislocated ankle remained in a 'poor, lame condition' for the rest of his life.

Some of Turner's histories illustrate how individuals other than patients became involved in the case. For instance, one man was injured during his flight from the bailiffs who were sent after him by his 'creditor'.[76] With moral sentiment, Turner recalled how the creditor, upon seeing the patient after the 'sad Accident ... freely forgave him his Debt' and even paid Turner to care for him. In another case, a man sharing a room at the Dolphin Inn without Bishopsgate was 'committed to the Compter' after summoning help for his 'Chamber-fellow' who had slashed his throat during the night. In intriguing detective-fiction style, Turner recounted the details under which he eventually healed the man's throat so that he could speak and inform officials that he had attempted his own life, and that the gaoled man was not an assassin. Rather, he regarded the gaoled 'stranger' as the sole reason for which he was still alive.[77]

Surgeon–Patient Communication

In many instances, Turner appears to have practised according to what Talcott Parsons described as a functionalist relationship between practitioner and patient.[78] Turner, as practitioner, wielded considerable authority over his patients. The patients accordingly submitted their bodies to the care of an all-knowing practitioner. At times, however, Turner heavily relied upon a patient's input in order to discern just how their disorders affected their lives. In such cases, Turner operated in more of a Foucauldian manner in which the power relation between surgeon and patient was not unidirectional. Rather, patients could wield an upper hand in negotiating their own care when they held knowledge that Turner needed to elicit in order to alleviate their concerns regarding a particular disorder.

Turner's case studies reveal some, although minimal, insight into the level of communication that existed between surgeons and their patients. Overall, Turner appears to have spent little if any time describing the actual diagnosis of surgical disorders with his patients. There was probably little need for this since both Turner and his patients were generally aware whether the incapacity was due to a visible swelling, fracture, prolapse, hernia, or ulcer. Surgical diagnosis was, therefore, at least on one level, much less ambiguous to sufferers than diagnosing internal disorders. Any commentary in his text about diagnostic uncertainty or differential diagnosis was intended for the edification of surgical readers rather than illustrating a point of discussion with patients.

Instead, Turner devoted significant space in his case studies to describing his discussions with patients over his intended course of therapy.[79] He frequently noted the need to obtain the patient's consent, or, in young patients, that of their parents, before proceeding along a specific line of treatment. In other words, it was the patient's right to accept or refuse surgical treatment. 'The sick Man has his choice', stated Turner. *Quod volenti non fit Injuria.* If it 'be the Choice of the Sick to die ... Piecemeal, or to rot ... alive, you are to forbear pressing upon him, let him have his Choice'. However, 'if he desires Life upon any Terms, and you know of no other way than by cutting off a Limb, you are to proceed in God's Name, and will be ... justified at his Tribunal' should the patient die.[80]

Turner received the consent of some patients easily, while others often needed a great deal of 'persuasion' and 'encouragement' on his part. Patients who had previously been 'exceedingly harrass'd' by pretenders for a 'long Time' were, Turner argued, 'more easily prevailed on to submit' to his specific recommendations.[81] However, even with these patients, Turner acknowledged it was difficult to get them to submit to cauterization, castration, or amputation. For these situations, he cautioned readers, one must 'put' recommendations to a patient in the 'mildest way' possible, and then allow them a 'Day or two to Consider thereof'.[82] Part of this time, he suggested, allowed the patient to mentally adjust or to prepare for the recommended operation. A surgeon's success, therefore, depended not only upon his technical prowess, but also on his ability to clearly communicate his intentions to potential patients, to steer them away from quacks, and to reassure them about the proposed course of treatment.

Turner was not universally successful in persuading patients to undergo painful surgical procedures. Some patients were so 'terrified at the Thought of an Instrument' that they 'chose rather to dispense with the Disturbance, than ... to be relieved thereof'. He obligingly accepted these patients' wishes.[83] In one instance, however, a patient 'acknowledged' after receiving treatment that she had been 'more terrify'd by the Idea she had formed' about the surgical procedure than she was 'pain'd by the Operation' itself.[84]

Although apparently sympathetic to his patients, Turner did not attempt to deceive them into believing surgery would be pain free.[85] Rather, he sought to overcome the stigmatization of pain associated with surgical procedures on two levels: morally and practically. He claimed that, at times, surgeons were unable to control certain 'Sundry Causes' of suffering in surgical operations. Pain arose, he argued, from 'the Fluxion of Humours, the hot and dry Intemperies of the Part, the exquisite Sense of the Same, the ill position of the Member, the Irregularity of the Patient'. He assured readers that surgeons were not 'delighted' by having to inflict pain upon their patients during surgical operations. Quite the contrary, he claimed that upon hearing the 'clamorous shrieks and Outcries of poor suffering' patients, a practitioner often became an 'almost equal Sufferer'.[86]

All 'too often', however, Turner noted that pain arose from the 'Ignorance of the Surgeon in not rightly managing the Bandage, or proportioning the Strength and heat of his medicines to the diseased Patient'.[87] On a practical level, Turner suggested to surgeons, giving examples in many case studies, different ways they could best alleviate pain and comfort their patients. Surgeons could, he argued, soften dressings with more liniment, provide the type of dressing that was 'easier to the Patient', and place fractured limbs in 'as easie a Position' as they could 'contrive'.[88] Additionally, he claimed women and children, or 'more particularly, a Woman with Child', should never be 'suffer'd to see your [cautery] irons'.[89] This equipment should be, he argued, kept 'in a Dish by the Bed-side' but 'out of [the patient's] sight'.[90] Any 'Fears' created by the 'smoak ... and hiss' of the irons would, he claimed, be 'lessen'd' within a few days of treatment.[91] As to the pangs of 'heat and sharpness' derived from many medications, Turner cautioned readers against beginning to deterge or cicatrize wounds and ulcers 'too early' before the site had been well digested.[92] Turner also urged readers to use a patient's outward expression of pain as a sign to modify treatment. For example, Turner withdrew the old dossils in one patient's wound only upon watching for signs of the patient's complaint of pain.[93]

Overall, Turner presented his experience with the art of surgery as a personal relationship between himself and his patients. Each patient's case was described as an individual segment of his surgical career. Above and beyond the patients' contribution to Turner's income or enhancement of his occupational and social level, Turner depicted them as humans in whose lives he had effected some change. By revealing these humane aspects of the surgical art to his readers, Turner deemed his work would 'serve, not only the present, but the succeeding Generation' as a moral guide to practise even after any particular procedures he advanced became outdated.[94]

This chapter has drawn upon myriad examples illuminating various aspects of the surgical art. The emphasis upon Turner's case studies is a step towards reconstructing a more complete account of surgical practice within a particular time period. As Turner's descriptions suggest, surgery involved much more than treating externally manifest disease. Instead, Turner and many surgical contemporaries concentrated upon the need to prepare and treat the whole body rather than just a local site of injury, inflammation, or irritation. Surgeons like Turner became involved in correcting the underlying, invisible causes of externally manifest disease as well as digesting wounds and reducing fractures. This extended realm of surgical treatment became the focus of another of Turner's writings, *De Morbis Cutaneis. Diseases Incident to the Skin.*

Notes

1 S. Sharpe, *Critical Enquiry Into the Present State of Surgery*, preface.

2 D. Turner, *Art of Surgery* (London: C. Rivington, J. Lacy and J. Clarke, 1725) vol. 2, 28. Henceforth, unless otherwise noted, my references are taken from this 2nd edition revised and expanded beyond the original 1722 publication. I previously discussed Turner's surgical career in 'Daniel Turner and the *Art of Surgery* in Early Eighteenth-Century London', *Journal of the Royal Society of Medicine*, lxxxvii (1994), 781-5. Two of the most helpful accounts which demonstrate the potential usefulness of case histories as historical documents are Guenter B. Risse and John Harley Warner's 'Reconstructing Clinical Activities: Patient Records in Medical History', *Social History of Medicine*, v (1992), 183-205, and Ortrun Riha's 'Surgical Case Records as an Historical Source: Limits and Perspectives', *Social History of Medicine*, viii (1995), 271-83. Additionally, Barbara Duden provided a remarkable analysis of the case record books of one eighteenth-century physician in *The Woman beneath the Skin: A Doctor's Patients in Eighteenth-Century Germany* (Cambridge: Harvard University Press, 1991).

3 Robert Darnton points out this missing element of history in his *The Kiss of LaMourette* (London: Faber and Faber, 1990), xix. John C. Rose and Milton Corn, 'Dr E. and Other Patients: New Lessons from Old Case Reports', *Journal of the History of Medicine*, xxxix (1984), 5.

4 Henry Robert Plommer included brief biographical details of each of these booksellers in his *Dictionaries of the Printers and Booksellers who were at work in England, Scotland, and Ireland, 1557-1775* (London, Bibliographical Society reprint, 1977).

5 For a discussion of the various works see P. K. Wilson's 'Vernacularisation vs. Vulgarisation'.

6 Daniel Turner, *The Art of Surgery*, 1722, vol. 1, Preface, 6-7, and the 1725, 2nd edition, vol. 2, p.438.

7 For example, see John Maubray, *The Female Physician* (London: J. Holland, 1724) or Nicholas Fontanus, *The Woman's Doctour* (London: J. Blague & S. Howes, 1652). Robert A. Erickson discussed the style of English midwifery texts is in 'The books of generation: some observations on the style of the British midwife books, 1671-1764', in P.-G. Boucé (ed.), *Sexuality in Eighteenth-Century Britain* (Manchester: Manchester University Press, 1982), 74-94.

8 L. Beier, *Sufferers & Healers,* 51-96, F.N.L. Poynter, *The Journal of James Yonge (1647-1721), Plymouth Surgeon* (London: Longman's, Green, & Co., 1963). W. Wood's 1679-1690 surgical casebook is found at the Royal College of Surgeons (England), MSS Tract A297 (3). Guenter Risse provided an extensive analysis of late eighteenth-century surgical patients and practice of The Royal Infirmary, Edinburgh in his *Hospital life in Enlightenment Scotland: Care and teaching at the Royal Infirmary of Edinburgh* (Cambridge: Cambridge University Press, 1986), esp. 119-239. Details of Richard Austin's and Charles Oxley's recorded observations at St Thomas' Hospital, Southwark form the basis of my 'Sacred Sanctuaries for the Sick: Surgery at St Thomas' Hospital (1725-1726)', *The London Journal,* xvii (1992), 36-53. Only two of the gentlemen, Mr Darnelli of the Penny Post Office, and Mr C.S., were specifically identified. He also treated one Gentleman's child.

10 D. Turner, *Art of Surgery*, vol. 2, 127.

11 P.K. Wilson, 'Sacred Sanctuaries for the Sick', 38-40

12 D. Turner, *Art of Surgery*, vol. 1, 378.

13 *Ibid.*, vol. 2, 380.

14 *Ibid.*, *Art of Surgery*, vol. 2, 193.

15 Roy Porter, *Health For Sale. Quackery in England 1660-1850* (Manchester: Manchester University Press, 1989), 136. As was concluded at the 13 October 1990 Society for the Social History of Medicine symposium on 'Accidents in History: Injuries, Fatalities and Social Relations', a study of the causes, consequences, and treatments of accidents in the 18th century awaits its author. Roy Porter has provided an impressive beginning to this underexplored area in 'Accidents in the Eighteenth Century', in Roger Cooter and Bill Luckin (eds), *Accidents in History: Injuries, Fatalities and Social Relations* (Amsterdam: Rodopi, 1997), 90-106.

16 F.N.L. Poynter, *Journal of James Yonge*, 80 and Dorothy Porter and Roy Porter, *Patient's Progress: Doctors and Doctoring in Eighteenth-*

century England (Cambridge, Polity Press, 1989), 170.

17 Concluding that Turner only bled the minority of his patients based solely on the numerical representations in Table 3.2, however, would be incorrect. Instead, these data must be interpreted in context with what was presented in the text.

18 D. Turner, *Art of Surgery*, vol. 1, 533. Joseph Binns also discriminated between which patients to bleed: L. Beier, *Sufferers & Healers*, 63.

19 D. Turner, *Art of Surgery*, vol. 1, 30-34.

20 Turner mentioned fees in only five other cases. The most elaborate 'contract' Turner described appears in his *Syphilis. A Practical Dissertation on the Venereal Disease* (London: J. Walthoe), 4th edn, 1732, 379. For £50 he agreed to dress a patient's head wound at Turner's house every day for a year. When the patient grew too 'feeble' to 'come out', Turner attended him 'for the same Stipend every other Day' at the patient's house. After a year, upon finding many more nodes appearing on his head, the patient found the 'Expense too great for his Income' and Turner agreed to dress the patient twice weekly for £40 per annum.

21 D. Turner, *Art of Surgery*, vol. 1, 402.

22 L. Beier, *Sufferers & Healers*, 62, described that purgatives were often administered for preventative as well as curative measures.

23 D. Turner, *Art of Surgery*, vol. 1, 51.

24 These remedies are also found in George Bate's *Pharmacopeia Bateana: or, Bate's dispensatory* (London: W. & J. Innys, 1770), 5th edn; a work to which Turner frequently referred his readers.

25 D. Turner, *Art of Surgery*, vol 1, 228. In D. Turner, *De Morbis Cutaneis* (London: R. Bonwicke, J. Walthoe, R. Wilkin, T. Ward, and S. Tooke, 1723), 2nd edn, 492, the author described how two children that he knew had been killed by overpurgation.

26 D. Turner, *Art of Surgery*, vol. 2, 372.

27 *Ibid.*, vol. 1, 534.

28 *Ibid.*, vol. 2, 85.

29 *Ibid.*, vol. 1, 275.

30 *Ibid.*, vol. 1, 16.

31 *Ibid.*, vol. 2, 39.

32 *Ibid.*, vol. 2, 14. See also Thomas Fuller, *Pharmacopeia Extemporanea* (London: B. Walford, 1710).

33 D. Turner, *Art of Surgery*, vol. 1, 127-8.

34 *Ibid.*, vol. 2, 50.

35 D. Turner, *De Morbis Cutaneis*, 213.

36 D. Turner, *Art of Surgery*, vol. 1, 39.

37 Turner adopted the common distinctions for the stages of healing: digestion, mundification (or detersion), incarnation, and cicatrisation.

38 D. Turner, *Art of Surgery*, vol. 1, 61-2.

39 *Ibid.*, 21.

40 Ned Ward, *The London Spy* (London: Folio Society Edition, 1960), 102.

41 See J. J. Keevil, 'Coffeehouse Cures', *Journal of the History of Medicine*, ix (1954), 191-5. As we know so very little about individual physicians' practices, I concur with W. F. Bynum's comment that the idea of a regular coffee house practice most likely arises by overgeneralizing from the few instances that are known. See W.F. Bynum, 'Health, Disease and Medical Care' in G.S. Rousseau and Roy Porter (eds), *The Ferment of Knowledge: Studies in the Historiography of Eighteenth-Century Science* (Cambridge: Cambridge University Press, 1980), 229.

42 D. Turner, *Art of Surgery*, vol. 1, 515.

43 *Ibid.*, vol. 2, 74.

44 *Ibid.*, vol. 1, 385, vol. 2, 364.

45 *Ibid.*, vol. 2, 141.

46 Turner described his preparation of these candles in *Syphilis*, 96.

47 D. Turner, *Art of Surgery*, vol. 1, 212.

48 *Ibid.*, 1722, vol. 1, 334.

49 *Ibid.*, vol. 1, 343.

50 *Ibid.*, vol. 1, 193-4.

51 *Ibid.*, vol. 1, 23.

52 Additionally, 4 unidentified physicians and 1 unidentified surgeon were mentioned as consultants.

53 Peter Earle, *The Making of the Middle Class: Business, Society and Family Life in London, 1660-1730* (London: Methuen, 1989), 150.

54 *Whitehall Evening Post*, as cited in Arnold Zuckermann's 'Dr. Richard Mead (1673-1754). A Biographical Study' (Ph.D. thesis, University of Illinois, Urbana, 1965), 268-269.

55 D. Turner, *Art of Surgery*, vol. 2, 287.

56 *Ibid.*, vol. 2, 328. Turner so admired him that he dedicated the second volume of the third and later editions of *Art of Surgery* to Ferne.

57 *Ibid.*, vol. 1, 215.

58 'The Rules Orders and Ordinances of "Barbers and Surgeons" of London', MSS A/2/1, 33.

59 D. Turner, *Art of Surgery*, vol. 1 (1722), 253.

60 *Ibid.*, vol. 2, 350-351. Turner did not describe any amputation, but referred readers to texts by La Vauguion, Le Clerc, La Charriere, Fabricius Hildanus, and Wiseman. Apparently, Turner rarely

performed amputations, a find corroborating recent historical reassessments that amputations were not as common as once claimed. See, for example, R. Porter and D. Porter, *In Sickness and In Health*, 106, L. Beier, *Sufferers & Healers*, 53, 70, and J.J. Keevil, *Medicine and the Navy*, vol. 2, 171.

61 D. Turner, *Art of Surgery*, vol. 1, 76.

62 N. D. Jewson, 'Medical Knowledge and the Patronage System in 18th Century England', *Sociology*, viii (1974): esp. 375-8.

63 D. Turner, *Art of Surgery*, vol. 1, 192, 210.

64 *Ibid.*, vol. 1, 288-289.

65 D. Turner, *Apologia Chyrurgica*, 1.

66 D. Turner, *Art of Surgery*, vol. 2, 22.

67 *Ibid.*, vol. 1, 154.

68 *Ibid.*, vol. 2, 52.

69 *Ibid.*, vol. 2, 89.

70 *Ibid.*, vol. 2, 83-3.

71 Of these, Turner secured permission to dissect seven of the bodies. In addition to a number of dissections described in the Royal Society's *Philosophical Transactions*, contemporary accounts of the dissecting 'Art' were detailed in the vernacular English translation of Michael Lyser's *The Art of Dissecting the Human body* (London: for Joseph Davidson, 1740) and Charles Nicholas Jenty's *A Synoptical Exposition of the Parts of the Human Body, as they are gradually met with in Dissection* in his *Course of Anatomico-Physiological Lectures on the Human Structure and Animal Oeconomy* (London; James Rivington and James Flecher), 1757, vol. 1, clxxxiii-ccxv. For a cursory survey, see Victor Robinson's 'Anatomical Dissection in the 18th Century', *Ciba Symposia*, iii (1941), 845-53.

72 D, Turner, *Art of Surgery*, vol. 1, 79.

73 *Ibid.*, vol. 1, 386.

74 *Ibid.*, vol. 1, 524.

75 *Ibid.*, vol. 2, 175.

76 *Ibid.*, vol. 1, 378-7. The man's biceps tendon had been ripped from its attachment as the patient caught his shoulder on a tenterhook jumping 'over the Rails in a Neighbour's Yard'.

77 *Ibid.*, vol. 1, 439-42. An affidavit was drawn up 'for each Witness to sign' which was used, together with the one Turner made himself 'before the Magistrate', to procure the 'poor Fellow's Release'.

78 Talcott Parsons' functionalist approach is discussed in Deborah Lupton's *Medicine as Culture: Illness, Disease and the Body in Western Societies* (London: SAGE Publications, 1994), 7, 89-90, 105-6

79 Lynda Payne examined Turner's professional relationship with his

patients as part of her analysis of the emotional distance that early modern practitioners chose to put between themselves and their patients. See her '"To lose foolish tenderness": Clinical detachment and its origins among medical men in early-modern England' (Ph.D. thesis, University of California, Davis, 1997).

80 Daniel Turner, 'Some modest Animadversions on Dr. Harris' *Dissertationes Medicae*, especially his thirteenth, *de Erroribus Chirurgorum*', appended to his *Art of Surgery*, vol. 1, 560.

81 D. Turner, *Art of Surgery*, vol. 2, 366.

82 *Ibid.*, vol. 2, 350-1.

83 *Ibid.*, vol. 1, 208.

84 *Ibid.*, vol. 2, 100. It remains unknown whether this was a common or rare experience.

85 For further insight into 'Pain in the Age of Enlightenment', see Roselyn Rey's *History of Pain* (Paris: Editions La Decouverte, 1993), 107-146.

86 D. Turner, *Apologia Chyrurgica*, 121-2.

87 D. Turner, *Art of Surgery*, vol. 2,18.

88 D. Turner, *Apologia Chyrurgica*, 93.

89 D. Turner, *Art of Surgery*, vol. 1, 528.

90 *Ibid.*, vol. 2, 377.

91 *Ibid.*, vol. 1, 166.

92 *Ibid.*, vol. 2, 20.

93 *Ibid.*, vol. 1, 498.

94 *Ibid.*, vol. 1, To the Reader.

4

Surgical Perspectives of the Body with a Special Focus on Skin

Historians have typically represented surgeons as treating a different domain of disease than physicians. Eighteenth-century physicians attended patients suffering from internal disorders such as fevers, gout, consumption, asthma, rheumatism, and palsies. Their armamentarium consisted primarily of internally administered medicine or physic. Alternatively, surgical texts described treatments for externally manifest diseases and disorders. Surgeons were instructed how to incise and dress tumorous swellings, reduce fractured bones and dislocated joints, repair ruptures and fistulae, amputate limbs and 'cut' for bladder stones. In addition, they frequently applied topical astringents, digestives, repellants, blisters, plaisters and poultices.

More noticeably than for practising physicians, the skin provided the basis of the mechanical handicraft of surgery. Eighteenth-century surgical treatises described particular mechanical operations which involved excising, incising, denuding, debriding, and injecting the skin. Some contemporary case histories placed so much emphasis on the external treatments and so little on the patients themselves, the writings suggest that surgery was more skin-oriented than patient-oriented.

Few popular or medical histories have focused upon the skin. When the skin has become the object of scrutiny, it is typically used to develop an understanding of racism and monstrosity (i.e., the 'other'), to lay the foundation for cosmetic or clothing histories, or to explain how minute ecosystems are dependent upon this living surface[1] (see Figure 4.1). To establish an historically appropriate cultural and medical context, this chapter discusses various popular and professional views of skin markings and diseases addressed in early eighteenth-century London.

Although many late seventeenth- and early eighteenth-century English surgical authors discussed skin disorders, only one author, Daniel Turner, elaborated at length upon the diseases which he claimed were 'incident upon the skin'. Turner's primary work on these diseases,

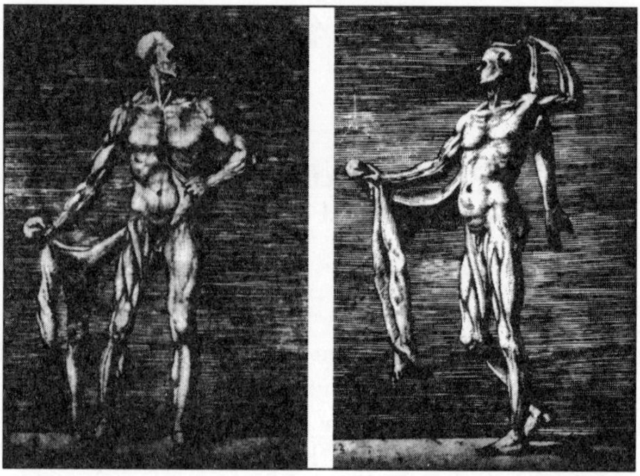

Figure 4.1

The skin has typically been removed from any discussion of anatomy just as it is removed from these male ecórché anatomical figures. (G. Bonasone, 15—; Wellcome Institute Library, London)

De Morbis Cutaneis (1714), not only describes contemporary treatments for these disorders, but it illuminates much of the importance skin and skin diseases held for surgeons in early eighteenth-century London.[2]

Rather than expound upon the contemporary skin disorders and their treatments, this chapter examines the ways that Turner's *De Morbis Cutaneis* illuminates how the skin represented or expressed a paradoxical barrier between the practices of physicians and surgeons. After briefly explaining contemporary views of the skin and the arrangement, content, and explicit intended readership of Turner's work, the chapter turns to Turner's representation of the skin as much more than the physical boundary separating the practices of surgery and physic. Specifically, his discussion of the therapeutic capacity of the skin was actually part of the contemporary dispute over the surgeons' right to administer internal physic. By focussing upon Turner's identification of the skin as a literal and rhetorical reference point to disease, new insight is provided about the surgical view of the body in Enlightenment London.

Visible Bodily Markings

Many popular Enlightenment ideas about skin markings and spots were carried over from the previous century.[3] Moles on the face, for example, as discussed in *Aristotle's Last Legacy* (1733), had long been thought to forecast 'bad Fortune'. Warts, devil's marks, and witch's tits, although no longer usable as court evidence in witchcraft trials, retained their diabolical association in folk belief.[4] A growing interest in physiognomy also focused attention upon facial skin markings on the face.[5] Like many Anglican clerics, physiognomists also proclaimed that the marks and expressions upon the face bore an outward reflection of the soul.[6]

Peculiar markings on a person's left cheek close to the nose were often publicly recognized as a shoplifter's brand. When no one would employ innocent individuals with similar natural markings, public outcry altered the form of punishment in 1705. Thereafter, such skin markings no longer forced innocent and convicted individuals into a 'life of crime' for mere subsistence.[7]

Blemishes on the face and hands of women were often associated with another illegal pastime: prostitution.[8] Some, like the harlots of Hogarth's engravings, covered their blemishes with 'beauty spots'.[9] Women not among this following 'resolv'd' to 'get rid' of any skin marking which their sweethearts might mistakenly perceive as a 'sign of sluttishness'.[10] Individuals 'poxed' or 'clapped' from prostitutes also became 'marked' in ways which led to much public jeering. The 'French Crown', for example, became a 'favourite literary *double entendre*' for baldness associated with the French Pox or syphilis. A deteriorated 'saddle-nose', the mark of long-standing syphilis, was frequently seen on passers-by as well as in contemporary drama and fiction.[11]

Parallel with or consequent to the rise of consumerization in the early eighteenth century, beauty became even more of a commodity than in previous centuries.[12] Beautifying the skin was particularly important among females. 'The female world', so the *Spectator* reported, was 'very busy among themselves in bartering for features' of beauty.[13] Turner corroborated this account, arguing that the 'fair Sex' set a 'higher value' upon beauty than anything else.[14] Men, too, were skin conscious. One gentleman whose face appeared rough, covered with pustules, and coloured with a 'flaming Redness', claimed himself too 'shy' to appear 'in the Ladies Company, and in public Assemblies'. After a local surgeon helped him recover his 'natural complexion', his 'Acquaintances' claimed that he 'seem'd to be a quite different Person' from what he had been.[15] Handbills posted throughout London advertised recipes for particular 'complexion waters' and 'Beautifying creams' to remove everything from redness, roughness, and wrinkles, to the 'Pits in the Face' from smallpox. Domestic self-help manuals also proffered 'secret' and 'well approved' preservatives for the skin alongside their preservatives for fruits and vegetables.

In addition to providing beautification remedies, popular writings also addressed three other skin concerns: the plague, smallpox, and the itch. Although most eighteenth-century Londoners had little if any personal experience with the devastating 1665 plague, anxiety over its potential recurrence was ever-present. Such anxiety reached a peak in 1719 when news reached London of an outbreak of the plague in Marseilles. Anglican ministers, including the Bishop of London, delivered both moral pronouncements and public precautions against its reappearance in England.[16] The public, as well as physicians and surgeons, had come to recognize palpable skin growths under the armpits or in the groin as plague-sores which were ultimately viewed as signs of impending death. Public fear was further exacerbated by the vivid accounts of the skin markings and related sequela from this disease in Daniel Defoe's popular *Journal of the Plague Year* (1722).

Smallpox also stirred significant public concern. When a 'servant-maid' of 'fine Skin and clear Complexion' discovered a 'Cluster of Pimples' on the skin of her thigh, she immediately 'acquainted' her mistress with her 'Fears of the Small-Pox'.[17] These fears may have ranged from the physical discomforts and high mortality of this disease, to the life-long disfigurement that many survivors suffered.[18] Stories abounded, like that of Nancy Jones, who, at nineteen, 'Struck misfortune' by 'catching' smallpox. The disease 'ruined' her 'pretty face' and her health, after which she was reduced to abject poverty and prostitution.[19] Many women, particularly young, marriageable middle- or upper- class women, sought extreme measures to preserve their beauty against this disease. Such effort is attested by one young Gentlewoman who, in 1723, when smallpox was 'more than usually Epidemical' in London, applied a 'defensative mask' endeavouring to 'save her Face'. Although this preventative measure preserved her facial beauty, it unfortunately 'bound the pores' of her facial skin, ultimately leading to her demise.[20]

A distemper known as 'The Itch' also troubled many Londoners. Historical accounts claim that the itch was one of the most prevalent skin diseases of the period.[21] Although some authors, like physician Richard Boulton, claimed it 'too well known to want any Description',[22] we can gain further understanding of this disorder through contemporary descriptions readily found in popular domestic manuals. Arabella Atkyns, pseudonymous author of *The Family Magazine*, described this disorder as 'a breaking out of pustules over the whole body, chiefly between the fingers, and about the joints, from a sharp humour, which causes itching, and thence scratching'. In some patients, the itch 'suddenly disappears', whereas in others, it 'return[ed] at stated seasons'.[23] Londoner Thomas Spooner argued that the itch was capable of undergoing a natural progression or transformation into scabies and eventually into that most 'malignant Distemper ... affect[ing] the External Parts of the Body', leprosy.[24] Public anxiety over this transformation created such a demand for treatment that, according to one contemporary, there was 'scarce an old woman ... without some Secret [remedy] for the Itch'.[25]

Like many diseases, the itch created awkward social and economic situations. Scratching the itch in public was not tolerated in polite society. Ned Ward, in his *London Spy* (1699-1703), pointed out the uncouthness of the Scottish and the Irish as people 'very much given to scratching and shrugging, as if they held lousiness no shame and the itch no scandal'.[26] Lancashire parish records indicate that the itch reached such proportions there that many local inhabitants were rendered unable to work.[27]

With an increasing social consciousness of beauty, a fear of particular skin disease and disfigurements, and an expanding middle-class wealth, the demand for protection of the skin and correction of visible markings grew as well.

Surgical and Medical Views of Skin Disease

Treatments for skin diseases were typically found in surgical writings. Among the 85 different English surgical treatises available in early eighteenth-century London bookstalls, Richard Wiseman's *Eight Chirurgical Treatises* (5th edn, 1719) and William Salmon's *Ars Chirurgica* (1698) provided considerable information on certain diseases of the skin.[28] James Cook, Alexander Read, John Moyle, and James Handley also commented on skin disorders, but in much less detail. Foreign authors including Charles Gabriel Le Clerc, Paul Barbette, Joannes Muys, and M. de La Vauguion discussed skin diseases in English editions of their surgical works as well. Typically, these authors discussed skin diseases within sections on disorders of the 'Head, Face, and Neck' and devoted special attention to disorders including erysipelas, herpes, scurvy, ecchymoses (i.e., bruises) and haemorrhoids. Of all these authors, only the self-proclaimed London physician William Salmon organized skin disorders within a major section of his work.[29]

Although these authors devoted some attention to skin diseases, none had, prior to Turner, compiled a work solely devoted to diseases 'incident' upon the skin. Turner published his key dermatological writing in 1714 and taxonomically divided disorders into two

Part 1: 'Inward' Origin		Part 2: 'Outward' Origin	
Ch.1	Leprosy History	Ch.1	Falling Out of Hair
Ch.2	Lepra Graecorum	Ch.2	Scald Head
Ch.3	Itch	Ch.3	Lousy Evil
	i. Local		
	ii. Scorbutic or Cacochymical		
Ch.4	Children's Scabs or Breakings Out	Ch.4	Diseases: Skin of Face
Ch.5	Herpes	Ch.5	Diseases: Skin of Hands & Feet
Ch.6	Erysipelas (St Anthony's Fire)	Ch.6	Diseases: Prepuce
Ch.7	Smallpox & Pestilential Eruptions	Ch.7	Haemorrhoids or Piles
Ch.8	Carbuncle or Cancer	Ch.8	Natural Passages Stopt
Ch.9	Other Cutaneous Diseases	Ch.9	Other Hurts Befalling
Ch.10	Twofold Perspiration	Ch.10	Burns
	i. Insensible		
	ii. Sensible		
Ch.11	Skin Colour Change	Ch.11	Bites of Venomous Creatures
	i. Chlorosis		
	ii. Yellow Jaundice		
Ch.12	Spots & Marks	Ch.12	Hurts of Venomous Insects
	Maternal Imagination		

Table 4.1
Contents of Daniel Turner's *De Morbis Cutaneis*

categories. In the first category, he grouped diseases such as leprosy, herpes, the itch, and smallpox which, according to his own account, arose 'inward[ly] but presented themselves externally'. In the second category, he described diseases or 'accidents' of an 'Outward' origin including the 'Lousy Evil', syphilis, burns, and venomous insect bites (see Table 4.1). Unlike the few earlier writings of skin disease which were regionally organized according to external diseases of the scalp, face, or body, Turner identified conditions as skin diseases more upon their appearance than upon their location or origin.[30]

Despite having made these distinctions, Turner argued that such clear delineations rarely exist in nature. For instance, Turner agreed with many contemporaries that leprosy was an internal disorder. Yet, he directed as much of his treatment towards improving the externally manifest presentation of the disease as to the internal cause. In this sense, leprosy was not exclusively regarded as either an internal or an external disease. Rather, the skin was not so much a direct component of the disease as it was a literal and rhetorical reference point to disease and its treatment.

Some of the diseases Turner described as 'Incident' upon the skin were also found in contemporary physicians' writings. In 1703, for instance, London physician Richard Mead wrote of the bites of vipers, tarantulae, and mad dogs in his *Mechanical Account of Poisons* (1702). He also reported on Giovanni Cosimo Bonomo's discovery that the itch was caused by the continual biting of 'cutaneous worms'.[31] Such a claim opposed the common idea that the itch was of constitutional origin. Mead, together with London physicians James Jurin, Thomas Nettleton, Richard Blackmore, John Arbuthnot, William Wagstaffe and Hans Sloane, also expressed concern over inoculation as a treatment for smallpox.[32] Physician Sir Richard Blackmore and surgeon William Beckett are both found elaborating upon the causes and treatment of scrofula.[33] The origin, spread, and treatment of syphilis were also addressed in contemporary medical as well as surgical writings.

In their diagnoses of 'internal' disorders, physicians were primarily attentive to symptoms such as the type of cough, location of pain, or duration of fever. Additionally, many also interpreted signs of these diseases from examining the skin. For example, yellow jaundice, green sickness, plethora, spotted fevers, and smallpox were diagnosed in part from the appearance of discoloured or marked skin. Some internal malignancies were also claimed to have been diagnosed and tracked from the sequential appearance of tumours and discolorations upon different regions of the skin. Overall, however, physicians limited their use of the skin as an indicator of disease without physically manipulating the bodily surface as part of their practice.

Pores and Policy

One tool of the Enlightenment – the microscope – allowed natural philosophers to reveal (or construct, depending upon your epistemological viewpoint) microscopic skin pores, thereby demystifying the mechanical operations of the skin. Although surgical authors had long discussed the anatomy beneath the skin, the structure of the skin itself had received little comment. This view began to change with London surgeon and anatomist William Cowper's publication of *The Anatomy of Humane Bodies* in 1698.[34] In this work, Cowper argued that the skin was not only the integument covering the internal anatomy, but that it was comprised of an anatomy of its own. He delineated five anatomical layers of the skin through the 'assistance of a microscope', and he argued that it was through a more thorough understanding of this anatomy that his contemporaries would come to know how the skin transported substances and juices outward and inward[35] (see Figure 4.2).

In the early decades of the eighteenth century, many – indeed, most – Collegiate physician authors offered explanations of internal physical mechanisms in their writings. Their approach to medical theory and practice was typically modelled upon Newtonian methods of mathematico-hypothetical deduction.[36] Some, however, including Turner and, later, Richard Mead and Edward Strother, refused to adopt Newtonianism as the basis of medicine. Instead, they urged fellow practitioners to re-examine the works of Thomas Sydenham, the 'English Hippocrates'. In particular, they stressed Sydenham's emphasis upon the diagnostic usefulness of observing outward signs and/or symptoms of disease.

Concurrent with the reexamination of Sydenham, William Cockburn, Jeremiah Wainewright, Francis Fuller, John Burton, and others revived an interest in the ancient Galenic non-naturals.[37] The

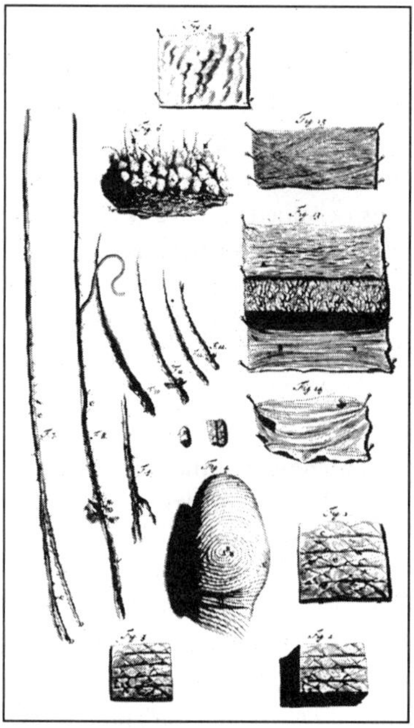

Figure 4.2
Skin and hair follicles from William Cowper's 1698 *The Anatomy of Humane Bodies* (Wellcome Institute Library, London)

non-naturals were thought to be the six causes of health and disease which were not dependent upon the nature or constitution of the body. They consisted of air, food and drink, motion and rest, sleep and exercise, retentions and evacuations, and the passions of the soul.[38] Turner, too, particularly in prescribing dietary regimens, advocated the use of remedies for regulating the non-naturals. He also emphasized the need for surgeons and physicians to monitor and regulate their patients' excretions and retentions, the fifth Galenic non-natural, by the regular use of purges and vomits as well as maintaining the patency of the skin's pores.[39] His explanation of the skin's ability to 'let forth superfluous humours' was explicitly drawn from physician James Drake's description of the five 'uses' of the skin and Cowper's anatomical and experimental study of the skin.[40] Turner, however, greatly expanded these accounts with his own observations of the skin's ability or power both to naturally heal many external wounds and to cure internal disorders.

Contemporaries claimed that microscopic skin pores served as the passageways responsible for the spread of contagion. The itch, for instance, was thought to be 'transmitted to a Person in sound health' after 'drawing on the Glove or Stocking, wiping on the Linen, or lying on the sheets' of an infected person. Such contact, it was argued, allowed the 'Contagion or Seminal Particle' to enter the body 'externally' via the pores of the skin whereby it travelled into the 'Glandules', where it 'vitiates' the texture of the body, 'corrupts' its juices, and 'raiseth the same Ferment ... [inside the body as] that from which it was propagated or derived'.[41]

Turner claimed that the precise aetiology or 'efficient Cause' of most internal distempers consisted of 'immaterial Beings' that were 'imperceptible' to the senses. Each skin pore, he continued, offered a 'sufficient [entry] Passage' for the 'cause' of apoplexy, epilepsy, 'convulsive and hysterical' disorders, and 'Pestilential' diseases, including the plague.[42]

Although blocking the pores might effectively prohibit the spread of this contagion, such treatments were also thought to produce the potentially fatal sequela of fevers. If physicians were to believe Thomas Sydenham, two-thirds of all internal diseases presented as fevers. Turner, a Sydenhamian disciple, extended his mentor's argument, and claimed that two-thirds of all fevers were due to 'Perspiration hindered' by clogged pores in the skin. As caretakers of fevers, physicians, so Turner claimed, must devote much of their practice to promoting the evacuation of noxious humoral fever-causing particles via bloodletting, purging, and, in particular, relieving blocked pores.[43]

A variety of methods was available for unclogging blocked pores. Turner, like many colleagues, used common diaphoretic (i.e., sweat provoking) remedies to promote the release of insensible perspiration.[44] Dislodging clogged skin pores was also a medical aim of the 'water cures', or hydrotherapy. Like his contemporaries George Cheyne, William Oliver, John Arbuthnot, Jeremiah Wainewright, John Quinton, John Smith, and Thomas Short, Turner recommended the bath as a treatment for several diseases 'Incident' upon the skin.[45] He also recommended the use of a 'flesh brush' for patients with leprosy in order to open any obstructed pores and cutaneous glandules, thereby allowing the internal 'lurking [leprous] Snake' to be 'carried off' with one's perspiration.[46]

Similar to the manner in which he described the skin's role in 'letting forth humours', Turner elaborated upon the skin's remarkable ability to take things in. Most particularly, he argued that the pores of the skin allowed 'Outward Remedies' to be transported inwardly, thereby effectively removing certain 'internal Maladies'.[47] Turner noted, for example, how purgative ointments rubbed on the 'Belly' were capable of effecting an evacuation from the bowels. He also recalled the efficacy of Thomas Willis' 'Ague-stopper' medicines which brought about their cures when applied to the wrist, feet or chest.[48]

Skin as a Therapeutic Medium

Many authors before Turner had claimed that externally applied medicines produced their effect within the body. Among those Turner acknowledged were Galen, Jean Fernilius, Gulielmus Fabricius Hildanus, Gregor Horstius, Franciscus Sylvius de la Boe, Guernerus Rolfincius, and Theophile Bonet.[49] In addition, Turner elaborated upon Thomas Willis' description that the effects were caused by 'sympathetic attraction'.

Willis used sympathy to account for the special 'sense' existing within the nerves and spirits which allowed or 'consented' for distinct parts to communicate.[50] Remote sympathy, for example, existed between the pregnant womb and milk-producing breasts. Continuous sympathy explained the similar role of the continuity or lining that existed between the mouth, the oral cavity, and the alimentary tract. Finally, contiguous sympathy allowed for communication between bodily parts in close proximity, for example the heart and the lungs, or the outer skin and the bowels.

By the 1720s, 'sympathetic attraction' was a popular explanation of the 'magical' powers produced by that popular panacea, the anodyne necklace.[51] And Turner, the practitioner probably most keenly attuned to abolishing quackery in London, took every precaution to distinguish his explanation of the therapeutic capacity of the skin from the 'ludicrous Argumentation' among the 'Toy-Medicine-Mongers' and dealers in 'Physical Baubles' who sold this necklace.[52] Therefore, instead of incorporating sympathetic attraction into his explanation, Turner relied upon Nehemiah Grew's experimental findings of the pores in the skin.[53]

Turner argued that externally applied medicines effectively treated 'inward' diseases due to their transport through the skin. 'Mint and Wormwood, with some ... Aromaticks' externally applied acted as effective anti-emetics; 'hot Epithemes laid upon the ... Abdomen' were effective treatments for the colic, 'Iliac Passion', and dysentery.[54] Some substances, however, appeared to be potentially harmful. He related two cases whereby children had died as the result of 'overpurgation' from 'rubbing in a little ointment upon their navels' as a treatment for worms.[55] Yet, he turned these cases to his advantage and argued that if such medicines were, after entering 'by means of cutaneous pores', able to 'excite such intestine Feuds', leading to the 'Destruction of the whole Animal Fabrick', medicines with a 'friendly or agreeable nature' would certainly be able to 'amicably allay the Storm or Hurrican [sic] raised [from disorders] within'.[56]

During the time Turner practised surgery, surgeons and physicians disagreed over whether surgeons had the right to administer internal medicines to their surgical patients. Although most surgeons and surgical reformers expressed no qualms over their traditionally perceived role of treating only external diseases, they argued that their patients were generally in need of internal as well as external medicines. External medicines applied alone on an ulcerated arm would 'do [the patient] no service', it was argued, 'without [also offering] Internal Medicine, that might correct the ill State of ... [the] Blood'. If patients were not allowed to 'conform to a proper [external and internal therapeutic] Regimen' many, like Turner, argued that surgeons were 'not likely to get much Credit, ... [nor] obtain a good and speedy Cure' for their patients.[57] Thus, to Turner, the issue put the surgeons' reputation at stake.

The physicians replied, claiming that previous legal statutes remained in force which specifically prohibited surgeons from practising physic. They diverted attention from the issue of using internal medicine to what they construed as an overall greater fallacy of surgical practice. In particular they noted the 'abuses' that occurred when surgeons had previously been left alone to tend the needs of wounded militia. In one example, the physicians argued that when five thousand sick and wounded sailors were 'put to Shore' at Portsmouth in 1689 and treated by surgeons, 'not above 500 returned to the Fleet'. Whereas, when physicians Lawrence, Smith, Dunn and Commins alone treated six thousand sick soldiers in the Army at Ireland, 'not above 130 dyed'.[58]

Unlike physicians' battles with apothecaries over the right to administer physic, which were officially resolved by the Rose case, no such settlement was reached between physicians and surgeons.[59] Some, like the anonymous author of *The Present State of Physick and Surgery in London* (1701), reiterated the argument that surgeons should 'perform all Chirurgical Operations, and have the sole application of external remedies; but [they] are [to be] restrained from selling, advising or administering the internal [remedies]'.[60] Some surgeons who practised outside of this proscribed therapeutic boundary, like Fenton Bynns, were charged with 'giveing internal medicines', and brought before the College of Physicians.[61] The physicians' resistance to the surgeons' encroachment upon treating diseases internally reinforced their use of the skin as a physical barrier between these occupations.[62]

Turner's 1714 *De Morbis Cutaneis* addressed this same argument at a later date from a different approach. He furthered the claim that surgeons had long been administering external remedies which produced internal effects similar to the internal physic offered by physicians. Specifically, he argued that the pores of the skin allowed externally applied medicines to be transported inward. Thus, through *De Morbis Cutaneis*, Turner urged the College of Physicians formally to extend the right for surgeons to administer internal medicines by acknowledging that the medicines surgeons already used were producing internal effects. As a practising surgeon, Turner had regularly administered internal medicine for 'surgical' or external disorders.

Turner's Cerate

Table 4.2 indicates the types of treatments Turner's patients received. These figures, compiled from 'scattered memoirs' of 'certain remarkable Occurrences' during Turner's twenty years in surgical practice, reveal several points. First, over one-third of the patients suffering from external diseases (i.e., those diseases typically treated by surgeons) received both internal and external remedies. Turner, for one, opposed the physicians' stance and administered internal medicines for some 'surgical' or external disorders.[63] Also of note is the relatively high percentage of patients with 'Internal' diseases who received externally applied remedies.

	I. Internal Diseases	II. External Diseases
% patients receiving internally administered remedies	73.3	36.6
% patients receiving externally applied remedies	70.0	73.2
% patients receiving both internal and external remedies	60.0	36.6
% patients whose treatments were not specified	13.3	22.0
% patients receiving Turner's Cerate	26.7	29.3

Table 4.2

Treatment Turner's patients received according to *De Morbis Cutaneis*

This table also shows that Turner treated over one-quarter of each group of patients with a specially compounded *Certatum de Lapide Calaminari*, colloquially known as 'Turner's Cerate'.[64] He promoted this compound primarily as a eupolotic (i.e., to 'cicatrize' or 'skin over' wounds and ulcers), claiming that after the 'Incarnation' of a wound, 'my Cerate ... will induce a Cicatrix (or scar), and finish the work'.[65] The cases discussed in *De Morbis Cutaneis* indicate he also found it effective for treating other skin conditions. For example, he used this cerate to hasten the suppuration of a boil, to heal 'corrosive ulcers' on the scalp, to treat a patient's serpigio on her knuckles, as well as to alleviate shingles, and erysipelas. Additionally, he used it to treat gunpowder burns, facial pustules and ulcerations of the prepuce and labia. He also found it effective in treating the remaining wound of an apprentice's ear which had been bitten off and swallowed in a drunken brawl, as well as the neck wound of a child who had been bled excessively with leeches. In one situation, Turner found the 'opportunity of making an Experiment' to test the efficacy of his cerate against the spirits of wine which the Gentleman patient's friend, a 'chymist', preferred. Upon treating each of the patient's bruised legs with a different compound, Turner found his cerate produced more favourable effects.[66]

In early eighteenth-century London, name brand remedies were trademarks of many local mountebanks and 'pretenders' of the medical and surgical arts. Typically, they were advertised as 'Infallible' cure-alls or panaceas, which were 'more like a miracle than a medicine'. However, many orthodox practitioners also promoted products they had developed, modified, or found particularly effective for treating certain disorders. Among these eponymous medicines were Mead's 'pulvis Antylisus', Sloane's medicinal chocolate, James' Fever powder, and Ward's 'Pill and Drop'.[67] Turner also relied upon his cerate for treating a relatively broad range of skin diseases. However, treating only twenty of the seventy-one patients described in *De Morbis Cutaneis* with his product was hardly promoting a panacea in the way of contemporary 'quacks'. Unlike the testimonial evidence proffered by many local 'quacks', Turner did not claim to have cured all of his patients' skin diseases with his cerate. Instead of a cure-all, Turner regarded the cerate as his 'Mite to the Surgeon's Treasury of Medicine'.[68]

Reception of *De Morbis Cutaneis*

Turner's *De Morbis Cutaneis* underwent four editions in two decades, and it spread abroad with translations into French in 1743, and later into German (1766)(see Figure 4.3).[69] Apart from the twelfth chapter in which Turner argued that a pregnant woman's imagination could be transferred to her unborn child, imprinting it with various marks and deformities – a stance which sparked a major pamphlet war between Turner and London physician James Blondel – Turner's discussion of skin disease met with little contemporary recognition.[70]

Nearly all historical accounts of English and international dermatology cite Turner's 'pioneering' work, *De Morbis Cutaneis.* Some even describe Turner as the 'First English Dermatologist'.[71] Typically, this work is represented as a critical piece of dermatological classification.[72] Retrospectively, this indeed may be true. But there was actually little mention of a taxonomy of skin disease in the English medical and surgical literature until Robert Willan's system of classification was introduced at the end of the eighteenth century.[73]

As such, there is little evidence beyond the mere arrangement of the work that suggests Turner viewed himself as a classifier of diseases 'incident to the skin'. He did not introduce a new nomenclature, or arrange diseases in new categories in the style of prominent nosologists François Bossier de Sauvages and William Cullen later in the century.[74] Nor did Turner alter commonly held associations between diseases such as the itch, scabies, and leprosy. It was not until the nineteenth century that remarks began to appear noting Turner as the first to offer a 'good description of the various species of herpes'.[75] Instead, Turner's work is more consistent with early eighteenth-century compilations of diseases of specific body parts such as the liver, the urinary bladder, and the spleen.[76]

Unlike bone setting, bladder stone cutting, and cataract couching, treating skin disease did not develop as a special branch of surgical practice in early eighteenth-century London. Nevertheless, the skin remained central to arguments of occupational territory between physicians and surgeons as neither group sequestered sole responsibility of treating skin diseases.

Turner received an *imprimatur* from the censors of the College of Physicians to publish *De Morbis Cutaneis* in 1712, only a year after he had quit surgery and had become a licentiate of the College. He dedicated this work to these censors, desiring to 'convince' Collegiate physicians that they had bestowed the 'privilege' to practise medicine upon 'no idle ... useless person'.[77] In this sense, he used this work to obtain official permission from his new colleagues to turn from the practice of surgery to medicine. Having been officially recognized as competent in both surgery and physic, an uncommon position for his time, Turner was a most suitable author to discuss diseases of the skin, the subject of interest to both realms of practitioners.[78] Thus crossing the occupational barrier from surgery to medicine with a discourse on the skin was a most symbolic choice of topic for Turner.

Overall, Turner appears to have used *De Morbis Cutaneis* to achieve two primary goals. First, he wanted to provide the College of Physicians with a convincing account of his capability of administering internal medicines (i.e., practising physic). And more significantly, to clearly and openly advocate, to both physicians and surgeons, the need for surgeons to administer internal medicines.

Retaining the Integrity of the Integument

The skin, to eighteenth-century practitioners, was more than a boundary delimiting the physical self. As we have seen, an

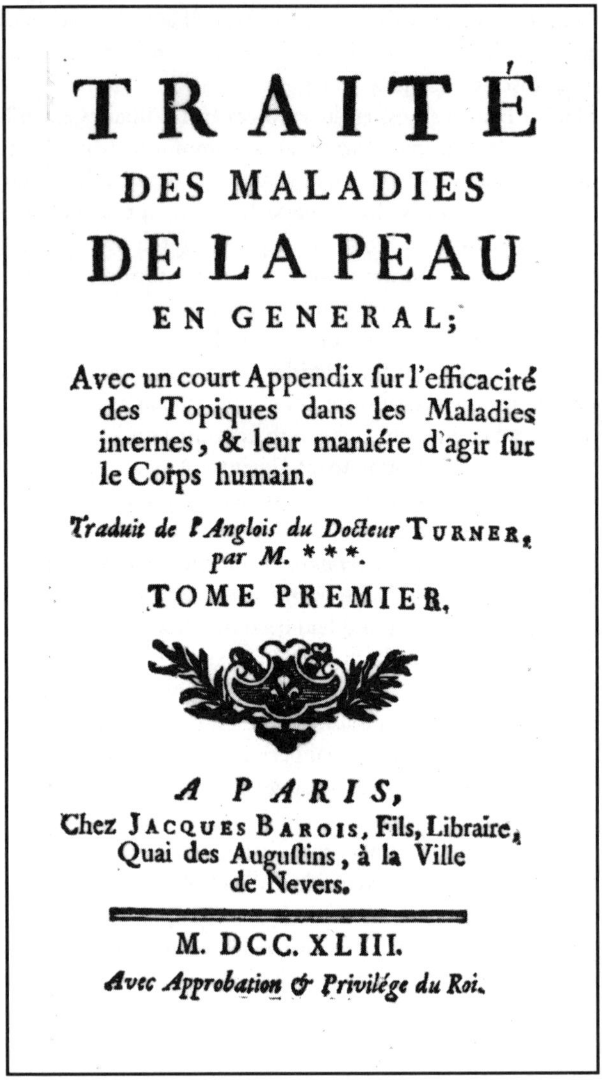

TRAITÉ
DES MALADIES
DE LA PEAU
EN GENERAL;

Avec un court Appendix ſur l'efficacité des Topiques dans les Maladies internes, & leur maniére d'agir ſur le Corps humain.

Traduit de l'Anglois du Docteur TURNER, *par M.* ***.

TOME PREMIER.

A PARIS,
Chez JACQUES BAROIS, Fils, Libraire, Quai des Auguſtins, à la Ville de Nevers.

M. DCC. XLIII.
Avec Approbation & Privilége du Roi.

Figure 4.3
Title page of the French translation of Turner's *De Morbis Cutaneis*
(Wellcome Institute Library, London)

occupational pluralism existed with both surgeons and physicians using the skin as a defining point of their practices. Yet they both relied upon the skin in their armamentarium against disease. In this physical, therapeutic sense, both surgeons and physicians viewed the skin as a penetrable barrier. However, the rhetorical and symbolic use of the skin as the border of professional practice actually remained an impenetrable barrier between surgeons and physicians throughout the eighteenth century.

Turner directed his reader's gaze from the layers of skin to the pores, literally an absence of skin. By doing so, he exemplified the goal of an anatomist: to visualize the previously invisible. Typically, dissection was the means by which anatomists displayed nature's secrets. Dissection allowed individuals, surgeons in particular, to view nature's parts for themselves, and to rationalize and interpret correlations between anatomical structure and physiological function.

For Turner, the skin encoded many messages. Skin pores provided a conduit connecting, and at times equilibrating, the inner and outer environments. The skin could also be 'read' in that an internal or otherwise invisible action could be interpreted through changes on the skin surface. Just as one judges his actions or communication with another by 'reading' the flushing or blushing of the skin, surgeons, too, could mediate their actions with their patients by 'reading' signs of internal activity written upon the skin. Although Turner, at least in one major writing, focused upon a specific part – actually the absence of part – he never lost sight of the whole. The skin was a contiguous covering which, only as a function of the whole, provided a therapeutic medium.

Notes

1 Recent scholarship includes David M. Stoll, *A Woman's Skin* (New Brunswick: Rutgers University Press, 1994); Marc Lappe, *The Body's Edge: Our Cultural Obsession with Skin* (New York: Holt, 1996); Ann DuCille's *Skin Trade* (Cambridge, Massachusetts: Harvard University Press, 1996); Armando R. Favazza's chapter on 'The Skin' in his *Bodies Under Siege: Self-Mutilation and Body Modification in Culture and Psychiatry* (Baltimore: Johns Hopkins University Press, 2nd edn, 1996); Arthur K. Balin and Loretta Pratt Balin, *The Life of the Skin* (New York: Bantam, 1997); and Rosemaire Garland Thompson (ed.), *Freakery: Cultural Spectacles of the Extraordinary Body* (New York: New York University Press, 1996). On the related topic of the medico-surgical sculpturing of the skin, see Elizabeth Haiken, *Venus Envy: A History of Cosmetic Surgery* (Baltimore: Johns Hopkins

University Press, 1997).

2 Daniel Turner, *De Morbis Cutaneis. A Treatise of Diseases Incident to the Skin* (London: R.Bonwicke, W.Freeman, T.Goodwin, J.Walthoe, M.Wotton, S.Manship, J.Nicholson, R.Parker, B.Tooke and R.Smith, 1714). Henceforth, unless otherwise noted, all citations are taken from the 'revised and very much enlarg'd' 2nd edn, 1723.

3 See later editions of the seventeenth-century *Aristotle's Last Legacy: or, His golden cabinet of secrets*, pt IV of *Aristotle's Works Compleated* (London: The booksellers, 1733), esp. 55-62. Roy Porter discussed the popularity of this work in 'The Secrets of Generation Display'd': *Aristotle's Master-piece* in Eighteenth-Century England', in R.P. Maccubbin (ed.), *Tis Nature's fault. Unauthorized Sexuality During the Enlightenment* (Cambridge: Cambridge University Press, 1987), 7-21. Excerpts from John Bulwer's account of facial markings in his *Anthropometamorphosis: Man Tranform'd; or, The Artificial Changling* appear in H.J. Norman's 'John Bulwer and his *Anthropometamorphosis*', in E.A. Underwood (ed.), *Science Medicine and History*, vol. 2 (London: Oxford University Press, 1953), 89-95.

4 Keith Thomas described these witches' and devils' marks in his 'canonical' *Religion and the Decline of Magic* (London: Penguin edition, 1973), 530, 667, and 687. Signs of pregnancy and prediction of sex interpreted from skin examination are also described by Thomas Forbes in *The Midwife and the Witch* (New Haven: Yale University Press, 1966), 48, 51-2, 54.

5 Roy Porter, 'Making Faces: Physiognomy and Fashion in Eighteenth-Century England', *Etudes Anglaises*, xviii (1985), 185-96; Barbara Marie Stafford, 'One Face of Beauty, One Picture of Health: The Hidden Aesthetic of Medical Practice', *Journal of Medical Philosophy*, xiv (1989), 213-30; and John Graham, 'Lavater's "Physiognomy" in England', *Journal of the History of Ideas*, xxii (1961), 561-72.

6 This issue was discussed in English popular literature of the seventeenth century, and returned as or remained a popular area of discourse for eighteenth-century authors as well. Graeme Tytler identified physiognomical aspects within eighteenth-century literature in *Physiognomy in the European Novel. Faces and Fortunes* (Princeton: Princeton University Press, 1982). See also John Liggett, *The Human Face* (London: Constable & Co., 1974), Patrizia Magli, 'The Face and the Soul', in M. Feher (ed.), *Fragments for a History of the Body*, pt 2 (New York: Zone, 1989), 87-127. Masaaki Matsushita discussed a most interesting East–West comparative view of physiognomy in his 'The Body as Visible Mind', a paper presented at the 22nd Taniguchi Symposium on the Comparative History of

Medicine East and West in Autumn 1997.

7 Frank McLynn, *Crime & Punishment in Eighteenth-Century England* (Oxford: Oxford University Press, 1991), 281.

8 An example is found in Ned Ward's urging to 'Have a care of your cheeks, you whoers; we shall have you branded next sesions so that the world may see your trade in your faces', *London Spy*, 118.

9 Hogarth visually depicted such markings in Plate III, The Inspection of his 'Marriage A-la-mode' (*c.*1742-43) and in the plates of 'A harlot's progress' (*c.*1730-32). Robert L.S. Cowley, in his 're-view' of Hogarth's narrative *Marriage A-la-mode* (Manchester: Manchester University Press, 1983), discussed the markings of prostitutes on pp. 81-99. Consistent with Ned Wards account, Cowley also noted that the 'F.C.' branded on the bosom of one woman likely stood for Female Convict or Criminal; the mark of a convicted prostitute, p. 87. See also N. F. Lowe, 'Hogarth, Beauty Spots, and Sexually Transmitted Diseases', *British Journal for Eighteenth-Century Studies*, xv (1992), 71-9.

10 D. Turner, *De Morbis Cutaneis*, 287.

11 For example, see Isaac Bickerstaff's 'Dissertation upon Noses' in *The Tatler*, no. 260. Herbert Silvette extracted many lines about syphilis from Restoration comedies in his *The Doctor on the Stage. Medicine and Medical Men in Seventeenth-Century England* (Knoxville: University of Kentucky Press, 1976), 82-234.

12 The importance of beauty, particularly among females, appeared in Hieronymous Mercurialis' *De Decoratione Liber*, 2nd edn (Venice: Junitas, 1601), and Alexander Read's *Chirurgorum Comes* (London: E.Jones for C.Wilkinson, 1687), 465-473. The keystone of consumerism studies remains Neil McKendrick, John Brewer, and J.H. Plumb, *The Birth of a Consumer Society: The Commercialization of Eighteenth-Century England* (London: Europa Publications, Ltd, 1982).

13 *The Spectator*, No.559, 25 June, 1714.

14 D. Turner, *Art of Surgery*, vol. 1, 318.

15 D. Turner, *De Morbis Cutaneis*, 253.

16 See, for example, the clergyman William Hendley's *Loimologia Sacra: or, A Discourse shewing that the Plague never proceeds from any first Natural Cause, but is sent immediately from God, and that as a Punishment to a People for their Sins* (London: T. Bickerton, 1721); and Edmund Gibson, the Bishop of London's *The Causes of the Discontents, In Relation to the Plague, and The Provisions against it, Fairly Stated and Consider'd* (London:, J. Roberts, 1721). Physician Richard Mead was enforced by the government to prepare written works on the plague for the benefit of the public. See Mead's *A Short*

Discourse Concerning Pestilential Contagion and the Methods used to prevent it (London: S. Buckley and R. Smith, 1720), which spurred other writings such as George Pye's *A Discourse of the Plague; wherein Dr. Mead's Notions are Consider'd and Refuted* (London: J. Darby, 1721).

17 D. Turner, *De Morbis Cutaneis*, 81.

18 Smallpox was reported on the Monthly Mortality Bills. Its prevalence in London during the eighteenth century has recently been investigated by John Landers. See his 'Mortality and Metropolis: the Case of London 1675-1825', *Population Studies*, xli (1987), 59-76, and John Landers and Anastasia Mouzas, 'Burial Seasonality and Causes of Death in London 1670-1819', *Population Studies*, xlii (1988), 59-83.

19 E.J. Burford, *Wits, Wenchers and Wantons. London's Low Life: Covent Garden in the eighteenth century* (London: Robert Hale, 1986), 117.

20 D. Turner, *De Morbis Cutaneis*, 103.

21 A. Fessler, 'Skin Diseases in 17th and 18th Century Lancashire Local History Document', *Bulletin of the History of Medicine*, xxvii (1953), 416, 418.

22 R. Boulton, *Rational and Practical Chirurgery*, 128.

23 Arabella Atkyns, *The Family Magazine* (London: J. Osborn, 1741), 71. The seasonality of the itch was also addressed in Thomas Spooner's *A Short Account of the Itch* (London: T. Child, 1714). Both of these popular works appeared in multiple editions.

24 T. Spooner, *Account of the Itch*, 4, 10-12.

25 D. Turner, *De Morbis Cutaneis*, 52.

26 Ned Ward, *The London Spy*, 1699-1703, as cited by David Piper, *The English Face* (London: Thames and Hudson, 1957), 155.

27 A. Fessler, 'Skin Diseases', 416.

28 For an account of the surgical writings available in vernacular English, see P.K. Wilson's 'Vernacularisation vs. Vulgarisation', 1169-72.

29 See Salmon's *Ars Chirurgica* (London: J. Dawks, 1698), 337-468. Daniel Turner regarded Salmon as the 'Ring Leader, or King of the Quacks' in his analysis of *The Modern Quack, or, Medical Impostor*, 2nd ed (London: Thomas Warner, 1724), 79.

30 Hieronymus Mercurialis' *De Morbis Cutaneis et Omnibus corporis Humani Excrementis Tractatus* (Venice, 1572), was discussed and reprinted in Richard Sutton's *Sixteenth Century Physician and His Methods. Mercurialis on Diseases of the Skin. The First Book on the Subject (1572)* (Kansas City, Missouri: Lowell Press, 1986). For a recent description of early skin classifications see Franz Ehring, *Hautkrankheiten. 5 Jahnhunderte wissenschaflicher Illustration* (Stuttgart: Gustav Fischer Verlag, 1989), 36-62.

31 Richard Mead, 'An Abstract of part of a Letter from D. Bonomo to Signior Redi, containing Some Observations concerning the Works of Humane Bodies', *Philosophical Transactions*, xxiii, No.283 (1702-3), 1296-9.

32 The standard authoritative account of treatment against smallpox at this time remains Genevieve Miller's *The Adoption of Inoculation for Smallpox in England and France* (Philadelphia: University of Pennsylvania Press, 1957). Adrian Wilson analysed political associations of the 1720s–1740s controversies over inoculation in 'The politics of medical improvement in early Hanoverian London', in A. Cunningham and R. French, *The Medical Enlightenment of the Eighteenth Century* (Cambridge: Cambridge University Press, 1990), esp. 24-34.

33 W. Beckett, *Free and Impartial Inquiry into the Antiquity and Efficacy of Touching for the Cure of the King's Evil* (London: J. Peele, 1732), and R. Blackmore, *Discourses on the Gout, a Rheumatism, and the King's Evil* (London: J. Pemberton, 1727).

34 William Cowper's work is discussed in Philip K. Wilson's 'William Cowper's Anatomy of the Human Skin', *International Journal of Dermatology*, xxxi (1992), 361-3. Like Cowper, Drake described the skin and included an illustrated plate of the skin's anatomy in his *Anthropologia Nova; or, A new system of Anatomy*, vol. 1 (London: S. Smith and B. Walford, 1707), 15-27 and figures I and II of Table 38 facing p. 73 of the appendix. Brief anatomical descriptions of the skin are also found in Blankaart's and Quincy's medical dictionaries.

35 P. K. Wilson, 'Cowper's anatomy of skin', 361-3

36 As many historians have explored specific aspects of Newton's influence upon medicine, I cite only three solid, useful sources: William Coleman, 'Mechanistic Philosophy and Hypothetical Physiology', *Texas Quarterly*, x (1967), 259-69; Anita Guerrini, 'James Keill, George Cheyne, and Newtonian Physiology, 1690-1740', *Journal of the History of Biology*, xviii (1985), 247-66; and Theodore M. Brown, 'Medicine in the Shadow of the *Principia*', *Journal of the History of Ideas*, xli (1987), 629-48.

37 Turner described the 'judicious Sydenham' as 'our modern Hippocrates' in *De Morbis Cutaneis*, 93. This use was consistent with many other authors' adulations. Writings on the non-naturals included Jeremiah Wainewright's *A Mechanical Account of the Non-Naturals* (London: R.Smith, 1707); Francis Fuller's *Medicina Gymnastica: or, A treatise concerning the Power of Exercise* (London: J. Matthews for R. Knaplock, 1705); and John Burton's *Treatise on the Non-Naturals* (London: A. Staples & J. Hildyard, 1738).

38 For a recent review of the use of the non-naturals in the eighteenth century see Antoinette Emch-Deriaz, 'The Non-naturals made Easy', in R. Porter (ed.), *The Popularization of Medicine 1650-1850* (London: Routledge, 1992),134-59.

39 Turner does not, however, appear to have kept 'Journals of Perspiration' in the Sanctorian method as that of Sir John Floyer in the latter's *Enquiry into the Right Use and Abuses of ... baths in England* (London: R. Cland, 1697).

40 D. Turner, *De Morbis Cutaneis*, iii. The other uses of the skin Drake mentioned were to touch, to defend underlying parts, to close the mouths of the vessels and glandules dispersed throughout the skin, and to give 'ornament and Loveliness' to the whole person (*Anthropologia Nova*, vol. 1, 12-14).

41 D. Turner, *De Morbis Cutaneis*, 49.

42 *Ibid.*, 496. Lester S. King discussed contemporary concerns of causality in 'Some Problems of Causality in Eighteenth Century Medicine', *Bulletin of the History of Medicine*, xxxvii (1963), 15-24.

43 The vast literature on fevers supports the 1719 Quincy *Lexicon* generalization that fevers, defined as an 'augmented Velocity of Blood', were claimed to have arisen from an 'almost infinite variety of causes', many of which created some humoral imbalance. John Quincy, *Lexicon physico-medicum; or, A new physical dictionary* (London: A.Bell, W.Taylor, and J. Osborn, 1719), 148.

44 D. Turner, *De Morbis Cutaneis*, 125. In eighteenth-century terms, insensible perspiration was the 'Steams and Vapours' which were 'exhaled' through skin pores in order to 'ventilate the blood', in contrast to sensible perspiration, or sweat. E.T. Renbourn discussed perspiration in both his 'The Natural History of Insensible Perspiration: A Forgotten Doctrine of Health and Disease', *Medical History*, iv (1960), 135-52, and 'The History of Sweat and the Sweat Rash From Earliest Times to the End of the 18th Century', *Journal of the History of Medicine*, xiv (1959), 202-27.

45 Turner prescribed use of the baths for patients with leprosy and the shingles in *De Morbis Cutaneis*, 31-33, 40, 82. Baths became increasingly fashionable as both therapy and an entertainment for London's middle and upper classes during this period. Charles F. Mullett reviewed many contemporary writings on the effects of baths and waters in his *Public Baths and Health in England, 16th – 18th Century* (Baltimore: Johns Hopkins University Press, 1946), esp. 20-31.

46 D. Turner, *De Morbis Cutaneis*, 31. Turner later cited Lord Verulam, Francis Bacon's claim that the regular use of a flesh brush promoted longevity. (See 504)

47 *Ibid.*, 491.

48 *Ibid.*, 496-7.

49 Two contemporaries whom Turner did not cite who also promoted the use of external remedies were Richard Boulton, *An Essay on External Remedies* (London: s.n., 1715) and Peter Kennedy, *An Essay on External Remedies Wherein it is Considered, Whether all the Curable Distempers incident to Human Bodies, may not be cured by Outward Means* (London: A. Bell, 1715).

50 Richard Y. Meier provided a clear account of 'Sympathy' in the neurophysiology of Thomas Willis in *Clio Medica*, xvii (1982), 103.

51 Francis Doherty's informative and entertaining review of this panacea, 'The Anodyne Necklace: A Quack Remedy and its Promotion', *Medical History*, xxxiv (1990), 268-93, was significantly expanded upon in *A Study in 18th-Century Advertising Methods: The Anodyne Necklace* (Lewiston, New York: Edwin Mellen, 1992). Similarly, Turner regarded 'Sympathetic Powder' useless other than as 'an Amusement'. D. Turner, *Art of Surgery*, vol. 1 (1725), 304. Cambridge science historian Patricia Fara provided a fascinating, in-depth interdisciplinary analysis of the multiple meanings of sympathetic attraction in her *Sympathetic Attractions: Magnetic Practices, Beliefs, and Symbolism in Eighteenth-Century England* (Princeton: Princeton University Press, 1996).

52 D. Turner, *De Morbis Cutaneis*, 492-3. According to Turner, Newton 'never intended' his 'great Principle of Attraction' to be 'thus abused' (494). Contemporary investigations into the power of attraction in medical theories were discussed in Geoffrey Bowles, 'Physical, Human, and Divine Attraction in the Life and Thoughts of George Cheyne', *Annals of Science*, xxxi (1974), 473-88.

53 Although the idea of a 'porous' skin may be found in the Hippocratic writings, Grew's microscopic identification of the skin pores factualized the earlier concept. N. Grew's 'Description and use of the Pores in the skin of the hands and feet' appeared in Royal Society's *Philosophical Transactions,* xiv, No.159 (1684), 566-7. Turner copied much of this account in *De Morbis Cutaneis,* 120-21.

54 D. Turner, *De Morbis Cutaneis*, 495. This method of transport, later identified as percutaneous absorption, is discussed in Frederick Reiss' 'Percutaneous Absorption, A Critical and Historical Review', *The American Journal of Medical Science*, cclii (1966), 588-602.

55 *Ibid.*, 492.

56 *Ibid.*, 493.

57 D. Turner, *Syphilis*, 4th edn, 120.

58 'The Physician's Reply to the Surgeon's Answer' (S.1: s.n., 1689-90), 3.

59 Harold Cook has extensively examined the disputes comprising the Rose case in his 'The Rose Case Reconsidered: Physicians, Apothecaries and the Law in Augustan England', *Journal of the History of Medicine*, xlv (1990), 527-55.

60 *Present State of Physick & Surgery in London* (London: Thos. Speed, 1701), 17.

61 Barber–Surgeons' Company of London, Court Minutes, MSS. 5257, 12 December 1690.

62 An example of this resistance is found in 'The Physicians Reply to the Surgeons Answer', 1689 or 1690.

63 D. Turner, *De Morbis Cutaneis,* 1714, Dedication.

64 Turner provided the recipe for this compound in *De Morbis Cutaneis*, 222.

65 D. Turner, *Art of Surgery*, vol. 2, 440.

66 D. Turner, *De Morbis Cutaneis*, 360-6. A. Lyell described this case in 'Daniel Turner, and the First Controlled Therapeutic Trial in Dermatology', 191-4.

67 R. Porter offered an extensive discussion of quack remedies in *Health for Sale: Quackery in England, 1660-1850* (Manchester: Manchester University Press, 1989), 99-117.

68 D. Turner, *De Morbis Cutaneis*, 396. He added that 'I am sure no ingenious Person will despise [his cerate] for its being less compounded and consequently less pompous than some others, or for that it is only a Tetrapharmacum'. Historians, with few significant exceptions, have been reluctant to analyse claims about the efficacy of particular treatments in earlier time periods. This work only considers Turner's judgments of the outcome of his therapy. Guenter B. Risse discussed the problems of judging efficacy in 'The History of Therapeutics', in W.F. Bynum and V. Nutton (eds), *Essays in the History of Therapeutics*, special issue of *Clio Medica*, xxii (Amsterdam: Rodopi, 1991), 3-11, and Andreas-Holger Maehle has made great strides toward answering some of these lingering historical questions. See, for example, Maehle's 'Pharmacological Experimentation with Opium in the Eighteenth Century', in R. Porter and M. Teich (eds), *Drugs and Narcotics in History* (Cambridge: Cambridge University Press, 1995), 52-76 .

69 Daniel Turner, *Traité des Maladies de la Peau en General* (Paris: J. Barois Fils, 1743); and Daniel Turner, *Abhandlung von den Krankheiten der Haut* (Altenburg: In der Richterischen Buchhandlung, 1766).

70 I have described and analysed this dispute in '"Out of Sight, Out of Mind?": The Daniel Turner – James Blondel Dispute over the Power

of the Maternal Imagination', *Annals of Science*, xlix (1992), 63-85.

71 Sir Archibald Gray initiated this appellation in 'Dermatology from the Time of Harvey', *Lancet*, ii (1951), 759. John Thorne Crissey and Lawrence Charles Parish have corrected this anachronism, revising it as 'protodermatologist' in *The Dermatology and Syphilology of the Nineteenth Century* (New York: Praeger, 1981), 8.

72 H.S. Purdon, 'Brief Historical Sketch of Dermatology, Classification of Skin Diseases, General Remarks on the Anatomy of the Skin', *Journal of Cutaneous Medicine*, iv (1871), 204; L.J.A. Loewenthal, 'Daniel Turner and *De Morbis Cutaneis*' 125-31; and R. J. Mann, 'Daniel Turner, the First British Dermatologist', 62-6. The most historically perceptive account is Alan Lyell's 1982 'Daniel Turner (1667-1740) LRCP London (1711) M.D. Honorary, Yale (1723) Surgeon, Physician and Pioneer Dermatologist', 162-70.

73 Robert Willan, *Description and Treatment for Cutaneous Diseases* (London: J. Johnson, 1798-1808). For a thorough review of nineteenth-century skin disease classifications, see Edward Bennet Bronson, 'The Classification of Skin Diseases', *Journal of Cutaneous Diseases*, v (1887), 371-81, 427-33. Fielding Garrison provided a brief survey of the skin as a functioning organ in his 'The Skin as a Functional Organ of the Body', *Bulletin of the New York Academy of Medicine*, ix (1933), 417-32.

74 See Julian Martin, 'Sauvages' nosology: medical enlightenment in Montpellier', in A. Cunningham and R. French (eds), *The Medical Enlightenment of the Eighteenth Century* (Cambridge: Cambridge University Press, 1990), 111-37; and Knud Faber, *Nosography in Modern Internal Medicine* (New York: Paul Hoeber, 1923), 1-27.

75 P.F.O. Rayer, *Theoretical and Practical Treatise on the Diseases of the Skin*, 2nd edn (1835), as cited by R.J. Mann, 'Daniel Turner', 65.

76 Jeremiah Wainewright, *An Anatomical Treatise of the Liver, with the Diseases Incident to it* (London: J. Clarke, 1737); William Rutty, *Treatise on Urinary Passages* (London: for T. Worrall, 1726); and Sir R. Blackmore, *Critical Dissertation upon the Spleen* (London: J. Pemberton, 1725).

77 D. Turner, *De Morbis Cutaneis*, 1714, Epistle Dedicatory.

78 Only four physician-contemporaries of Turner have been identified as having 'turned over' from the practice of surgery: Caleb Coatesworth (1688), Stephen Hall (1708-9), John Bamber (1724) and Francis Douce (1735). Similarly, few apprentice-trained apothecaries 'turned' to medicine as official licentiates. I have only identified three during this period in William Munk's *Roll of the Royal College of Physicians of London*, vol 1 & 2 (London: The

College, 2nd edn, 1878), John Colbatch (1696), John Turner, no relation (1708), and James Sherard (1732). Edmund King exploited his royal connections and received a 'Lambeth degree' in 1671, thereupon turning from practising surgery to physic. As Lawrence Stone has demonstrated in 'Social Mobility in England', 29-33, many tradesmen turned from one trade to another solely for potential financial gain. However, individuals rarely made an official turn from the practice of surgery to the practice of physic. The major obstacle to such a move was that surgery was an apprenticed trade whereas physic was typically entered upon completing a university education.

5

A Culture of Reform

Reform permeated London's societal infrastructure during the late seventeenth century. John Wilkins, William Petty, and others promoted various 'projects' to reform and improve London society and its inhabitants for the 'National good'.[1] Political dissidents, chiefly radical Whig nonconformists, allegedly plotted their own reform against Charles II's restoration.[2] Relatedly, prevailing Anglican High Church Tory structures were destabilized as Low Church latitudinarians (i.e., free-thinking, theologically liberal Anglicans) increasingly gained authoritative positions within governmental and intellectual arenas.[3] The ministry used the calamities of the 1665 plague and 1666 fire to prompt people to rethink their morals. Thomas Vincent, for example, decreed these disasters represented 'God's Terrible Voice' against Londoners for their sins.[4] The need for moral reform was also evident in Thomas Brookes' preachings that

> God had matter enough against the seventy thousand that died in the Plague, and certainly there is no man that hath been a sufferer by this late dreadful fire, but upon an easy search into his own heart and life, he may find matter enough to … satisfy himself that, though God has turned him out of his habitation, and burnt up all his comfort around him, yet he had done him no wrong.[5]

Antecedents of the eighteenth-century Societies for the Reformation of Manners were, according to some historical accounts, evident among the Religious Societies of the 1670s and 1680s.[6] This urge for reforming morals and manners was, for many Londoners, as much a part of restructuring the capital's living environment as were the newly built brick houses and improved water and sewage transport systems. There was 'never known such a trade', so Defoe claimed, as the rebuilding of the capital during the 'seven years' following the plague and fire. It has been estimated that the fire destroyed 90% of London's settlements within the walls. Thus, during his boyhood, Daniel Turner had the opportunity to witness the contributions various tradesmen made towards the piecemeal rebuilding and reforming of the capital. He experienced a London in which reform was a daily visible activity, and, for the devout, a daily personal activity as well. This chapter explores several reform measures to which Daniel Turner devoted considerable thought throughout his life.

'The Greatest Lies can be Invented': Mechanists as Enemies

Theoretical writings predominated in the medical literature of early Enlightenment London. Many of these medical theories were formulated in light of mechanistic philosophy. For instance, readers approaching John Clarke's bookshop at 'The Bible' under the Royal Exchange in 1732 would have found approximately three-fourths of the available medical works representing some mathematical or mechanical-based medical theory.[7] British medical writers including Archibald Pitcairne, Richard Mead, George Cheyne, James Keill, James Jurin, William Cockburn, Henry Pemberton, and Nicholas Robinson used mechanically based deductive arguments in their explanations of animal oeconomy (i.e., physiology) and physic. For instance, they explained consumption, jaundice, and fevers in terms of forces, powers, and causes adopted from natural philosophical writings.[8] Newton was their model, and the exchange of theories between the College of Physicians and the Royal Society was fostered by men like Hans Sloane and James Jurin who served as leading figures of both groups.[9] Furthermore, members of these groups shared antiquarian and literary connections, political and religious allegiances and, for some, royal privileges as well.

An analysis of the arguments and constituencies of physicians who opposed these theoretical medical writings is wanting. This section only begins to explore this under-researched area by focusing upon the anti-theoretical medical writings of one contemporary, Daniel Turner. The authors whom Turner regarded as his opponents are identified, and the basis of the type of medical practice he preferred – a patient-oriented approach – is discussed. Additionally, Turner's use of similar rhetoric when discussing mechanical medical physicians and quacks is explained. Although anti-theoretical sentiments pervade all of Turner's writings as a physician, they are most pronounced in his works on syphilis (1717 & 1739), fevers (1727), and the power of a pregnant woman's imagination to deform or mark her foetus (1714, 1727-30). Therefore, this account of Turner is primarily based upon these works.

According to Turner, his writings provoked 'Resentment' from many medical colleagues who deemed him an 'Enemy to learning'.[10]

If 'learning' to these physicians implied only a study of theoretically based medicine, then Turner was indeed an enemy. Among those he identified as adversaries were: John Woodward, the physician and antiquary who claimed that all physical disorders stemmed from impaired mechanical digestion or blocked secretion of digestive juices; John Colbatch, the 'acidophile' who claimed 'our Stomachs could never abound with too much Acid'; and the 'Alkalinus', John Radcliffe, who argued alternatively that acids were the 'chief Enemy of English Constitutions'. Turner also denounced the 'pyrophylus' Richard Morton's claim that all diseases originated from a 'venom or poisonous ferment' which 'seized [up]on the animal spirits'.[11] He also disregarded John Quincy's 'geometrical reasoning' and opposed Nicholas Robinson, that 'Standard Bearer' of Newtonian medicine, who argued that 'Sickness ... [was] nothing else but a Disorder' in which the 'Equilibrium [of solids or fluids] is destroy'd' thereby turning 'the Balance [of Nature] to one side or the other'.[12] Turner ridiculed a number of other leading English iatro-mathematicians who claimed that by using mathematical principles, the causes and treatments of medical disorders could be reduced to a 'certain Rule'.[13]

Instead, Turner adopted the belief that medical practice was to be guided solely by experience, 'without regard to any Theory or Hypothesis whatever'. It is 'One thing', he argued,

> to talk of Cures, which may be enterpris'd by the Ratios of Quantities, increased Momentums, by calculating the Diameters of ... Vessels, comparing the given Force at the Heart, with the reciprocal Resistance at the Sides of those Vessels, and their Angles of Incidence; computing also the exact Degrees of Viscidity in the Fluids ... therein circulating. And it is a quite different thing to perform the Cure, from a constant and sedulous Observation of the same Disease.[14]

The pathway of a disease was not, he claimed, *a priori* predictable according to any certain natural laws of physics. For physicians were not, according to Turner, like natural philosophers who were free to apply rules 'to Bodies inanimate, or putting simple Fluids into ... Balance ... [or] counting ... Pressures or Impulses'.[15] Rather, they were dealing with human lives. Physicians, he asserted, must not 'sacrific[e] Mens Lives' for the sake of some 'meer [sic] Hypothesis'.[16]

Turner: A Sydenham Disciple

Turner represented himself as facing a formidable opposition. After emphasizing the overwhelming prevalence of theoretical writings to his readers, he claimed that the greatest 'Difficulty' lay in their 'choice of Guides'.[17] "Tis our great Misfortune, that those Gentlemen' who work in making a 'sufficient number of Observations' enabling them to detect Nature's role in disease are 'for the most part silent; and the writing Task falls chiefly to the Theorists who being big with some Hypothesis, are impatient till they are delivered thereof, or to the mercenary Scribes, who write for their own and their Booksellers Profit'. How else 'has it fallen out', Turner queried, that 'for almost a Century, ... England [produced] but one Sydenham?'[18]

To illustrate his anti-theoretical stance, Turner explicitly advocated the ideals of Thomas Sydenham, the 'English Hippocrates' (see Figure 5.1). Specifically, he directed his readers' attention to the sufferers of disease rather than to the underlying theoretical

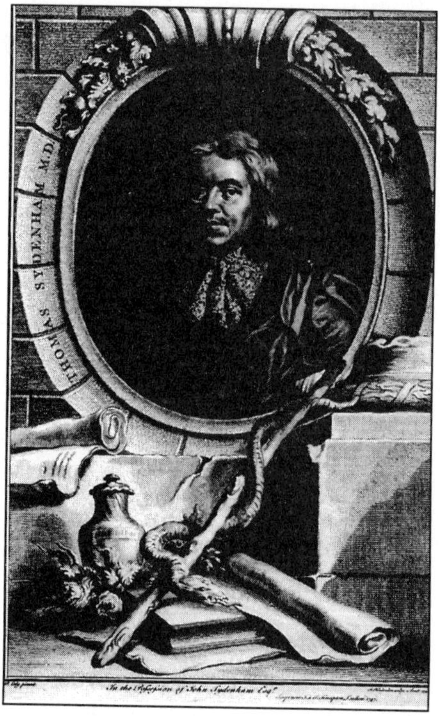

Figure 5.1
Thomas Sydenham, 1624-1689
(J. Houbraken, 1746, after Mary Beale, 1672;
Wellcome Institute Library, London)

constructs of disease.

Concurrent with many physicians' adulation of Newton, the writings of Thomas Sydenham appear to have gained something of a revival in the 1720s.[19] The seventeenth-century Sydenham sought to dispel the belief that theories and hypotheses could afford any true understanding of the cause, and consequently, the treatment of disease. 'How we can cure diseases whilst we know nothing of their causes, gives us no trouble' claimed Sydenham, for 'It is not by the knowledge of causes, but by ... experience, that the cure of the majority of diseases is accomplished'.[20]

Historian Andrew Cunningham has argued that post-1690 adherence to Sydenham was indicative of support of the 'Good Ol' [Cromwellian] Cause'.[21] Unlike Cromwellian supporters, Turner despised 'radical whig' ideals; however, his embroiled polemics against fellow Jacobites Pitcairne, Keill, Freind, and later Ward, suggest that his criticisms of these 'Hypothetical Schematists' were based on more than recognizable partisan politics.[22] Indeed, Turner argued that part of the 'character' of a physician was not to 'meddle ... in Party Quarrels or Disputes'.[23]

Unlike physicians Cheyne and Woodward, and later Mead, Strother, and others who openly turned to Sydenham consequent to their mid-life anti-theoretical crises, Turner's Sydenhamian leanings were laid early in his life. At the heart of Turner's conviction, he claimed that the theories of the "mechanicians" not only failed to offer practical aid, but that by adhering to them, physicians actually brought their patients much harm. Moreover, the concerns of the patient were being entirely neglected. 'I dare say', Turner argued, that 'the Patient will be equally thankful for his Cure, though you should be sometimes at a Loss for the Modus, or Mechanism, by which the Disease was ... produced'.[24]

Turner backed his Sydenhamian argument regarding the patient's concerns with case studies illustrating how 'mechanicians' had bled, purged, and sweat their fever patients to death. Similar results were to be expected, he argued, by administering medicines according to a 'rule' without considering the patient's age, constitution, or observing the effects of previous treatment. Instead, Turner instructed his readers to consider each patient's treatment individually in the manner of Sydenham and Hippocrates. He explained that treatments were best guided by observing nature's actions rather than relying upon some rule. For example, upon finding a patient 'no worse than the Day before, and the Day following in the same Condition, [Turner] thought it his Duty still to [a]wait [Nature's] Motion, fearing [that], by intermeddling, he should do some Hurt'.[25] Letting Nature show the physician 'what way ... to take' was, Turner claimed, the best route to 'steer ... safe ... the medical Compass'.[26]

One of Turner's opponents, London physician-author Thomas Morgan, stated in his 1735 *Mechanical Practise of Physick* that 'to declaim against mathematical theorems' is to say that 'medicine is grounded upon no Principle at all'. If, for instance, such theorization were abandoned, he argued there would be 'no difference between a Physician and a Quack but a Diploma'.[27] Such reasoning was strictly antithetical to Turner's. Turner was not promoting blind empiricism, but rather what he termed 'rational empiricism'.[28] It was, he claimed, through a physician's capability of 'Reasoning' upon his observations of the 'Operations' of 'Nature', 'back'd with a true Knowledge of the Structure of the Parts' and a 'thorough acquaintance with *Materia Medica*' rather than using *'arithematical calculi'* that we 'distinguish a Physician from a Quack'. The latter, he claimed, being 'ignorant of the Nature and Seat of the Disease, prescribes his Medicine ... at random'.[29]

Identifying a Quack

Just how were quacks identified? From the patient's viewpoint, distinguishing between qualified and unqualified practitioners was, as Roy Porter has lucidly recounted, quite difficult.[30] Turner's explication in *The Modern Quack*, however, suggests that he was familiar with the intricate details of the well-polished ploys and tactics of local mountebanks. Quacks, like the mechanist physicians, typically followed certain methods, and Turner claimed he wanted to help the public understand and avoid these methods.

The methods of mechanists and quacks succeeded, Turner argued, because of the 'wild ... Ideas' most people shared about their bodies. The 'Generality', he claimed, had the 'Notion of their Stomach ... as a Bason to receive' and their 'Bowels ... as a Pipe ... to convey off what is left ... thus if any ... Stop happens to the first, a lusty Vomit will Pump all up again, or a strong Horse-drench forcing down the [stopped] Plug'. Should they believe the 'Offence' had gotten 'farther into the Blood', the public proceeds to 'roast' their 'Patient with some burning Cordial or Spirits, ... to force a ... Sweat'.[31] Reasoning about the body in a mechanical way was not exclusive to mechanical physicians, but was, at least to some extent, also shared by the public.

To point out further fallacies, Turner drew attention to the similarities between the patter of a quack and the rhetoric of a mechanical physician. He denounced Newtonian mechanist, Nicholas Robinson's 'prophesy' that actions of the solid and fluid components of the body were due to an inherent 'electrical attraction'.[32] He noted that quack practitioners used similar arguments in promoting the sale of that very popular panacea, the anodyne necklace.[33] To illustrate what he recognized as further similarities between the mechanists and the quacks, he explained that quacks had borrowed natural philosophical terms such as physical, chemical, electrical, magnetic, pneumatic, hydraulic, and hydrostatic to describe the special 'powers' of their remedies. Although some have argued that quacks used these terms in an attempt to gain legitimacy,[34] from Turner's view, the use of this terminology only served to legitimize their reputation as quacks (see Figure 5.2).

Turner further argued that both quacks and mechanists followed methods which were based upon false principles. He warned readers that either swallowing the bait of an impostor or swallowing medicine which was administered only according to some 'hypothetical' or 'mechanical' theory held the same potential for destroying patients. Thus his anti-theoretical writings, like those exposing quackery, were guided to educate readers to understand and avoid particular methods.

Quacks: Professional Adversaries and the 'Common Enemy of the Public'

In addition to the variously trained orthodox practitioners of surgery, contemporary accounts suggest that 'thousands' of 'quacks' also practised surgery in London, the city hailed as 'the best Quack-Market in the Kingdom'.[35] According to Roy Porter, the term 'quack' was tossed around rather casually in the Enlightenment.[36] Among those whom contemporary surgeons labelled as quacks were the barbers, apothecaries, midwives, and bone-setters who practised outside of their authorized realm of care. The oculists who set bones, the bone-setters who 'breathed' veins, and the barbers who practised surgery were, regardless of any benefit they may actually have provided society, viewed by many orthodox surgical practitioners as quacks.

Besides these brands of quacks, contemporary writings such as *The Modern Quack, the Quacks Unmask'd,* and *The Life of… A Sham-Prophet Doctor* would have us believe that the most numerous impostors were those who, without any surgical or medical training, offered their services through self-advertisement.[37] There was 'scarce a Street, Lane, Court, Alley or other Building' in London, it was claimed, where these 'Intruders have not shamefully crept in'.

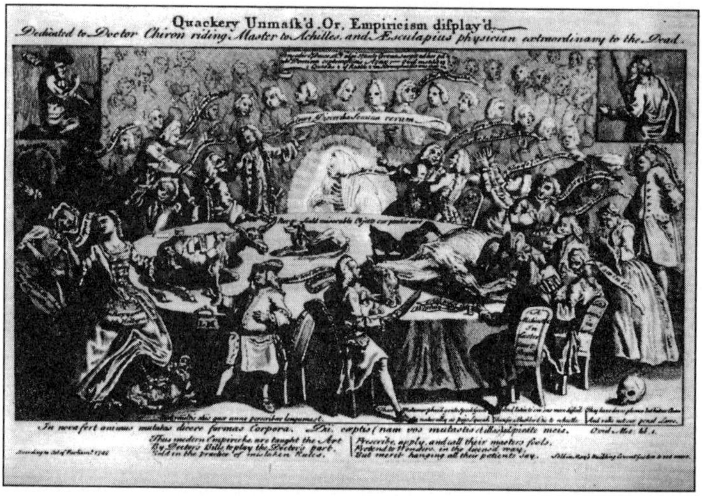

Figure 5.2
Gathered around a large table in a dissecting room are 18th-century medical practitioners of dubious repute including Baron Schwanberg, Dr Bateman, Benjamin Okel, G. West, Dr Caru, John Williams, the 'Bugg Doctor', Matha Misaubin, the seller of the anti-venereal pill, Dr Rock, Robert Turlingham, and J. Barrow (1748, Wellcome Institute Library, London)

Handbills advertising their treatments were posted at the entrances of all public 'thorow-fares', on corner-houses, and on 'Pissing-Post[s]'.[38]

Quacks had been depicted as a problem to London surgeons for centuries. Surgical author Thomas Gale, for instance, criticized unskilled surgical practitioners in his 1564 *Certain Works of Chirurgerie* as did John Securis in his 1566 *A Detection and Querimonie of the Daily Enormitics and Abuses committed in Physick*.[39]

During the 1690s, fellows of the Royal College of Physicians divided over their recognition as to who represented acceptable, qualified, expert practitioners. The growing city needed more practitioners to maintain the health of the populace. The 'ancient fellows' of the College opposed the 'new College' fellows' attempts to expand the definition of expert practitioner. In addition, the 'new College' fellows, including Edward Tyson, deplored their 'ancient fellow' colleagues' attempts to assume the sole authority over what comprised quality medical practice.

'New College' fellows, as Harold Cook has elucidated, developed a medical agenda that recognized surgeons, and especially apothecaries, as delivering quality 'medical' care in London.[40] Their persistence ultimately led to the 'decline of the Old Medical Order' and the establishment of a New Order which promoted more liberal, empirical medical practices. The concomitant competitive marketplace practice met the desire of both the New Order and the public. It also created an environment in which control over 'quack' practitioners became increasingly difficult.

By the late 17th century, Daniel Turner was among the most vocal surgical authors urging action against the quacks practising his trade.[41] Beginning with his 1695 apologetic writings of surgery through to his 1735 attack of Joshua Ward's pill and drop, Turner declared the dangers Londoners faced from local medical impostors. The numerous written advertisements and oral harangues of bonesetters, lithotomists, oculists, barbers, and especially the 'petticoat practitioners' had, he claimed, ultimately brought only misery to their patients. Not only had such impostors cost their victims much money, but they had, according to Turner, also cost many Londoners their lives.

London was, so Turner claimed, 'most abominably put upon' as an 'Abundance of its Inhabitants' were 'maimed and undone through the Countenancing [with] great Numbers of Ignorant, ill designing' pretenders of surgery.[42] 'Every Art has had its Adversarys', Turner claimed, but 'methinks 'tis very strange' that surgery, the art which 'gives Sight to the Blind, Hearing to the Deaf: Sets together ... disjoynted and broken Bones, and reduses [sic] the Frail Structure of Humane Bodys to their wonted Health and Vigour, should have so much as one [adversary], amongst the most barbarous part of mankind'.[43]

Among these adversaries, Turner 'accounted' street mountebanks as the most 'Common Enemy of the People' (see Figure 5.3)[44]. Not only for the 'Time he cheats ... [people] of [during] which [they] should otherwise be employed', but the mountebank also preyed upon people's money. Money which, Turner argued, was 'better thrown to Swine'.[45] He disparaged bone-setters as 'Man-slayers',[46] and claimed it was 'very rare' to meet a patient that had not been 'spoyl'd' by the hands of some ignorant 'petticoat practitioner'.[47] However, Turner's chief accusations were directed against the barbers. 'It's almost a Rarity', he argued, 'to find one of their Poles without a Frame of Porringers, or some other signal of their Pretension to Chyrurgick Practice'. He claimed they readily 'Bleed [patients], cut Issues, treat Apostems, apply Plaisters, Pultisses [sic] and Fomentations',[48] yet they were actually 'such a Stranger to Chyrurgery' that they could not give a 'discerning Querist a satisfactory definition of either Wound or Ulcer'.[49] Moreover, the 'very Notion of a Barber-Surgeon' seemed, to Turner, to 'countenance the Arrogance' of most apprenticed barbers.[50]

Concurrent rumblings against barbers overstepping the limits of their practice also occurred within the Barber-Surgeons' Company. The tension between barbers and surgeons elevated to such a point that in 1684, the surgeons pleaded for Charles II to separate the Company. The barbers, according to the surgeons, were so 'ignorant of the Science and Faculty of Surgery' which they claimed they commonly practised, that the barbers 'hinder[ed] and [did] not promote the order for which they were united'.[51] This attempt at separation was unsuccessful, and similar pleas were voiced throughout the first half of the eighteenth century. (See Appendix 2 for another attempted surgical reform.)

Many of these 'Roguish Imposters' practised, according to Turner, without any formal training. Others, however, chiefly through the want of 'private Lucre', set themselves up in practice after

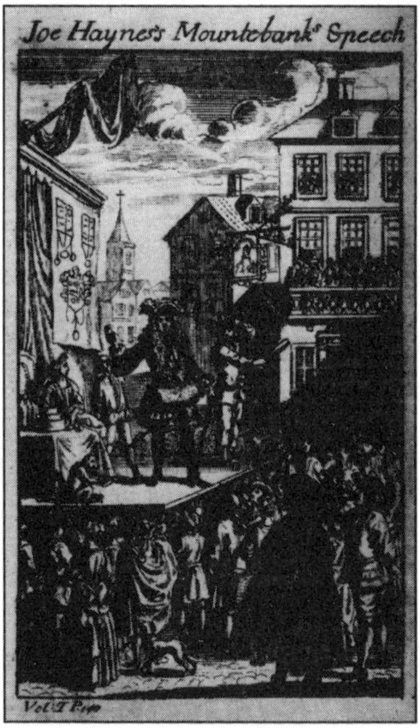

Figure 5.3
Well-known itinerant mountebank, Joe Haynes, selling his wares from a stage to a large audience assembled in the town square
(Wellcome Institute Library, London)

only a 'Year, two, or three' of apprenticeship to some barber or apothecary, and purchased the protective 'screen' of an ecclesiastical licence.[52] The only 'Journey work' this type of quack pursued, he argued, involved 'diligently conning over his Grandmother's receipt-[or recipe] book'.[53] Similarly, Turner identified those 'brought up' in either physic, pharmacy, or surgery who attempted to 'intermeddle' in all three as 'Cosin-German [sic] to a quack'.[54] Each 'Transgressor' should, he argued, be 'look'd on as a kind of false Brother by the rest, and ... a Trespasser ... on the Law of Nature' by 'doing as he would not willingly be done unto'.[55]

One contemporary complained how 'monstrous' it was to see 'that Mob of Empirics' including barbers, farriers, and mountebanks 'overreach and bubble the People both of their Lives and Money'.[56] Turner depicted surgery as having been degraded into a 'Sanctuary or Refuge for decay'd Tradesmen'.[57] Turner claimed people 'of Sense, at least' did not choose a scrivener to make their clothes, a tailor to write their will, or a shoemaker as their spiritual guide, yet he found it 'hard to account' why people 'often [en]trusted' all three of these trained tradesmen with their bodies.[58] 'One would think', Turner complained, that surgery was the easiest Art to perfect for 'a meer Pretence ... will carry a man very far into the good Opinion of other People'.[59]

Reform – like that undergirding the city of London – was also needed to stabilize the infrastructure of surgery. He argued that society would remain plagued with quackery until 'Men can make a more clear distinction' between an 'ingenious [surgical] Artist' and the 'Artless Pretender'.[60] In order to clarify what he saw as distinguishing features, Turner sought to 'undermine the Foundation' of the 'Infamous Impostors' or quacks. This was the goal of his 1695, *Apologia Chyrurgica. A Vindication of the Noble Art of Surgery* (see Figure 5.4). With surgical precision, he claimed he would 'dissect their pernicious Principles, and lay open the treachery and impiety of their Dealings'.[61] In this way, he believed his *Apologia* offered a 'most necessary piece of service' not only to his chosen trade, but to the public good as well.

Turner offered vivid, lengthy descriptions in minute detail of well-polished ploys and tactics used by London quacks he claims to have observed. These detailed verbal pictures of practice set his *Apologia* apart from most previous and contemporary accounts of quackery. He hoped these extensive accounts would make surgeon readers aware of the typical traps local quacks used to ensnare their victims. If readers had no personal experience attending cases of this 'abuse', Turner urged them to consider the 'Great Number of those

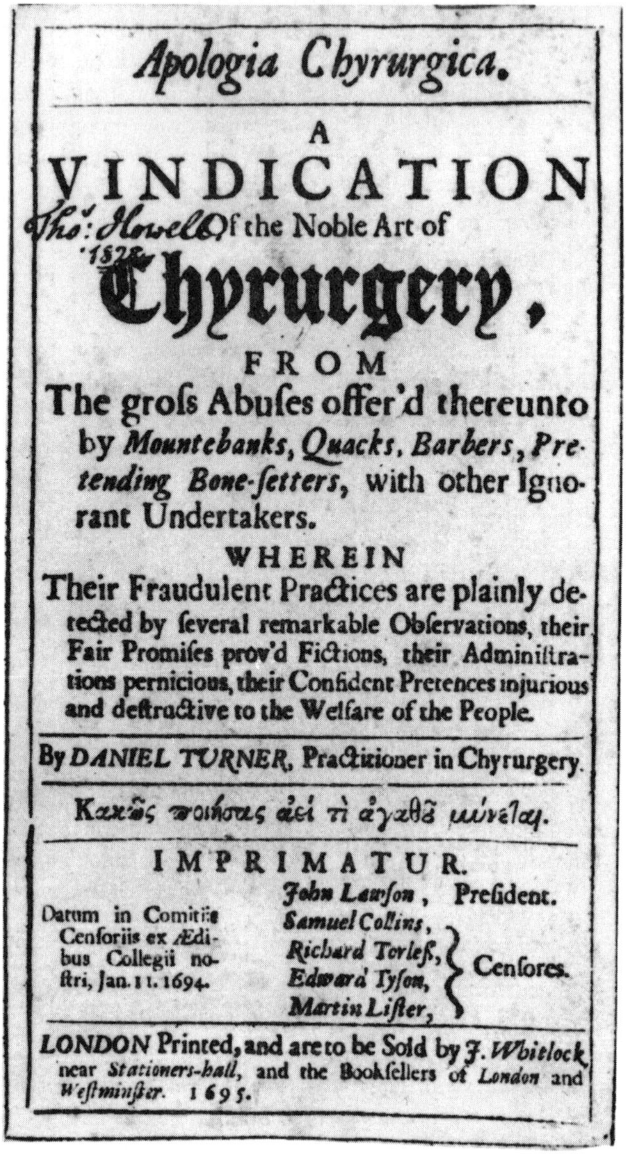

Apologia Chyrurgica.

A

VINDICATION

Tho: Howell Of the Noble Art of

'1828

Chyrurgery,

FROM

The groſs Abuſes offer'd thereunto by *Mountebanks, Quacks, Barbers, Pretending Bone-ſetters,* with other Ignorant Undertakers.

WHEREIN

Their Fraudulent Practices are plainly detected by ſeveral remarkable Obſervations, their Fair Promiſes prov'd Fictions, their Adminiſtrations pernicious, their Confident Pretences injurious and deſtructive to the Welfare of the People.

By *DANIEL TURNER*, Practitioner in Chyrurgery.

Καλῶς ποιήσεις ἀεί τι ἀγαθὸ μένειν.

IMPRIMATUR.

Datum in Comitiis Cenſoriis ex Ædibus Collegii noſtri, Jan. 11. 1694.

John Lawſon, Preſident.

Samuel Collins, *Richard Torleſs*, *Edward Tyſon*, *Martin Liſter*, Cenſores.

LONDON Printed, and are to be Sold by *J. Whitlock* near *Stationers-hall*, and the Bookſellers of *London* and *Weſtminſter*. 1695.

Figure 5.4

Daniel Turner devoted his first published work, *Apologia Chyrurgica* (1695), to exposing the methods of quackery. (Wellcome Institute Library, London)

Deplorable Misfortunes' in hospitals whose conditions were, so he claimed, singularly derived from the 'injuditious Management of some Unlearned Empiric, or Ignorant Old Woman'.[62]

Nothing within the records of the Barber-Surgeons' Company indicates that Turner was selected to document the abuses of the 'Present State' of surgery. Rather, his 'inspection' into 'the business' of quackery appears to have owed its origin to his own surgical practice.[63] As mentioned in Chapter Three, Turner claimed it was 'very rare' that he met a patient who had not already been ruined by some 'ignorant and foolish' quack.[64] Indeed his own practice provided him 'many opportunities' to inspect and treat the 'Abuses' derived from the hands of empirics.[65]

Not only did Turner crusade to expose quackery, but he also outlined a specific plan to reform its 'shameful' state. Other authors had argued that quacks deserved 'Slight and Contempt'[66] but Turner deemed the 'simple Detection of the Fraud, without coercion upon the Delinquent' was 'insufficient' both as an attempt to 'rectify this Disorder, and [to] secure the People from being thus … sacrificed'.[67] Instead, Turner urged the 'representatives' of the Barber-Surgeons' Company to take the matter of reform 'into their serious Consideration'.[68]

Specifically, Turner suggested they pass an Act whereby 'no Person shall presume to practise, till He had first past an Examen, and was found fit to be entrusted with the Care of the Diseased Subject'.[69] He regarded the Governors of the Court of Assistants as the most 'proper Arbiters of sound and artful Practice'.[70] Seeking similar support as that of 'new College' physicians, Turner argued that the old guard of the Barber-Surgeons' Company needed 'Incouragement' from a higher magistracy to more effectively control the 'gross Enormities Committed under a Pretence of [surgical] Practice'.[71] With the endorsement of the like-minded reformer, Edward Tyson, Turner argued that ultimately there was 'no better way' to overcome the 'unspeakable Damage accruing to [the public by their] … unlimited Toleration of Ignorant and Unskillful Persons' in surgical practice than to 'obtain an ACT of Parliament for its future Prevention'.[72] Once such reform was obtained, so Turner claimed, the city of London would find a 'Diminution in the Bills of Mortality: Every Parish therein would be less burthen'd with their Sick and Lame, and those renowned Hospitals, [would] perhaps [be] capable of receiving all that should be presented'.[73]

Contemporaneous with, and likely precipitated by Turner's

proposed reforms, the Barber-Surgeons' Company re-examined their by-laws. Their first actions, undertaken in 1697, identified which laws were still 'usefull' regarding 'male-practice' [sic].[74] Within a year, a committee of the Court undertook the specific task to determine whether 'all persons exercising Barbery & Chirurgery' were doing so 'within the limitts' of the by-laws.[75] If cases of abuse were found, they were empowered to inflict the 'penaltys mentioned in the By laws' according to the severity of 'male-practice' in each case.

Despite the general climate of reform, few individuals were actually charged with 'male-practice' and brought before the Court. In 1697, Peter St Hill was charged with 'practising Chyrurgery being not qualified'. Several barbers, including the barber of the Archbishop of Canterbury, were also charged with unrightfully extending their practice of barbery to include surgery.[76] That same year, Turner specifically complained against the surgical 'mal practice' of Peter Perkins.[77] Although Perkins was 'summoned' before the Court, it is, as in the aforementioned cases, unknown whether any disciplinary actions were taken.

Leaders of the Barber-Surgeons' Company were not exempt from following the Company's by-laws. On 21 October 1700, it was ordered that due to the 'ill management' of examinations while in the office of master of the Company, i.e., having 'acted contrary to the establishment of the Corporation', the past master of the Company be 'expel'd' from the Court of Assistants. At the following Court of Assistants meeting, 7 November 1700, the committee claimed to have found 'upon their inquiry that [the past master] had committed diverse crime[s] against the Constitution of the Corporation in certifyeing Chirurgeons & Chirurgeons' mates to bee qualified ... that were not duely examined in Court & approved of by two of the Examiners at least'. The Court declared that the past master be 'for ever discharged from being one of the Examiners' of the Company, and 'discharged from being any longer one of the Court of Assistants'. The past master of the Company in question was Thomas Lichfield, Daniel Turner's own master.[78] After having suggested that the Company implement more stringent examination procedures in his 1695 *Apologia*, it is ironic that Turner, five years later, witnessed his own master removed from the Court of Assistants for not upholding the Company's newly enforced examination procedures which Turner himself had suggested.

Despite having trained under a man later convicted of a form of surgical 'mal practice', or perhaps fuelled by this experience, Turner continued his anti-quackery crusade throughout his life. Eight years following his *Apologia*, Turner reiterated his view of reforming 'vulgar' surgical practice by singling out and penalizing each 'pseudo-chirurgus' in *The Present State of Chyrurgery*.[79] Later writings, however, suggest that Turner came to envision the direct removal of all surgical impostors as too idealistic. Instead, he modified his crusade to combat what he claimed could be more realistically achieved. Specifically, he sought to improve the level of care which qualified surgeons could offer and to prevent the public from falling prey to vulgar practitioners. Turner argued that the public would take notice of this improvement and gravitate towards qualified practitioners. Thereby, within a few years, vulgar practitioners would be eliminated as competition. To ensure the success of this process, Turner reminded public readers about what types of practices to avoid in his 1718 *The Modern Quack*.

Atheists as Enemies

Publicizing about mechanists and quacks appears to have been linked to Turner's private religious convictions. Although these convictions are not so explicit in his published writings, Turner elaborated upon his religious beliefs in his private devotional, 'Religio Medici Reformata'.[80] Borrowing only the title from Sir Thomas Browne's well-known work, Turner's writing more closely parallels the commonplace *The Whole Duty of Man*.

The Whole Duty of Man is the devotional guidebook which religious historians have claimed best symbolized Restoration High Anglicanism.[81] This work was designed to establish a 'set form' of religious worship or catechism through which one could, by living according to its precepts, 'avoid heresy' and gain salvation.[82] To achieve this benefit, one was expected to confess one's sins according to an 'authorized' format. Only through this regular 'Method of Devotion' did High Anglicans like Turner believe the 'corruption' of man would be 'cured'.[83]

The rhetorical style of Turner's devotional, apart from the catechism, is consistent with his polemical writings against quacks. This finding is particularly noteworthy considering that Turner claimed to have compiled this work for private use 'In his closet'. As such, it provides suggestive evidence that Turner's inner struggles were closely related to the struggles against enemies in his outer or 'professional' world. This finding reaffirms Richard Holmes' view that in biographically representing a life, the 'public and private life do … make sense of each other'.[84]

Consequent to the Glorious Revolution in 1688, Anglicanism

underwent a series of reforms. The ensuing years, as historian Margaret Jacob has documented, saw an increasing spread of Whig latitudinarian ideals to the pulpits, the Parliament, and the governing bodies of the Royal Society and the College of Physicians.[85] These tolerant, liberal Low Churchmen formed much of the platform on which the following generation of Newtonianism was based.

One primary distinction between Low and High Church Anglicans at this time was the role they attributed to the Creator. Many latitudinarians envisioned a natural religion in which God was removed or displaced from the central position of their depictions of nature. Economic historian, Peter Earle clearly described this view in his reconstruction of the world of Turner's contemporary, Daniel Defoe: 'God had created Nature; but now Nature had taken over from her creator and God Himself was obliged to conform to the natural laws of His own creation'. The basis of this 'natural religion' was not so much God as it was reason.[86] This position became pronounced through the 'argument from design' as expressed in the growing body of physico- and astro-theological writings as well as in the renowned Boyle lectures delivered between 1692 and 1714.[87]

Turner, however, did not subscribe to this belief of a natural religion. Rather, he argued that his contemporaries had, by their use of that 'aequivocal term Nature', strengthened the 'Boundary' between medicine and religion.[88] By doing this, he claimed, these physicians were true separatists from the Church. Specifically, having separated the Creator from discourse on nature, they had, he argued, made their initial step towards atheism. As had been argued by many in preceding centuries, Turner charged that 'too many of [his] own profession' lacked a true faith in God. Although they may 'possibly ... acknowledg[e]' the 'general Providence ... of that Being which created [nature], in ... support of the Mundane Fabrick', Turner claimed they gave 'very little reason by their words or actions' that they do not 'deny' the Creator's existence altogether.[89]

Turner's conviction that most physicians were atheists was shared by many writers in the popular press. A 1707 issue of *The Weekly Comedy*, for instance, claimed that 'Physicians ... are generally accounted atheists'.[90] However, as historian Michael Hunter has convincingly argued, atheism was a rhetorical term used to mean 'Godless' in a rather broad and loose sense in early modern England.[91] 'Believers' who challenged God's 'active supervision of the world' were but one example of those who were called atheists.[92] Many people appear to have used 'atheist' as a condemnation of anything that was, in their view, unorthodox. To identify Turner's specific target for the label of 'atheist', it is necessary to reconstruct some of Turner's religious views.

The sparsity of socio-historical religious writings covering this period prevents a full contextualization of Turner's beliefs within London's religious milieu.[93] Some basic points about Turner, however, allow me to build the foundation of his religious beliefs. Turner was a High Church Anglican. His devotional is filled with animosity for all separatists from the Church. These separatists included Low Churchmen as well as the growing number of 'enthusiasts' in a variety of sects.

To Turner, God was omnipotent and omnipresent. Life, as he described it, was generated and maintained only through the direct intervention of the Creator. The impetus which he considered underlay all internal bodily workings was attributed to the 'invisible hands' of the divine providential Creator. Turner also regarded that Nature's healing 'power' within humans stemmed from God. Humans were, he described, 'only passive' beings guided as Nature dictates.[94] He accepted that Nature's actions attested to God's presence, but he argued they revealed nothing about God Himself. No one, Turner claimed, can 'know or acquaint Himself, with that holy Ardour, or fervency, of Spirit, ... that attends the Devout Supplicant'.

This view is consistent with his discussion of mechanical physicians. These physicians' attempts to experimentally investigate what end was being sought, that is, the final cause of all bodily action, was, to Turner, futile.[95] For these causes, he concluded, were knowable 'only to the Creator', and 'impenetrable' to human understanding.[96] Likewise, no one could become, using Turner's words, 'enlightn'd, to see through the end of all' living things and discover the Creator's 'Wisdom, Power, and Goodness' until his or her 'Entrance into the [Heavenly] Sanctuary'.[97] In this sense, Turner claimed that God was the 'only mathematical Physician'.[98]

Pretenders in Religion and Medicine

During the time in which Turner described medical quacks being rampant in London, religious pretenders were also prevalent. 'There are Quacks in Divinity, as well as in Physick', so *The Entertainer* reported in 1717 (see Figure 5.5). 'Spiritual Mountebanks, Inspired Merry-Andrews, Interlopers, [and] Invaders of Spiritualities' were claimed to have commonly gained more 'Popular Applause' than 'those who really deserve[d] it'.[99] Turner particularly denounced the enthusiasts who, he claimed, 'made a business of praetended

Inspiration' by using a 'Fitt of … misguided Zeal … [to carry] them into one of their supposedly divine Raptures'. He also disapproved of the 'dismal and tremendous consequences of the delusions' spread by the Anabaptists, the Adamists, the Melchiontes, the Georgians, and the Menoists.[100] Most emphatically, he renounced the 'fals prophets' James Naylor, Tobias Venner, John Mason and the 'French Prophets' who had more recently threatened English Anglicanism with their separatist beliefs.[101] Turner's depiction of the contemporary 'prophets' as pretenders who claimed themselves privileged with divine inspiration was consistent with his characterization of the medical pretenders who claimed themselves privileged in holding cures. The harm the religious pretenders inflicted, however, was considerably greater as their 'delusions' held dismal consequences on an eternal scale.

Religious pretenders were, to Turner, as deceptive in offering practical aid as were quacks of medicine and surgery. His rhetoric against the separatists of the Church and the unorthodox medical practitioners was remarkably similar. Turner employed the same tactics to abolish the false 'Apostolic Messengers' of religion as he had used to overpower the medical impostors in his *Modern*

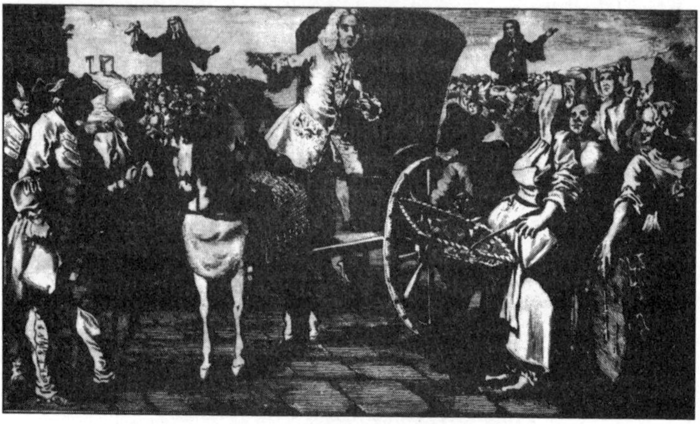

Figure 5.5

Dr Richard Rock, itinerant medical vendor at Kennington Common. Rock was well known around St Paul's and Covent Garden for his 'anti-venereal, grand, specifick pill'. Dissenting founders of Methodism, John and Charles Wesley are also pictured in the background. (1743, Wellcome Institute Library, London)

Quack. First, he explained the need to 'distinguish' between the 'pretence to extraordinary Illumination' and the 'plain and simple Truths' set forth in the authorized 'Sacred Writings'. In particular, he warned that those who claimed divine inspiration or prophecy often stood behind a façade of 'Gesture, Tone or [an] Ecstatic Way of pronunciation'.[102] Medical quacks supported similar façades before the gullible public.[103] Second, Turner claimed that if people would 'reflect' upon their own experiences, they would clearly see that all the recently professed prophecies had passed unfulfilled. Similarly, the expectations which quacks built around their products also, according to Turner, passed with no avail. Third, Turner warned people not to be misled or to 'abuse' their 'Prepogative Reason' which is 'bestowed upon us that wee may distinguish Truth from Error'. Fourthly, Turner begged 'readers' to 'weigh' in their minds how the truly 'instructive' learned Anglican clergy offer 'Design[s]' for 'holy Living, ... good Life, ... [and] Christian Faith ... without assuming this unwarrantable Privilege of Inspiration'.[104] He claimed that by comparing the 'convoluted tales' of the prophets with the sacred writings which were 'free of ornamental Insinuation ... [and] Ensnaring Sophistry', the impostors' façades would be destroyed, and the false 'Apostolic Messingers' exposed for the pretenders he claimed them to be.[105] Turner's arguments in both his religious and medical writings were appeals to the public to use their common sense to discriminate between 'quackery' and 'truth'.

Notes

1 Michael Hunter discussed Wilkins' universal language proposal and Petty's political arithmetic within the context of contemporary discourse in *Science and Society in Restoration England* (Cambridge: Cambridge University Press, 1981), 113-35. See also Umberto Eco's chapter, 'John Wilkins', in *The Search for the Perfect Language* (Oxford: Blackwell Publishers, 1997), 238-59. Peter Gibbons provided several examples of projects designed to benefit the health of the English in 'The Medical Projectors, 1640-1720', *Journal of the History of Medicine and Allied Sciences*, xxiv (1969), 247-71. Glyndwr Williams discussed another example of contemporary 'projects' in '"The Inexhaustible Fountain of Gold": English Projects and Ventures in the South Seas, 1670-1750' in John E. Flint and Glyndwr Williams (eds), *Perspectives of Empire: Essays Presented to Gerald S. Graham* (New York: Barnes & Noble, 1973), 27-53. W. H. G. Armytage discussed a number of other 'projects' in *Four Hundred Years of English Education*

(Cambridge: Cambridge University Press, 1970).

2 Ronald Hutton brilliantly described the actual reforms which occurred prior to James II's accession in 1685 in *Charles the Second: King of England, Scotland and Ireland* (Oxford: Clarendon Press, 1989), esp. 357-445.

3 See, for example, James R. Jacob and Margaret C. Jacob, 'The Anglican Origins of Modern Science: The Metaphysical Foundations of the Whig Constitution', *Isis*, lxxi (1980): 251-67, and Margaret C. Jacob, *The Newtonians and the English Revolution 1689-1720* (Hassocks, Sussex: The Harvester Press, 1976), esp. 72-100, 143-61.

4 Thomas Vincent's provocative 1667 *God's Terrible Voice in the City* stimulated much contemporary discussion over the extent to which man's immoral living had instigated these disasters. F. Bastian claimed this important work was also the crucial source for Defoe's *Journal of the Plague Year*. See Bastian's *Defoe's Early Life* (Towanda, New Jersey: Barnes & Noble Books, 1981), 18-31, and 323, footnote 33.

5 In his 1670 *London's Lamentations: A Serious Discourse Concerning that Late Fiery Dispensation that Turned Our (Once Renowned) City Onto a Ruinous Heap*, Thomas Brookes identified many sins which he claimed were responsible for the 'heavy judgement' of the fire including gross and practical theism, luxury and intemperance, excessive worldliness, extortion, deceit, bribery, insolent and cruel oppressing of the poor, rejecting or condemning the Gospel, lying, fornication, 'going after strange flesh', profanation of the Sabbath, profaneness, lewdness, blindness and wickedness of the clergy, and the sins of the rulers as they abuse, mock and despise the messengers of the Lord. As cited in John Bedford's *London's Burning* (London: Abelard-Schuman, 1966), 147-8.

6 T. C. Curtis and W. A. Speck, 'The Societies for the Reformation of Manners: A Case Study in the Theory and Practice of Moral Reform', *Literature & History*, no.3 (1976), 45.

7 According to an advertisement for Clarke's books bound following D. Turner's *Art of Surgery*, 4th edn, 1732.

8 Turner discussed mechanists' descriptions of jaundice and consumption in his *Discourse on Fevers* (London: John Clarke, 1739), 108-09, and 287, respectively. Newton's influence on fever discourse is found in the works of Archibald Pitcairne, Richard Mead, George Cheyne, and John Freind. See for example William Coleman, 'Mechanistic Philosophy and Hypothetical Physiology', *Texas Quarterly*, x (1967), 263; R.J.J. Martin, 'Explaining John Freind's *History of Physic*', *Studies in History and Philosophy of Science*, xix

(1988), 406; and Anita Guerrini, 'Isaac Newton, George Cheyne and the "Principia Medicinae"', in R. French and A. Wear (eds), *The Medical Revolution of the Seventeenth Century* (Cambridge: Cambridge University Press, 1989), 227-8. Theodore M. Brown discussed the mechanists' argument in his 'The Mechanical Philosophy and the "Animal Oeconomy": A Study of the Development of English Physiology in the Seventeenth and Early Eighteenth Century', (Ph.D. thesis, Princeton University, 1968). Newton's prominence over mechanical medicine diminished in the decade following his death and iatromechanism became increasingly eclectic.

9 Anita Guerrini has studied Newton's influence on contemporary medical writing. See, for example, her 'Archibald Pitcairne and Newtonian Medicine', *Medical History*, xxxi (1987), 70-83, 'Isaac Newton, George Cheyne and the 'Principia Medicinae", 222-45, and 'Newtonianism, Medicine and Religion' in Ole Peter Grell and Andrew Cunningham (eds), *Religio Medici: Medicine and Religion in Seventeenth-Century England* (Aldershot, Hampshire: Scolar Press 1996), 293-312.

10 D. Turner, *Discourse Concerning Fevers*, 90.

11 *Ibid.*, 14-15, 18-20, 23-4.

12 *Ibid.*, 34, 37-8, 55-6. Turner also referred to 'Mathematical Medicine' in the dedication of his *Syphilis*.

13 D. Turner, *Discourse Concerning Fevers*, 81.

14 D. Turner, *Syphilis*, preface.

15 D. Turner, *Discourse Concerning Fevers*, 1st edn (1727), 58.

16 *Ibid.*, 28-9, and D. Turner, *Art of Surgery*, vol. 2 (1725), 75.

17 D. Turner, *Discourse Concerning Fevers*, 89.

18 *Idem.*

19 Andrew Cunningham rightly argued this revival was primarily orchestrated by Boerhaave. See his 'Thomas Sydenham: Epidemics, Experiment and the "Good Old Cause"', in R. French and A. Wear (eds), *The medical revolution of the seventeenth century* (Cambridge: Cambridge University Press, 1989), 189.

20 Thomas Sydenham, *Medical Observations Concerning the History and Cure of Acute Diseases*, as cited by Lester King, *The Road to Medical Enlightenment 1650-1695* (London: Macdonald, 1970), 127. Donald Bates provided the most thorough account of Sydenham on 'method' in his 'Sydenham and the Medical Meaning of "Method"', *Bulletin of the History of Medicine*, li (1977), 324-38. Also see Kenneth Dewhurst, *Dr Thomas Sydenham (1624-1689): His Life and Original Writings* (London: The Wellcome Historical Medical Library, 1966), esp. 60-7.

21 Andrew Cunningham, 'Thomas Sydenham: Epidemics, Experiment and the "Good Old Cause"',189.

22 D. Turner, *Discourse Concerning Fevers*, 45 and preface. Anita Guerrini described how some Tory physicians ascribed to Newtonian theory in her 'The Tory Newtonians: Gregory, Pitcairne and their Circle', *Journal of British Studies*, xxv (1986), 288-311, as did Bruce Lehman in 'Physicians and Politics in the Jacobite Era', in Eveline Cruickshanks and Jeremy Black (eds), *The Jacobite Challenge* (Edinburgh: John Donald, 1988), 74-91.

23 D. Turner, *Discourse Concerning Fevers*, 329.

24 D. Turner, *Syphilis*, 1732, preface.

25 D. Turner, *Discourse Concerning Fevers*, 215.

26 *Ibid.*, 13.

27 Turner quoted this passage from Morton in his *Discourse Concerning Fevers*, 98.

28 D. Turner, *Syphilis*, in his dedication to Richard Blundell.

29 D. Turner, *Discourse Concerning Fevers*, 103.

30 Roy Porter, 'Before the Fringe: Quackery and the Eighteenth-Century Medical Market' in R. Cooter (ed.), *Studies in the History of Alternative Medicine* (Basingstoke: Macmillan Press, 1988), 1-26. Alison Klairmont Lingo's noteworthy research into contemporary French quackery appeared as 'Empirics and Charlatans in Early Modern France: The Genesis of the Classification of the 'other' in Medical Practice', *Journal of Social History*, xxx (1996-7), 583-603.

31 D. Turner, *The Modern Quack*, dedication. Lemuel Gulliver, perhaps the most popular 'physician' of the period portrayed practitioners offering similar accounts of the effects of vomits, purges and clysters in his *Travels into Several Remote Nations of the World* (London: Benjamin Motte, 1726), Part 4, Ch. 6, 87-8.

32 D. Turner, *Discourse Concerning Fevers* (1727), 43-4.

33 D. Turner, *Syphilis* (1732), 119. F. Doherty reviewed the clamour brought about by this one 'remedy' in 'The Anodyne Necklace', 268-93.

34 R. Porter, *Health For Sale*, 102.

35 [D. Turner], *The Modern Quack, or Medicinal Impostor* (London: J. Roberts, 1718), 89.

36 R. Porter, *Health for Sale*, 1-2.

37 See, for example, P. Coltheart, *The Quacks Unmask'd* (London: The author, 1727).

38 D. Turner, *Apologia Chyrurgica,* 39 and D. Turner, *De Morbis Cutaneis*, 312. Keith Thomas cited similar claims in his *Religion and the Decline of Magic: Studies in Popular Beliefs in Sixteenth- and*

Seventeenth-Century England (Harmondsworth; New York: Penguin Books, 1978), 14.

39 As cited by L. M. Beier, *Sufferers & Healers*, 39. For a full account and many examples of seventeenth-century quackery see Beier's complete section on 'Unlicensed Healers', *ibid.*,19-32.

40 H. Cook, *Decline of the Old Medical Regime*, 210-53.

41 Later surgeons' accounts to dispel quackery appear in Matthias Gottfried Purmann's *Chirurgia Curiosa* (London: D. Browne, 1706) and James Handley's *Colloquia Chyrurgica: or, The Whole Art of Surgery Epitomiz'd*, 4th edn, (London: A. Bettesworth & C. Hitch, 1733), preface.

42 D. Turner, *Apologia Chyrurgica*, 26-7.

43 D. Turner, *Present State*, 27.

44 D. Turner, *Apologia Chyrurgica*, 25.

45 *Idem.*

46 D. Turner, *Art of Surgery*, vol. 2, 123 and D. Turner, *Present State*, 77-105. Roger Cooter discussed the practice of bone setters from a later period in his 'Bones of Contention? Orthodox Medicine and the Mystery of the Bone-Setter's Craft' in W.F. Bynum and Roy Porter (eds), *Medical Fringe & Medical Orthodoxy 1750-1850* (London: Croom Helm, 1987), 158-73.

47 D. Turner, *Present State*, 106-31. Roy Porter described the practices of several of these female in 'Female Quacks in the Consumer Society', *History of Nursing Journal*, iii (1990), 1-25. A. L. Wyman provided a more balanced account of female practitioners in 'The Surgeoness: The Female Practitioners of Surgery 1400 – 1800', *Medical History*, xxviii (1984), 22-41.

48 D. Turner, *Present State*, 9.

49 D. Turner, *Apologia Chyrurgica*, 29.

50 *Ibid.*, 51. J. F. South, among others, reminds later generations that there was never an official fusion of the two callings, barber and surgeon. See his *Memorial of the Craft of Surgery in England* (London: Cassell & Co, Ltd, 1886), xii.

51 Leo M. Zimmerman, 'Surgery', in Allen G. Debus (ed.), *Medicine in Seventeenth-Century England* (Berkeley, California: University of California Press, 1974), 58.

52 D. Turner, *Modern Quack*, 151.

53 D. Turner, *Apologia Chyrurgica*, 39-40.

54 D. Turner, *Modern Quack*, 57.

55 *Ibid.*, 3. Officially moving or 'translating' between trades was common in the early eighteenth century. Between five to forty non-surgeon apprentices of the Barber-Surgeons' Company were annually

translated to other non-surgical trades. Moving unofficially from an outlying trade into surgery, however, lay beyond the normal occupational diversity Margaret Pelling so lucidly described in 'Occupational Diversity', 484-511. Rather, this turn between trades likely represented aspirations, as Lawrence Stone described, of attaining more solid financial security and/or greater social esteem (i.e., an upwardly mobile social status): 'Social Mobility in England', esp. 29-33.

56 Anonymous, *Medicina Flagellata: or, The Doctor Scarify'd* (London: J. Bateman and J. Nicks, 1721), xi-xii. Charles A. Stonehill, Jr, Andrew Block and H. Winthrop Stonehill attribute this work to Dr Chene (George Cheyne?) in *Anonyma and Pseudonyma,* vol. 2 (London: C. A. Stonehill, Jr., 1926), 1382.

57 D. Turner, *Apologia Chyrurgica,* 132.

58 D. Turner, *Modern Quack,* To the Reader.

59 D. Turner, *Apologia Chyrurgica,* 132.

60 *Ibid.*, 1-2. The physician Walter Harris described a 'Real' practitioner as 'cautious, Delibrate, and Prudently Timorous' whereas a 'quack' was 'Rash, Inconsiderate, and Stiffly heady in every thing he does'. *Pharmacologia Anti-Empirica; or, A Rational Discourse of Remedies both Chymical and Galenical ... Together with some Remarks on ... the Most Notorious Impostures of Diverse Empiricks and Mountebanks* (London: for R. Chiswell, 1683), esp. 317-18.

61 D. Turner, *Apologia Chyrurgica,* 1-2.

62 D. Turner, *Present State,* 5-6.

63 D. Turner, *Apologia Chyrurgica,* 54.

64 D. Turner, *Present State,* 106-31.

65 D. Turner, *Apologia Chyrurgica,* To the Reader.

66 D. Turner, *A Remarkable Case in Surgery,* vii.

67 D. Turner, *Modern Quack,* Dedication.

68 D. Turner, *Present State,* 8.

69 *Idem.*

70 D. Turner, *A Remarkable Case in Surgery,* i.

71 D. Turner, *Present State,* 15.

72 *Ibid.*, 23.

73 *Ibid.*, 9.

74 Court Minutes, MS 5257 (6), vol. 12.

75 *Idem.*

76 *Idem.*

77 *Idem.*

78 *Idem.* Within half a year, Lichfield's death was noted in the Court Minutes (24 July 1701).

79 For a brief overview of the contemporary 'vulgar' surgical writings, see P. K. Wilson, 'Vernacularisation vs. Vulgarisation', 1169-72.

80 D. Turner, 'Religio Medici Reformata', British Library, MS 14404.

81 Long neglected in historical accounts, John Spurr has recently analysed the influence of *The Whole Duty of Man* in his *The Restoration Church of England, 1646-1689* (New Haven: Yale University Press, 1992), 279-330. Richard Allestree and Henry Hammond were both integral to the composition and propagation of this work, as discussed by John W. Packer in *The Transformation of Anglicanism 1643-1660, with special reference to Henry Hammond* (Manchester: Manchester University Press, 1969), 42. For a similar contemporary devotional see *The True Church of England Man's Companion in the Closet:, or, A complete Manual of Private Devotions* (London, 1728). Turner explicitly followed the prescripts of *The Whole Duty of Man*, having copied the catechism into his own private devotional for daily use.

82 J. W. Packer, *Transformation of Anglicanism*, 143. See also J. Spurr, *The Restoration Church in England*, 283, 295.

83 J.W. Packer, *Transformation of Anglicanism*, 51.

84 R. Holmes, *Footsteps*, 175.

85 M. C. Jacob, *Newtonians and the English Revolution*, esp. 143-200. Alternative views have been raised by Geoffrey Holmes, 'Science, reason and religion in the age of Newton', *British Journal for the History of Science*, xi (1978), 164-71, and Colin A. Russell, *Science and Social Change 1700-1900* (London: MacMillan Press, 1983), 52-68. John Spurr further challenged Jacob's view in his '"Latitudinarians" and the Restoration Church', *The Historical Journal*, xxxi (1981), 61-82. See also W.M. Spellman, *The Latitudinarians and the Church of England* (Athens, Georgia: University of Georgia Press, 1993)

86 Peter Earle, *The World of Defoe* (Newton Abbot: Readers Union Limited Edition, 1976), 35.

87 See, in particular, William Derham's *Physico-Theology: or, A Demonstration of the Being and Attributes of God, from His works of Creation* (London: W. Innys, 1714) and *idem.*, *Astro-Theology: or, A Demonstration of the Being and Attributes of God, from a Survey of the Heavens* (London: W. Innys, 1715). Clarence Glacken summarized these and similar contemporary writings in his *Traces of the Rhodian Shore: Nature and Culture in Western Thought from Ancient times to the End of the Eighteenth-Century* (Berkeley: University of California Press, 1976), 415-26. See also John Hedley Brooke, *Science and Religion: Some Historical Perspectives* (Cambridge: Cambridge

University Press, 1991), esp. 117-91.

88 D. Turner, 'Religio Medici Reformata', f. 3.

89 *Ibid.*, ff. 4 and 3.

90 Cited in K. Bryn Thomas' *James Douglas of the Pouch and his Pupil William Hunter* (London: Pitman Medical Publishing Co., 1964), 15.

91 Michael Hunter, 'The Problem of 'Atheism' in Early Modern England', *Transactions of the Royal Historical Society*, 5th ser., xxxv (1985), 138. See also Michael Hunter and David Wooton (eds), *Atheism from the Reformation to the Enlightenment* (Oxford: Clarendon Press, 1992).

92 *Ibid.*, 141.

93 G. V. Bennett's essay, 'Conflict in the Church', in G. Holmes (ed.), *Britain after the Glorious Revolution*, 5th edn (London: Macmillan, 1984), 155-75, has, for many years, set a foundation of religion in society for other writers. More recently, attention has been drawn to religion in English society in works such as Peter Harrison's *Religion and the 'Religious' in the English Enlightenment* (Cambridge: Cambridge University Press, 1990); James E. Bradley's *Religion, Revolution, and English Radicalism: Nonconformity in Eighteenth-Century Politics and Society* (Cambridge: Cambridge University Press, 1990) and J. Spurr, *The Restoration Church of England.* See also John Gascoigne, 'Anglican Latitudinarianism, Rational Dissent and Political Radicalism in the late Eighteenth Century', in Knud Haakonssen (ed.), *Enlightenment and Religion: Rational Dissent in Eighteenth-Century Britain* (Cambridge: Cambridge University Press, 1996), 219-40. For specific ties between medicine and religion, see Andrew Wear, 'Religious Beliefs and Medicine in Early Modern England', in Hilary Marland and Margaret Pelling (eds), *The Task of Healing: Medicine, Religion and Gender in England and the Netherlands, 1450-1800* (Rotterdam: Erasmus Press, 1996), 145-169, and William Birken, 'Dissenting Tradition in English Medicine of the Seventeenth and Eighteenth Centuries', *Medical History*, xxxix (1995), 197-218.

94 D. Turner, 'Religio Medici Reformata', f. 5b. Passive obedience was also the dictate of High Anglican endurance to the threats against Stuart succession.

95 *Ibid.*, 10.

96 D. Turner, *Discourse Concerning Fevers*, 59.

97 D. Turner, 'Religio Medici', 5 and opposite 4.

98 D. Turner, *Discourse Concerning Fevers*, 92.

99 *The Entertainer*, No. 7, 18 December 1717, as reprinted in *The Entertainer. Containing Remarks upon Men, and Manners, Religion, and Policy* (London: J. Osborn, 3rd edn, 1734), 40. Historian Mark

Jenner also points to the similar language between religious enthusiasts and quacks in the seventeenth and eighteenth centuries. See his 'Quackery and Enthusiasm, or Why Drinking Water Cured the Plague', in Ole Peter Grell and Andrew Cunningham (eds), *Religio Medici: Medicine and Religion in Seventeenth-Century England* (Aldershot, Hampshire: Scolar Press, 1996), 331.

100 D. Turner, 'Religion Medici Reformata', f. 6b.

101 Hillel Schwartz described the socio-cultural tensions raised when three Huguenot 'prophets' appeared in London in 1706 and spread their millenarian views in his exhilarating *The French Prophets. The History of a Millenarian Group in Eighteenth-Century England* (Berkeley: University of California Press, 1980).

102 D. Turner, 'Religio Medici Reformata', f. 6.

103 Roy Porter, 'The Language of Quackery in England, 1660-1800' in Peter Burke and Roy Porter (eds), *The Social History of Language* (Cambridge: Cambridge University Press, 1987), esp. 79-95.

104 D. Turner, 'Religio Medici Reformata', ff. 7-8.

105 *Ibid.*, f. 6

6

Dispute over the Power of the Maternal Imagination[1]

Mary Toft's Imagination

One of the Enlightenment's greatest challenges between quackery and truth erupted in Daniel Turner's London. In November 1726, Mary Toft became the 'general Talk of the Town' in London for having, it was rumoured, been delivered of sixteen rabbits. These claims provoked responses from premier London physicians including Sir Richard Manningham and James Douglas; surgeons William Cheselden, Thomas Braithwaite, and Phillipus van Limborck; and male-midwives William Giffard and John Maubray. Sergeant Surgeon Claudius Amyand, together with Cyriacus Ahlers and Nathanael St André, surgeons to George I, also became involved with the case. Toft was removed from her home in Godalming, Surrey, and sent to Guilford and eventually to London. In London, the Duke of Richmond, the Duke of Montague, Lord Baltimore, and Samuel Molyneux, a natural philosopher and private secretary to the Prince of Wales, personally investigated Toft's claims. Interest in the 'rabbit breeder' extended to the monarch who was provided with an anatomical demonstration of the 'facts' on 26 November 1726. Within a fortnight, Toft confessed her fraud.[2]

At least fifteen pamphlets and songs appeared at the time satirizing Toft's mass deception. Many of these depicted her surgical and medical attendants as gullible and credulous. The medical attendants were also parodied in engravings, including one by Hogarth (see Figure 6.1), and in a Drury Lane play. Toft was vilified as a cheat for securing animal parts and leading her attendants to believe she had delivered the animals naturally. She had long accounted for the rabbits by explaining that while thinking she was with child, she was startled by a rabbit while working in the fields. She soon began to crave rabbit for a meal, but was unable to catch one. Her longings were further increased by a dream about rabbits, yet they remained unfulfilled.

Only a few of the popularized versions of Toft's case gave her longing more than casual mention. One such pamphlet entitled *The*

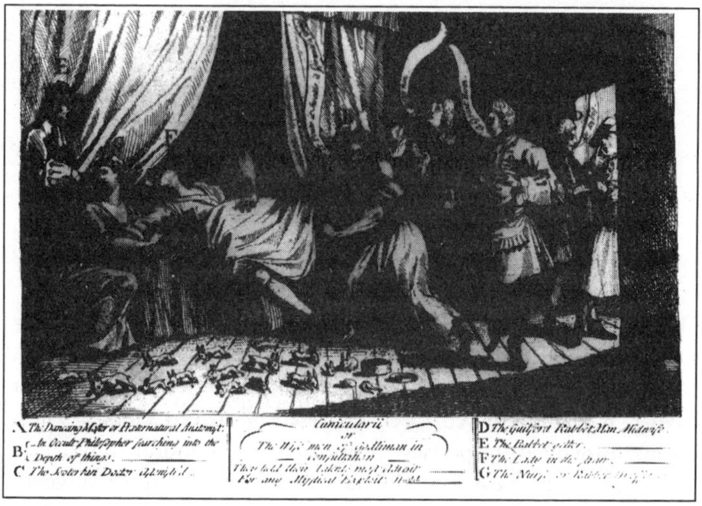

Figure 6.1

'Cunicularii, or the Wise Men of Godliman in Consultation', William Hogarth, 1726. Identified principal characters are A: Nathanael St André, B: Samuel Molyneux, C: John Maubray, D: John Howard, E: The 'Rabbet Getter', F: Mary Toft, G: The Nurse or 'Rabbet Dresser' (Wellcome Institute Library, London)

Strength of Imagination in Pregnant Women Examined appeared in London in May 1727. The anonymous author (James Blondel) identified himself as a member of London's College of Physicians and claimed to have written the work in response to the delusion created by the 'Cheat at Godalming'.[3] However, Daniel Turner deemed *The Strength* to be an attack upon his own work, 'Spots and Marks of a diverse Resemblance imprest upon the Skin of the Foetus, by the Force of the Mother's Fancy', first published as chapter twelve in his 1714 *De Morbis Cutaneis*.[4] In September 1729, Turner responded to Blondel's pamphlet with *An answer to a pamphlet on the Powers of Imagination in Pregnant Women*.[5] Later that year, Blondel issued a second work, *The Power of the Mother's Imagination over the Foetus Examined*, in which he identified himself. This work prompted Turner's final reply, *The Force of the Mother's Imagination upon the foetus in utero still further considered* (1730).[6]

Toft's case was far from the first to incite controversy over whether a pregnant woman's emotions, cravings, or imaginings could mark or deform her foetus. Earlier examples discussing the possible consequences of an expectant mother's imagination are found in Greek writings, others in the Bible.[7] Although convictions about the power of the maternal imagination have long been considered popular folk belief, many medical, religious, and philosophical authorities also supported this view.[8]

By the early eighteenth century, many medical authors dismissed the idea that children's physical markings, resembling such things as fish scales, or limbs deformed in the shape of bear claws resulted from a mother's wayward imagination, fright or cravings.[9] Yet, Turner and Blondel's dispute of the late 1720s drew unprecedented attention to this concern. This chapter examines the arguments presented by Turner and Blondel and discusses probable reasons for their differences. Two primary points of their disagreement will be analysed: the identity of the imagination, and the process of generation. Then, the authors' endeavours to gain public appeal will be examined. Finally, the responses which this dispute provoked in the periodical literature, and in English and Continental commentaries which appeared later in the century are discussed.

Turner and Blondel on the Mother's Imagination

James Blondel presented the whole issue of the power of the mother's imagination as a 'vulgar error', scorning the credulity of the medical practitioners involved in Toft's case.[10] Nothing 'can be more scandalous', he exclaimed, 'than to suppose, that those Whom God Almighty has endow'd, ... with so many charms ... [and] an extraordinary Love and Tenderness for their Children ... [are made to] bread [sic] *Monsters* by the Wantonness of their Imagination'.[11] In order to disprove this 'vulgar error', he designed an argument based 'partly by Reason, and partly by Anatomy'. Blondel acknowledged that circumstances such as falls, accidents, irregular diet, dancing, running, riding, excess laughter and frequent sneezing had caused some mothers to damage the 'Prosperity of the *Foetus*' and miscarry.[12] Sudden surprise or strongly expressed anger or grief were also, on occasion, capable of producing similar results.[13] Yet, he noted, most women experience various emotions or longings at some time during their pregnancy without producing marked children. Furthermore, many mothers of marked or deformed children claimed to have endured an entirely peaceful pregnancy. Blondel therefore concluded that the imaginationists' claim was based on recognizing some irregularity upon the child after birth (*ad hoc, ergo propter hoc*). He further noted the imaginationists' inconsistency in attributing the same defect to opposing causes. For example, he surmised that if a pregnant woman either craved or had 'a great Aversion' to mussels, she was 'reputed to run a vast Risque' for delivering a child marked with a resemblance to that shellfish somewhere on the body.[14]

Blondel provided alternative explanations of the ape-like, frog-faced and bear-clawed children described in literature. For instance, he recounted Nicolas Malebranche's tale, in which a boy was born with bones 'broken, in the same Places where Malefactors are broke[n upon the rack]'. Unlike Malebranche, who attributed the cause of this condition to an expectant mother having witnessed such an event, Blondel argued that 'Tis very probable, this young Man ... [was] troubled with the Rickets, [such that] the Bones of the *Carpus* and *Tarsus* had never come to their full Perfection [*in utero*], but did remain *Cartilaginous*, [so that] the Ligaments ... relaxed, and the Articulations ... [appeared] loose ... upon the least Touch'.[15]

Blondel also re-examined a biblical example which had been frequently used to prove the power of imagination. *Genesis* 30: 25-39 recounts Jacob's revenge against Laban. Laban, who had offered Jacob the mottled offspring from his flock, removed all the sheep with spots and speckles, provoking Jacob to devise a plan to produce mottled sheep. Jacob stripped the bark from some branches, giving them a ring-streaked appearance, and placed them by a water trough. He anticipated that when the ewes, in heat, came to drink, they would see the streaked branches and be inclined to produce marked offspring. Blondel claimed that this tale exemplified the 'Axiom of Logick' which stated that an argument which proved too much, proved nothing.[16] Blondel further argued that the 'Diviners' (i.e., Bible translators) during the reign of James I had been 'guided more by their Prejudices, than by the Original [Hebrew]'. Preferring, he said, the pristine over 'all the Commentators in the World', Blondel identified the inconsistencies between the 'Authorized' version and his own translation.[17] He surmised that the ewes in 'that hot Country' had been taught a 'Trick ... in Expectation of their Victuals', so that they 'could have no water, except [when] they drank it, where the part[l]y-coloured Rods [i.e., dappled branches] were placed'. Although this colour may have become 'very pleasant to them', their offspring resulted only from a 'natural ... Inclination towards the speckled Rams [in] preference to the others'.[18]

Blondel credited other imaginationists' fables to the 'Ignorant People's' lack of judgement, and the 'tale-monger's ... Enthusiasm and Bigotry', as well as attempts of 'Cruel Mothers' to move 'Charity and Benevolence' to finance their 'lazy and indolent' lives.[19] As evidence, Blondel urged his readers to consider why 'Irregularities ...

occasioned by the Strength of Imagination ... appear more on the Body of Beggars, than ... [on] any other people?'[20] He also claimed that the only reason so many midwives and physicians supported the imaginationists' view was to cover up mistakes made during the childbirths they attended.[21]

Blondel claimed that the irregularities seen on children appeared 'over and over again' in such a similar pattern that he proposed all such claims could be compiled into a 'catalogue' under four classes.[22] First, some marks were caused by variation in the number and combination of body 'Particles'. For example, blemishes may have been formed by superficial blood vessels appearing through the surface of the skin, when the blood was more 'rarified' in summer, as opposed to winter when it was more 'concentrated'. Second, distempers could arise from obstructions *in utero*. For instance, he cited hydrocephalus [i.e., fluid-filled cerebral ventricles], in which obstructions 'turn[ed]' humours to favour one part of the brain instead of another part of the body. Third, foetal growth could be disproportionately interrupted by an 'Obstruction of some vessels' which would deplete the 'Nutrition' of dependent parts, thereby hindering development. Finally, any extreme force or violence upon the body of the uterus sometimes created such a convulsion that 'two or three *Ova* ... [were] intermixed ... to make an odd and monstrous Combination'.[23]

In 1729, Turner responded to Blondel's *Strength* with *An Answer*, repeating much of the argument contained in his original 'Spots and Marks' first published in 1714. In the earlier work Turner had described the 'great Influence' which passions such as joy, anger, sorrow and fear had over the 'Blood and nervous Fluid, or animal Spirits, and consequently [over] the whole body'.[24] Like the passions, Turner described how the imagination could induce 'great [physical] Changes and Alterations'. He culled forty case histories from classical and contemporary sources, in which markings, deformities or diseases were attributed to the 'Fancy' or 'Force' of imagination.[25] Of the cases, thirty-six specifically pertained to pregnancy. For example, one case attributed a girl's extreme hairiness to her mother's 'unhappy ruminating' over a picture of the hirsute St John the Baptist.[26] Another case described a cat-headed girl who was delivered from a mother who had been frightened during her pregnancy by a cat jumping onto her bed.[27] A third, which had occurred in London, involved the child of Sir 'J.B.' whose 'Lady [then with child, was] frightened at the unexpected View of a Beggar's stump Arm upon her Coach Door'. Following this incident, according to Turner's account,

Lady B. was 'brought to Bed of a Child ... wanting one of its hands'.[28] Other deformed children were presented as evidence of the potential for maternally marking a foetus. Turner also repeated accounts describing the variegated markings (medically known as *Naevi sive Maculae Maternae*) on infants which arose from a pregnant woman's craving for various fruits or longing for red wine.

As 'Spots and Marks' was part of Turner's surgical textbook for treating skin disease, he guided readers through the treatment of various external disorders. On treating of 'fruitshaped excrescences' which arose from the maternal imagination, Turner instructed his readers that it was 'necessary to consider the Part on which they are seated, to what Parts adjoining, and with what communicating: What vessels they may be fed by: What Compass they take, [and] how deep they enter'.[29] Once this was determined, the growths could then be tied off at their stalk or 'pedicule' and cut away, but only during 'the Season when they look palest, lie flattest and softest, and are least troublesome'.[30] He argued that these tubercles and spots, 'like the Fruits they resemble, have their Times of bloom, ripening and languishing, tho' never quite dying or falling off [by] themselves'.[31] Illustrative of his treatments, Turner presented three cases in which he had achieved success surgically removing facial markings from children. Turner reported the mothers' testimony that these markings, shaped like a raspberry, a currant, and a shrimp, had resulted from particular unfulfilled longings which they had respectively experienced during pregnancy.

Enlightenment Londoners had acquired a taste for accounts of human monstrosities.[32] Members of all classes regularly gathered at 'raree' shows to see various freaks of nature.[33] The social elite frequently sponsored private exhibitions of nature's aberrations, while the intellectual elite discussed probable origins of monsters before such august bodies as the Royal Society.[34] Many natural philosophers had turned their attention to analysing the underlying forces and powers of natural phenomena such as gravity, light, meteors, and earthquakes, whereas supernatural marvels, miracles, and magic still remained 'in vogue' among London's populace.[35]

Given this setting, it is surprising that Turner's discussion in 'Spots and Marks' received scarcely any notice when first published.[36] The issue of folk beliefs about pregnancy was not seriously raised until the Toft case took place twelve years later. Unlike contemporary disputes within the College of Physicians which were often intraprofessional and divided along political lines,[37] the Toft case involved both professional and public beliefs. Physicians and surgeons were scorned by fellow practitioners for having been duped by a country woman's tale about her pregnancy. Blondel sought to re-establish the reputation of his profession by discrediting the maternal imagination as only a folk belief with no physiological basis.

Blondel had become a licentiate of London's College of Physicians in 1711. Reputedly born in Paris in 1665, he studied medicine at the University of Leiden, receiving his medical degree in 1692.[38] His later medical writings reveal his support of iatro-mechanical theories, similar to those taught in Leiden and later espoused by many London physicians.[39] Little else, however, is known about his life other than his Huguenot affiliations.[40]

Turner's professed intolerance of separatists from the Anglican Church would likely have set him against a dissenting Huguenot like Blondel.[41] However, Turner more likely took offence at Blondel's 'dogmatic' proclamation that medicine should be based upon particular theories or hypotheses. This disagreement with Blondel's iatro-mechanical arguments is central to their entire dispute.

Similar in format to Newton's *Principia*, Blondel's work began with a set of propositions (see Table 6.1).[42] He argued that once these propositions were 'all put together', they would 'amount ... to a full *Demonstration* of his thesis'.[43] In his *Answer*, Turner selectively criticized Blondel's 'hypothetical' deductions. He claimed that Blondel's propositions were

> no more to the Matter in hand, than if you had told us, that if we take three or four Strands of equal length, and lay them in the proper Position, they will make either a *Triangle* or a *Quadrangle*; but if any one of the three or ... four be longer or shorter than the rest ..., neither [figure] ... will be *equilateral*, and so deduced this Ergo, that *the Mother's Imagination can not mark the Body of her Infant*.[44]

He explained that no hypotheses were needed to account for the consequences of the maternal imagination other than that 'our Maker [had] placed such a relation between certain Causes and their Effects'.[45]

Blondel, on the other hand, represented the imaginationists' belief as being irrational and mathematically unsound. He postulated that for every 100,000 pregnant women, at least 25,000 of them were 'exposed to the Danger and Fury of Imagination'. Yet, only three hundred children would appear 'stampt with any tokens' of their mothers' imagination. Of these three hundred children, he estimated that one half were born to women who were unexposed to wayward thoughts during their pregnancies. From these approximations,

1. By IMAGINATIONISTS, I mean those, who believe in the Power of the Mother's Imagination over the Foetus.
2. There's no *Solutio Continui* without Force or Violence.
3. Imagination must act by some means.
4. Passion, in respect of the Mind, is a Modification of Thoughts, but Motion in Respect of the Body.
5. Passions act upon the Body by accelerating, or diminishing the velocity of Blood, and Spirits.
6. Imagination cannot act beyond the Sphere of the Soul, and of the Body.
7. There is no sensation without Nerves.
8. Nerves being once divided can never reunite.
9. A Ligature, or a Pression upon a Nerve, or a Blood Vessel, makes them useless, so long as it lasts.
10. The longer is an Artery, the slower is the Motion of Blood, at the Extremity of the Vessel.
11. The Rudiments of all Plants and Animals are from the Beginning of the world.
12. Conception is independent on the Mother's will.
13. The ovum is for a long Time in the Fallopian Tube, and in the Uterus without Adhesion.
14. The Foetus has a sensation, and a circulation of the Blood independent on the Mother.
15. Deformities ought to be less amazing than the vast Number of regular Bodies.

These propositions were listed in Blondel's *Power*, and had previously appeared in similar form in *Strength*. The earlier work also contained the proposition: 'There are not in the World, two Atoms, that be both alike'.

Table 6.1
Blondel's propositions

Blondel calculated the numerical odds against an effect of the force of imagination were 24,850:150 (or 166:1).[46]

Turner responded to these criticisms with *The Force*. He rejected Blondel's arithmetical argument as mere 'guess Work, or frivolous Supposition', reaffirming that even if the 'smallest Number [of people] ... carry the most indubitable Marks or *Signatures* ... they may well be the Objects of our Admiration, and justify the Power ... [of] the *Mother's Imagination*'.[47] He hoped that his readers would accept the '*Facts* [of the mother's imagination] we see before our Eyes, altho we cannot [wholly] account for their Modus', rather than to 'absolutely ... deny them, or pretend to account for them by some mere *Hypothesis*'.[48]

Identity of Imagination and its Power

Twentieth-century historians, philosophers, literary critics and psychiatrists acknowledge that the imagination intrigued Enlightenment English authors, but no consistent philosophical basis accounted for its invocation.[49] For instance, poet and satirist Joseph Addison popularized Lockian ideas in his 'Pleasures of Imagination' (1712). Robert James' *Medicinal Dictionary* on the other hand described the imagination using Aristotelian terminology as did *Chambers Cyclopedia*.[50] Remnants of Cartesian views can be found in some Enlightenment medical writings on imagination, but most authors incorporated Newtonian concepts into their works. An explicit example of Newtonian borrowing was that of the self-proclaimed London physician Thomas Morgan who, in 1725, defined the passions, including the imagination, according to the Newtonian equation of a force equal to the product of nerves (body) and the animal spirits (acceleration).[51] As the titles of Turner's and Blondel's writings suggest, the Newtonian language of 'Force' or 'Power' held both literal and rhetorical significance.[52]

In his own definition, Turner claimed that imagination acted similarly to the passions. Blondel denied this, and began *The Strength* purporting 'to determine What is Passion, and how, and where it affects the Body'.[53] He explicitly borrowed the Lockian definition that passion 'In Respect of an intellectual Being, is a modification of Thoughts; in respect to a corporeal Being, [a modification of] Motion'.[54] Blondel used this definition to distinguish between passions which affected the mind versus those which affected the body. Although both Turner and Blondel claimed that some passions could produce bodily effects, Blondel specified that the action of the imagination was confined to the mind. He then sought to establish the conditions by which passions were capable of producing physical effects. He claimed that strong mental attention to a particular object, whether with 'Desire' or in 'Abhorrence', was insufficient to produce any change in the body since the blood or spirit flow remained localized within the brain. Any impassioned longings or cravings during pregnancy were, he argued, like the imagination and other 'intellectual' thoughts, 'Scene[s] ... confined within the Mother's mind'.[55] The body, he claimed, could only respond physically to a violent passion which was mentally received as a 'sudden change'. For instance, fright could 'violently' accelerate the flow of blood and spirits throughout the body. This altered flow, he continued, resulted from the 'Mind' detecting a distinct change, i.e., making a judgement between an 'Object ... which we are used to, and an extraordinary one'.[56] Body and mind, according to Blondel, operated in a dualistic manner.

Employing Lockian ideas, Blondel refused to accept that comparing objects and events was an innate 'species' of understanding. Instead, he argued that some 'Ratiocination' was required for making such judgements. Foetuses, so he claimed, existed in a 'Limited' developmental state, whereby they were unable to reason logically. They were both 'unacquainted with … objects that disturb the Mother' and incapable of making any 'Reflexions' upon them. Consequently, even if a pregnant woman experienced a violent passion, her foetus was unable to 'sense' any change, and therefore it was protected from harm.[57]

Unlike Blondel, Turner claimed that imagination could produce both mental and physical effects. His view of the imagination as a 'Faculty of the sensitive [not rational] Soul', together with his mechanical explanation of its actions, explicitly followed the expositions of the seventeenth-century physician, Thomas Willis.[58] In his account of the working imagination, Turner identified the '*Image* of the thing desired or fear'd, being constantly represented to the mind' as the '*formal Cause*' of imagination. He also noted that when an individual was 'excited at the Appearance of the Object', the 'Appetite' was stirred so as to incite 'local Motion' of the 'Blood and nervous Fluid' in 'some Part of the Brain'.[59] Having generated such a 'power', the images or 'Species' which had been sensed and impressed 'upon the outward Organs' were, 'by a most quick Irradiation of the nervous Fluid[,] delineated inwards ... apprehending all the ... corporeal Things according to their external Appearance'.

To explain the specific process in which a likeness of the image was produced upon the foetus, Turner drew upon the Galenical writings of the physican, Thomas Fienus. In his *De Viribus Imaginationis* (1608), Fienus had explained that the imagination induced 'real changes' in the body solely by stirring the emotions. Such rarefied emotions were 'transformed' from the mother's body to the foetus, and the impressed immaterial 'species' from the mother's imagination became expressed as a result of the imagination's conformative power. Turner, like Fienus, argued that only the malleable foetus, and not the adult mother, was susceptible to any impressed 'species' from the imagination.[60]

Blondel used a deductive Newtonian approach to sustain his hypotheses regarding the maternal imagination. As his list of propositions illustrates (Table 6.1), Blondel claimed all life was reducible into atoms.[61] This reductionist argument echoed that of other iatro-mechanists who removed or displaced God from a central position in their depictions of natural phenomena.

Like Blondel, Turner also described the imagination as being 'transacted by mechanick Laws'.[62] But Turner accepted these mechanical explanations only to a point, beyond which he resorted to nature as the explanation or cause of action. Underlying his mechanistic terminology, Turner accounted for the imagination acting by a hidden, vital, spiritual, unknowable ultimate 'Cause' which, he claimed, had been provided by the Creator. For example, Turner described how 'Springs and Wheels' intermeshed between the 'sensitive Soul and nervous Fluids' acted through the intervention of 'Nature', to open 'little Doors of the Nerves, and conduct ... certain Spirits to [them]'.[63]

It has been argued that by the end of the 1720s, following Newton's death, the mechanical explanations of invisible actions were gradually giving way to more 'quasi-vitalistic' theories.[64] Turner possibly drew on this vitalist outlook when arguing that humans were guided as Nature dictated. He claimed that Nature's role in internal physical workings was akin to the force underlying the 'effects of the Magnet'.[65] It was this same immaterial force, he argued, which drew the mother's imagination to the foetus.[66] Turner's emphasis on an underlying immaterial substance, existing in both mind and body, was in distinct contrast to Blondel's mind-body dualism.

Turner and Blondel also disagreed over who was reliable as an authority on the imagination. Turner's reliance upon Fienus' and Willis' descriptions exemplifies his adherence to earlier authoritative doctrine. This appreciation is also seen in the numerous case histories he selected from ancient or classical writings. Blondel ridiculed the imaginationists' use of 'ancient' authority, noting that they were 'obliged' to place their arguments in 'old Antiquity or in remote Places' since such outrageous examples were not to be found in modern literature.[67]

Although distinguishing Turner's adherence to traditional doctrine from Blondel's espousal of Newtonian science allows some differentiation between the two physicians, it would be inaccurate to designate this dispute as a controversy between 'the Ancients and the Moderns'.[68] For Turner also used terminology and 'quasi-vitalist' ideas consistent with contemporary modern medical writers. Moreover, he challenged the use of mathematical or hypothetical reasoning as evidence. Such a challenge, particularly when emphasizing the role of observation, was, as historian Theodore Brown has shown, beginning to gain much support from the leading 'modern' figures of the College of Physicians by the mid-1720s.[69]

Turner and Blondel also disagreed over their reliance upon experiment. Blondel used experiment to mean demonstrable evidence or proof suggesting a Newtonian borrowing. He accepted 'nothing but what is certain and known, or demonstrable by Experiments'.[70] This contrasts with the imaginationists' accounts which, he said, were based upon 'Quibbles and Puns, Suppositions and *Canterbury* Stories'.[71]

Turner did not distinguish between the evidence offered by 'experiment' versus 'experience'. For example, he described each case history as an 'experiment' and collectively referred to them as 'experience'.[72] Relatedly, he represented these collective cases as multiple verifications of the 'truth'. The 'greatest part' of the cases, taken from Hippocrates, Galen, Malebranche, Fienus, Boyle and other authorities, had, so Turner claimed, been 'undeniably attested and unquestionably recorded'.[73] Turner argued that these men, like gentlemen of his own time, were to be taken on the 'credit' of their word.[74] Should we, Turner enquired, 'discredit all ancient History ... [regardless of] how well or sufficiently ... [cases were] attested at the times they fell out, and credit nothing we have not seen, or cannot warrant from the Testimony of our own Senses?'[75] He added that if the conjoined twins who were recently paraded around London would have been 'presented one hundred Years past, it ... [would] have been reckoned by Dr B[londel] as a Fiction'.[76]

Turner's apparent indiscriminate use of 'experiment' and 'experience' also distinguishes what he and his opponent accepted as proof. Blondel defined experience as the 'Knowledge of a Matter of Fact' drawn from 'a sufficient Number of Observation[s]'. To qualify as valid, such observations must relate to 'several Branches of the Fact in question'. Additionally, they should be 'clear, and intelligible, and grounded upon the Testimony of our Senses, and not depending upon occult Qualities, Suppositions, Conjectures, Hear-says, and Casualties'. For example, he argued that no credence should be given to reports from the anatomist and physician, Thomas Bartholin, whose writings he characterized as a 'Net [catching] any Thing communicated ... good or bad, without any Distinction'.[77] Instead, observations must be 'Uniform, and not contradictory', and procured 'in such a Number, as to over-ballance all Objections, or Counter-Observations, by a vast Disproportion'. Testimony from 'Hear-say, ... [i.e.] second or third Hand' was 'to be received with a great deal of Caution'. Blondel argued that the cases from Heliodorus, whom Turner had cited, were an admixture of 'Fable[s]' and fact, aimed only to 'beautify his work'.[78]

Rather than relying upon the Ancients, Blondel urged his readers to set each case history within the period in which it was written. Credit given to witnesses unknown to the observer should diminish 'In Proportion of the Distance of Places and Times' of the occurrence. Reliable witnesses must be 'true, honest, and without any Interest to cheat'. Additionally, they must be 'Judicious' and 'neither credulous, nor prepossest, nor too hasty' in their judgement. Finally, 'Witnesses are not to be trusted, if it be discovered, that, at any Time, they have been found to be false'.[79] By using such guidelines to examine the imaginationists' arguments, Blondel assured his readers that their 'impartial judge[ment]' would find his arguments to hold the truth.

Reproductive Generation and Foetal Development

Although Turner organized his writings around the mother's imagination, Blondel argued that reproductive generation was the central issue.[80] Historians of reproduction have represented preformationism as the predominant generation theory of the 1720s.[81] This theory proposed that the embryo was existent in a fully preformed, yet miniature state prior to conception. Arguments arose between preformationists over whether the preformed entity existed in the ovum (ovists) or in the sperm (animalculists).[82]

Blondel was a preformationist, and claimed that ovism and animalculism both held 'a great Deal of Truth ... *partly* grounded upon many undisputable Experiments'. Citing the disparate experimental findings of Rene de Graff and Antony van Leeuwenhoek, Blondel proposed to 'reconcile' their conclusions about formation.[83] Specifically, he claimed that 'they all agree ... that the

Parts of the *Foetus* are existent somewhere before conception'.[84] Blondel also employed the *emboîtment* theory.[85] This theory stated that the embryonic forms of all living beings had been in existence since the beginning of time. Smaller and smaller forms of each species were incased or embodied within the generative seed *ad infinitum*. Development occurred by an increase in the size of a pre-existent embryo. Blondel argued for the consistency of preformation by using mechanism and design.[86] He placed the active role of the Creator back to the 'Beginning of the World'; the time, he claimed, when the 'Rudiments of all Plants and Animals' were formed.[87] Providence had guided generation along a determined path since then. This path was consistent with Blondel's mechanistic view that Nature operated in a uniform, clockwork fashion. Conception was predetermined, and thus, dependent upon general providence. No creative or vital force was necessary to explain each individual creation.

Blondel expanded the *emboîtment* argument to support his proposition that 'conception is independent of the mother's will'. He claimed that just as a woman cannot, by her fancy or imagination, promote or delay conception, withhold nourishment from her embryo, or select the sex, number, colour, size, strength, or resemblance of her child, 'it is not within her power to disfigure it either'.[88]

Turner rejected preformationism. He claimed that both the ovist and the animalcular theories of generation were 'unsatisfactory' and rather 'ambiguously ... concluded'.[89] To highlight the ambiguity, Turner argued that neither animalculists nor ovists had fully accounted for the presence of 'mixed generations'. He noted that regardless of whether the male or the female was thought to provide the essential seed, neither theory could account for mixed breeds such as mules. Therefore, the generation must be, he claimed, the result of contributions from both male and female seed.[90]

Unlike typical opponents of preformation, Turner did not espouse epigenesis.[91] Rather, he explicitly adopted the argument of his contemporary, James Drake. Drake, a London physician and Tory pamphleteer, refused to accept preformationism due to a lack of animal, specifically human evidence.[92] To account for individual variation and deformities seen in humans, Drake invoked the mother's wayward imagination and the 'plastick power' of nature. This power had been described in various ways by seventeenth-century British luminaries including Ralph Cudworth, Matthew Hale, Henry More, Robert Boyle, George Rust, and William Harvey.[93] Although discussion of this power had declined by the 1720s, both Turner and Drake used it to explain foetal development.[94] According to Turner, humans were 'only passive' beings, dependent upon individual guidance by the Creator's 'Invisible hands'.[95] This guidance was, he noted, especially necessary at the beginning of life. For it was precisely at this time that the 'Plastick Power' of nature first intervenes, and the Creator moulds the 'Dough' or 'Paste' into human form.[96] Turner's claim that all humans were individually moulded during their gestation distinctly opposed Blondel's view of preformed, predetermined embryonic beings. On these grounds he concluded that the ovists' and animalculists' attempts to explain the operations of generation were futile.

Maternal-Foetal Circulation

In addition to their differences over theories of generation and the role of the Creator, Turner and Blondel also disagreed over the anatomical relationship between the mother and the foetus. Turner argued, adopting London anatomist William Cowper's description, that blood circulated between the mother and the foetus. This blood flow was established, he continued, during the early stage of pregnancy.[97] Blondel, however, argued that since 'before Pregnancy, the [mother's] Veins and Arteries of the *Uterus* are all matched together', one simply does not find '*idle* uterine Vessels, to joyn with those of the *Placenta*' during pregnancy.[98] He concluded that the placenta was solely of foetal origin, and was in no way connected to the uterus. He postulated that the uterus was merely an elastic container in which the developing foetus took 'Lodging for a short time',[99] thus no connecting circulation to the foetus was necessary. Turner, further disputing Blondel's claim, cited works by contemporaries including James Keill, James Drake, and John Freind in support of his view that foetal nourishment was totally dependent upon inter-connected circulations.[100]

Blondel also provided additional 'evidence' corroborating his own argument. He explained that the vessels which appeared to tortuously wind around the uterus had been laid out and adapted to 'check the Violence of the Blood' that reached the area.[101] Nature had taken 'great Care ... [to] preserve the *Ovum* against the *Impetus* of the Blood and of the Spirits'.[102] This vascular arrangement, he claimed, provided additional proof that independent circulations existed. Were it not so designed, he argued, birth itself would present an 'eminent Danger, [because] so much Blood ... would discharge in a short Time' such that the mother's life would be in jeopardy.[103]

Blondel added a list of quantitative proofs, noting that there was 'not ... an equal Number of Pulsations' between 'the Mother's Pulse, and ... the Umbilical String'.[104] Having combined rational, anatomical and experimental evidence, Blondel claimed to have 'proved' that no blood circulated between the mother and the foetus. He presented a similar argument against any nervous connection, and concluded that no pathway existed through which any maternal passions could be transported to the foetus.

Turner responded to Blondel's claims with contrary evidence. He reported that an acquaintance in London 'who has a large Share in the Practice of Deliveries' informed him that 'very little variation' existed between the maternal and foetal pulses.[105] But even if variations were found in individual cases, Turner reminded readers that it was 'well known' that one's pulse is, at times, 'different ... [between the] two Wrists'.[106]

At a time when, according to one historian, enthusiasm and philosophical predilection were the criteria which readers used to distinguish among theories of reproductive generation, Turner's and Blondel's dispute was more than an argument between a rationalist and an empiricist.[107] Their disagreements often originated from their different choices and interpretations of evidence, particularly as to whether that evidence was derived from experiment or from personal experience.[108] This different use of evidence significantly altered their explanations of similar case histories.

Appeal to the Public

Unlike the discussions and demonstrations in the closed meeting halls of the Royal Society and the College of Physicians, Blondel and Turner staged their dispute in public. Such polemical pamphlet warring was not uncommon in early eighteenth-century London.[109] Unlike lengthy books, pamphlets were quicker to print, lighter to distribute, cheaper to purchase, and easier to digest in a short period; all of these factors allowed authors to reach a wider audience. Turner and Blondel reserved the final judgement of their dispute for their readers.[110] Like contemporary advertisements for specific remedies, their pamphlets aimed to persuade the public. However, Turner and Blondel waged their war over medical beliefs and philosophies rather than a particular type of treatment or practice.[111]

The arguments and aims of Turner and Blondel appear similar to those in contemporary pamphlets. *Fog's Weekly Journal* of 1729 claimed that political pamphlets were written either to 'disabuse the Publick' of any 'false notions' with which they might 'be posses'd', to 'deceiv[e] and impos[e]', or to serve some 'particular Set of Men'. In the first case,

In his quest for public support, Turner devoted particular attention to Blondel's explication of the biblical passage on Jacob's sheep. This 'Textuary', Turner argued, exemplified how Blondel could alter a 'plain, natural, and genuine Construction' into one which 'for the most [part was] confus'd, perplex'd and unintellible [sic]'.[121] Turner denounced Blondel's translation, calling it 'irrelevant', and claimed it was typical of the way Blondel misrepresented the entire maternal imagination issue. 'What [a] pitiful *spoiling* of a *Text*', Turner observed, 'What a jumbled Story furnish'd out of two as plain Verses [as] are to be met with in the sacred *Pandects!*'[122] Appealing especially to any religious readers, Turner represented Blondel as sacrilegious for having tampered with the word of God.

Aftermath of the Battle

The extent to which the public actually exercised any adjudicatory role is unknown. In part, this stems from our lack of understanding 'who read whom' during this period.[123] Turner's and Blondel's use of pamphlets, however, appears to have effectively advertised their names and medical campaigns which, despite the personal slanders, perpetuated the reputations of both authors. Although their readership remains unknown, sources suggest that 'Dr Blondel's dispute with Dr Turner made no small noise' for decades.[124] 'N.M.', a Grub Street journalist, claimed their dispute caused such a commotion that he urged 'Waste-paper merchant', James Jones, to 'speedily interpose, and reconcile [these authors] ... who have poured out such a profusion of learning and logic, ... that it is feared, they will soon intirely [sic] exhaust, not only the argument, but themselves'.[125]

The responses which this dispute continued to provoke from the public and from fellow professionals demonstrated that, unlike the Toft case, there was no immediate resolution of the imagination issue. Both Turner's and Blondel's arguments continued to gain support for many years. The London physician John Mauclerc sustained Blondel's argument for more than a decade after Blondel's death in 1734.[126] Nearly forty years later, Blondel's claims were still explicitly supported. The author of a 1772 *Essay on the Force of Imagination in Pregnant Women* argued that if mental longings were actually conveyed from the mother to the foetus, children's deformities would have been much more varied. Since women think so often about their clothing, the author argued, the imprinted markings upon their children should 'depend on the reigning fashion'.[127] Another author, Isaac Bellet, followed Blondel's argument and claimed to have 'proved, by incontestable arguments, drawn from both reason and experience that it is a ridiculous prejudice to suppose it possible for a pregnant woman to mark her child' via her imagination.[128]

Turner's argument also received support. A report in *Gentleman's Magazine* of 1735 claimed it uncanny that the mother of a young boy whose skin annually turned to a dusky yellow colour and was subsequently shed 'can't remember any Fright' during her pregnancy.[129] This case history and other similar reports were abridged from the Royal Society's *Philosophical Transactions.*[130] Extraordinary childbirths attributed to a mother's wayward imagination were also featured in the popular literary tales of Martinus Scriblerus, Peregrine Pickle, and Tristram Shandy.[131]

The concept of imagination remained a controversial subject in medical, scientific, and literary writings throughout the Enlightenment. Consider, for example, the attempts of two widely recognized authors to quantify the force and intensity of imagination. David Hartley discussed one view of imagination and his own doctrine on mental phenomena in his *Observations on Man* (1749).[132] James Long also discussed connections between images and actions in his *Enquiry into the Origin of Human Appetites and Affections* (1747).[133]

Reproductive generation, the other major component of the Turner–Blondel dispute, also remained both a controversial and popular area of investigation. Disputes over preformationism became increasingly pronounced later in the century,[134] when new experimental evidence was adduced in favour of epigenesis.[135] In light of this experimentation, some physicians and natural philosophers re-examined the question of whether the mother's imagination could affect embryological development.[136] Although few authors specifically referred to Turner or Blondel, they continued to address concerns about generation similar to those which had been raised in Turner's and Blondel's dispute.

Turner's and Blondel's influence spread beyond London. Turner's *De Morbis Cutaneis,* including his chapter on 'Spots and Marks', was translated into French (1743) and German (1766). Blondel's 1729 pamphlet was printed in French (1737), Dutch (1737), German (1756) and Italian (1760).[137] The frequent citations of these works in Continental disputes over the power of imagination attest to their international appeal.[138] Lengthy quotations from the Turner–Blondel dispute also appeared as one of the remarkable, newsworthy, international events reported in the popular publication, *The Jewish Spy.*[139]

Aristotle's Works, the Study of an Anachronism', in J. Woodward and D. Richards (eds), *Health Care and Popular Medicine in Nineteenth Century England* (New York: Holmes and Meier, 1977), 56-88.

9 For example, Johann Conrad Brunner, in 1683, criticised Johann Conrad Peyer's belief that maternal influences were capable of marking the foetus. See F.J. Cole, *Early Theories of Sexual Generation* (Oxford: Clarendon, 1930), 57-8, 61. Francesco Maria Nigrisoli also argued against the common belief in the power of the maternal imagination in his *Considerazione Intorno alla Generazione de' Viventi* (Ferrara: B. Barbieri, 1712), 5.

10 Blondel, *The Strength*, title page. Blondel's use of 'vulgar' in the sense of the common people is similar to Thomas Browne's discussion of such errors in his *Pseudodoxia Epidemica: or Enquiries into Vulgar and Common Errors* (London: T. H. for E. Dod, 1646). Browne did not, however, include the power of the mother's imagination as an erroneous belief.

11 Blondel, *The Strength*, Preface.

12 *Ibid.*, 10.

13 *Idem*, 10.

14 *Ibid.*, 14. J. Du Plessis described and illustrated the contemporary case of a child born 'in all respects like a Lobster' due to its mother's longing when not able to pay the 'Exorbitant Price' asked for such a fish in Leadenhall market. See his *A Short History of Human Prodigious & Monstrous Births of Dwarfs, Sleepers, Giants, Strong Men, Hermaphrodites, Numerous Births, and Extream Old Age &c.,* British Library, Sloane MS 5246, f. 13.

15 Blondel, *The Strength*, 28-29. As later described, Blondel was a Huguenot. Following the principles of his faith, Blondel would likely have opposed Malebranche's attempt to reconcile Cartesian physics and philosophy to the Catholic doctrine. See T.L. Hankins, 'The Influence of Malebranche on the Science of Mechanics during the Eighteenth Century', *Journal of the History of Ideas*, xxviii (1967), 193.

16 Blondel, *The Strength*, 34.

17 Blondel's preference of a strict scriptural interpretation rather than supposition is indicative of a sustained influence of Frederick Spanheim, his Leiden Professor of Theology. See F.L.R. Sassen's 'The Intellectual Climate in Leiden in Boerhaave's Time', in G. Lindeboom (ed.), *Boerhaave and his Times* (Leiden: E. J. Brill, 1970), 2-3. Blondel's appreciation of his instructor is identifiable by the dedication of his medical thesis, *Disputatio Medica Inauguralis de Crisibus* (Leiden: Abraham Elzevier, 1692), to Spanheim.

18 Blondel, *The Strength*, 34-6. According to the biographical entry in Ollivier and Raige-Delorme Dezeimeris' *Dictionnaire Historique de la Médecine*, vol. 1 (1828), 418, Blondel was well versed in the Dead Languages, particularly Hebrew, and he wrote a large number of theological works. Reeve, in 'Conceptions', 97 claimed some aspects of Blondel's account were 'more accurate than any I have found in the commentaries'. Samuel Kottek, in his 'La Force de l'Imagination chez les Femmes Enceintes: A Propos d'un Texte Biblique Apporté par J. Blondel en Illustration à ce Théme Controversé', *Revue d'Historie de la Médecine Hebraique*, xxvii (1974), 43-8 elaborates upon Blondel's Biblical citations.

19 *Ibid.*, 20, 22.

20 *Ibid.*, 21. He further recommended such deceitful vagrants to be tried by the 'Coventry Act'. Although J. Du Plessis, in *Short History of Human Prodigious & Monstrous Births*, f.52 described how deformed children were often left to beg on the streets, he also tells of one poor London couple who got a 'Hansom Lively Hod [sic]' from showing, for money, the lifeless skeleton the wife reputedly delivered.

21 Blondel, *The Strength*, 14.

22 *Ibid.*, 95.

23 *Ibid.*, 94-106.

24 Turner, 'Spots and Marks', 105. For example, he described that when people experience sorrow, 'their Spirits move slow and dull, both in the Brain and into the *Praecordia* [around the heart], hence from their languid Influx, the Circuit of the Blood is retarded through the Ventricles'. *Ibid.*, 104.

25 Turner's examples were drawn from such classical authorities as Aristotle, Pliny, and Soranus, together with more contemporary sources including Ambroise Pare, Thomas Bartholin, Joannes Schenkius, and Robert Boyle.

26 Turner, 'Spots and Marks', 114. This case was also included in the works of Schenkius and Pare.

27 *Ibid.*, attributed to Bartholin.

28 *Ibid.*, 116. 'J.B'. was most likely the MP, Sir James Bateman (1660-1718), from Soho Square, London.

29 *Ibid.*, 122.

30 *Idem.*

31 *Idem.*

32 C.J.S. Thompson, in *The Mystery and Lore of Monsters* (London: Williams & Norgate, 1930), 63 claimed that London was the Mecca for every variety of monster, and Colin Clair in *Human Curiosities*

Enlightened England', *Eighteenth Century Studies,* iii (1969), 108-9; Marjorie Nicolson, 'The Scientific Background of Swift's "Voyage to Laputa"' reprinted in her *Science and the Imagination* (Hamden, Connecticut: Archon Books, 1976), 110-54; and Lester King, *The Philosophy of Medicine: The Early Eighteenth Century* (Cambridge, Massachusetts: Harvard University Press, 1978), 152-81. J.J. MacIntosh provided a prelude to this era in 'Perception and Imagination in Descartes, Boyle, and Hooke', *Canadian Journal of Philosophy,* iii (1983), 327-57. Additionally, the philosophical usage of imagination over several centuries has been addressed by James Engel, *The Creative Imagination: Enlightenment to Romanticism* (Cambridge, Massachusetts: Harvard University Press, 1981). For variations of the early descriptions of imagination, see C.E. McMahon, 'The Role of Imagination in the Disease Process: Pre-Cartesian History', *Psychological Medicine,* vi (1976), 179-84, and C.E. McMahon and J.L. Hastrup, 'The Role of Imagination in the Disease Process: Post-Cartesian History', *Journal of Behavioral Medicine,* iii (1980), 205-17. 'The Imagination and Psychological Healing' has recently been addressed by S.W. Jackson in *Journal of the History of Behavioral Sciences,* xxvi (1990), 345-58.

50 Philip Shorr noted that many marvels, including children born alive without heads, were discussed in *Chambers' Cyclopedia.* Yet he added, 'in all fairness to the cyclopedist', that some of the more questionable ancient marvels had been omitted. *Science and Superstition in the Eighteenth Century: A Study of the Treatment of Science in Two Encyclopedias of 1725-1750* (New York: Columbia University Press, 1932), 110.

51 Thomas Morgan, *Philosophical Principles of Medicine* (London: J. Darby & T. Browne, 1725), 365-95, as cited by G.S. Rousseau, 'Science and the Discovery of the Imagination in Enlightened England', 124. See also Morgan's *Mechanical Practice of Physick* (London: T. Woodward, 1735), 220-1.

52 Turner's use of 'Power' of Imagination in 'Spots and Marks' and *The Force* in his 1730 work implied, as will be discussed, an immaterial impetus, whereas the implications of Blondel's use of the terms 'Strength' and 'Power' remain uncertain. Such terms were consistent with his adherence to 'Newtonian' doctrine. Given Blondel's displayed talent as both a scholar and wit, he may have used these terms as a parody upon Turner's titles. As such, it supports Simon Schaffer's claim that a Newtonian language was often used 'for specific pugnacious purposes'. See 'Newtonianism', in R.C. Olby, *et al.* (eds),

Companion to the History of Modern Science (London: Routledge, 1990), 617.

53 Blondel, *The Strength*, 52.

54 Blondel included this as his fourth proposition listed at the beginning of *The Strength.*

55 Blondel, *The Strength*, 54.

56 Blondel, *The Power*, 101.

57 Blondel, *The Strength*, 51, 94.

58 See R.G. Frank, 'Thomas Willis and his Circle: Brain and Mind in Seventeenth-Century Medicine', in G. S. Rousseau (ed.), *The Languages of Psyche: Mind and Brain in Enlightenment Thought* (Berkeley: University of California Press, 1990), 107-46. A. Meyer and R. Heirons earlier elaborated 'On Thomas Willis's Concepts of Neurophysiology' in *Medical History*, ix (1965), 1-15, 142-55. See also W. F. Bynum, 'The Anatomical Method, Natural Theology, and the Functions of the Brain', *Isis*, lxiv (1973), 445-68. For a biographical overview of Willis, see J. Trevor Hughes, *Thomas Willis 1621-1675. His Life and Work* (London: Royal Society of Medicine Services Ltd, 1991).

59 Turner, 'Spots and Marks', 106-7.

60 *Ibid.*, beginning on 120. Thomas Fienus described this particular action of the imagination in *De Viribus Imaginationis* (Louvain: G. Rivius, 1608). Turner also drew upon Fienus' account, implicating the role of imagination in 'producing almost every kind of disease', namely, squinting, stuttering, smallpox, and the plague (110). For a further outline, translation, and description of Fienus' writing, see L.J. Rather, 'Thomas Fienus' (1567-1631) Dialectical Investigation of the Imagination as Cause and Cure of Bodily Disease', *Bulletin of the History of Medicine*, xxxi (1967), 349-67. Earlier descriptions of powers of the imagination are discussed in M.W. Bundy, *The Theory of Imagination in Classical and Medieval Thought* (Urbana, Illinois: University of Illinois, 1927).

61 Blondel, *The Power*, x. For a recent, concise survey of atomism see Martin Tamny, 'Atomism and the Mechanical Philosophy', in R.C. Olby, *et al.* (eds), *Companion to the History of Science* (London: Routledge, 1990), 597-609.

62 Turner, 'Spots and Marks', 53-4.

63 *Idem.*

64 Guerrini, 'James Keill, George Cheyne, and Newtonian Physiology', 248-9. T. Brown claimed that Turner, an 'articulate skeptic [of materialism] in the junior ranks of the College during the 1710s', had already adopted mechanical explanations which incorporated an

argument was akin to that used to support epigenesis in the preceding century.

91 Epigenesis, an alternative explanation to preformation, proposed that embryos arose, after fertilization, from a homogeneous living matter which gradually unfolded in a regularly observed order and combined to form the full foetus.

92 Drake had argued that the 'Existence of a form'd Animal in the *Ovum* has never been prov'd, but suppose'd only from Analogy ... to the Seed of Plants'. Additionally, he claimed that animalcules 'may only be Particles of a mixt Fluid in motion'. See his *Anthropologia Nova*, vol.1, 352. Theodore Brown has claimed that Drake's generation arguments were directed against the preformationist theory of the Newtonian mathematico-physician, Archibald Pitcairne. See 'The Mechanical Philosophy and the "Animal Oeconomy"', 269. Historian Estelle Cohen is currently assessing the writings of James Drake, particularly his sister, Judith Drake's contributions to his output.

93 W.B. Hunter, 'The Seventeenth Century Doctrine of Plastic Nature', *Harvard Theological Review,* xxxxiii (1950), 197-213. He noted that this theory had provided 'a convenient explanation for the production of monsters', 209.

94 Turner, *The Force*, 103.

95 Turner, 'Religio Medici Reformata', 6.

96 Turner, *Answer*, 97-8.

97 W. Cowper, *Anatomy of Humane Bodies*, see Table 54 and its explanation. Cowper described this blood flow as bidirectional.

98 Blondel, *The Power*, 123.

99 Blondel, *The Strength*, 47.

100 Turner, *The Force*, 105-10, 112-15.

101 Blondel, *The Strength,* 121.

102 *Ibid.*, 114. Furthermore, Blondel argued, following William Harvey's claim, that since the 'most violent of all' passions, that of coitus, did not cause the ovary to swell or alter the generative process in any way, any lesser passion would not be transmissible either.

103 *Ibid.*, 124.

104 *Ibid.*, 123.

105 Turner, *Answer*, 153.

106 *Ibid.*, 154.

107 Charles W. Bodemer, 'Embryological Thought in Seventeenth Century England', in Charles W. Bodemer and Lester S. King (eds), *Medical Investigation in Seventeenth Century England* (Los Angeles: William Andrews Clark Memorial Library, University of California,

1968), 3.

108 Joseph Needham made this claim in 'Limiting Factors in the Advancement of Science as Observed in the History of Embryology', *Yale Journal of Biology and Medicine*, viii (1935), 15. Although Blondel specified reason as one component of his argument and Turner gathered empirical detail, a lack of a clear distinction between the two protagonists supports Andrew Wear's claim that rationalist/empiricist divisions more likely represent an historical categorization than an historical fact. See Wear's 'Medical Practice in late Seventeenth- and Early Eighteenth-Century England: Continuity and Change', in Roger French and Andrew Wear (eds), *The Medical Revolution of the Seventeenth Century* (Cambridge: Cambridge University Press, 1989), 304. Indeed, Turner praised London surgeon Richard Blundell for having 'Declined Mathematical Argumentation ... [and] invoke[d], rather a rational Empiricism'. See the dedication in Turner's *Syphilis*.

109 See D. Harley, 'Honour and Property', 138-64. Adrian Wilson, 'Politics of Medical Improvement', 7, 8, also discusses the uses of pamphlets as '*appeals* for public support'. H. Schwartz described a contemporary appeal for a wide audience by religious groups in his *The French Prophets*.

110 N.D. Jewson first discussed the public's role in determining the care and medicines they received in his provocative 'Medical Knowledge and the Patronage System', 369-85. Roy Porter has also argued that part of a physician's success at this time depended upon 'public favour', and has documented how physicians' arguments were addressed to the public. See 'Laymen, Doctors, and Medical Knowledge in the Eighteenth Century: the Evidence of the *Gentleman's Magazine*', in R. Porter (ed.), *Patients and Practitioners* (Cambridge: Cambridge University Press, 1985), 311; and D. Porter and R. Porter, *Patient's Progress*, 102. Marina Benjamin has also discussed the role of the patient as judge in 'Medicine, Morality and the Politics of Berkeley's Tar-Water' in A. Cunningham and R. French (eds), *The Medical Enlightenment of the Eighteenth Century* (Cambridge: Cambridge University Press, 1990), esp. 176-80.

111 Medical practitioners regularly confronted 'quack' remedies in attempts to dispel any mystery about 'miraculous' curative powers the remedies were claimed to have held. See for example, F. Doherty, 'The Anodyne Necklace', 268-93.

112 *Fog's Weekly Journal*, Saturday, 30 August 1729.

113 Turner, *The Force*, 137.

131 Additional cases of extraordinary childbirth from this period are discussed in G.S. Rousseau's 'Pineapples, Pregnancy, Pica, and *Peregrine Pickle*', in G.S. Rousseau and P.G. Boucé (eds), *Tobias Smollett: Bicentennial Essays* (New York: Oxford University Press, 1971), 93-94.

132 David Hartley, *Observations on Man*, part 1 (London: J. Leake & W. Frederick, 1749). Hartley's elucidations of vibrations and mental phenomena are more fully addressed in T. Mischel's '"Emotion" and "Motivation" in the Development of English Psychology: D. Hartley, James Mill, A. Bain', *Journal of the History of Behavioral Science*, ii (1966), 124-9.

133 [James Long], *An Enquiry into the Origin of Human Appetites and Affections* (London: W. Wood, 1747). For further discussion, see C. McMahon's 'Images as Motives and Motivators: A Historical Perspective', *American Journal of Psychology*, lxxxvi (1973), 472.

134 For example, the Haller–Wolff debate as brilliantly analysed by S. Roe in *Matter, Life and Generation.*

135 F.J. Cole, *Early Theories of Generation*, 53. Yet ovists continued to battle animalculists. The evidence which ovists Albrecht von Haller, Charles Bonnet, and Lazzaro Spallanzani gathered showed that the female was chiefly responsible for *in utero* development. It was used, by some, in support of the imaginationist's argument.

136 For example, it has been claimed that William Hunter questioned each pregnant woman in a 'large' London lying-in-hospital whether anything had 'specially affected' her mind during pregnancy, and he recorded the answers. After many years of collecting this information, Hunter had not found 'one instance' suggesting a relation between the woman's answer and any 'abnormal structure' of the child when delivered. John Brown, 'Notes and Observations on Maternal Impressions' (M.D. thesis, Glasgow, 1887-1888), 3. Hunter scholars, however, have not uncovered any evidence to support that such experimentation occurred. (As related in Wellcome Institute Inquiry RQ No. 817b, 6 December 1983.)

137 D. Turner, *Traité des Maladies de la Peau en General*, and D. Turner, *Abhandlung von den krankheiten der Haut.* James Blondel, *Dissertation Physique sur la Force de l'Imagination des Femmes Enceintes sur le Fetus*, translated by Albert Brun (Leyden: Gilbert Langerack and Theodore Lucht, 1737); J. Blondel, *Natuurkundige verhandeling: Wegens het Vermoogen der Inbeelding van Zwangere Vrouwen op Haar Vrucht*, translated by Jan van der Hulst (Rotterdam: Hermanns Kentlink, 1737); and J. Blondel, *Drey Merkw Urdige Physikalische Abhandlungen von der Einbildungskraft*

der Schwangern Weiber, und Derselben Wirkung auf ihre Leibesfrucht (Strasbourg: Amand Konig, 1756); and J. Blondel, *Dissertazione della Forza dell'Imaginazione delle Donne Gravide Sovra il Feto* (Ferrara: Francesco Gardi, 1760).

138 N. Lemery, and J.B. Winslow, *Memories Academie Royale des Sciences,* xxxiii (1733), xxxviii (1738), and xl (1740). Ignazio Vari, *Discussione 'Ragionamento del Sig. Dottore Ignazio Vari ... al Sig. Dottore Lucio Bonaccioli'* in J. Blondel, *Dissertazione della Forza dell'Immaginazione* (Ferrara: Francesco Gardi, 1760), 175-212.

139 A letter from Aaron Monceca to Isaac Onis quoted at length from the Turner-Blondel dispute in Jean Babtiste de Boyer, Marquis d'Argens, *The Jewish Spy,* vol. 4 (Dublin: Oli. Nelson and H. Saunders, 1753), letter 69, 95-109.

140 George Louis Leclerc Buffon, *Oeuvres completes de Buffon,* vol.1 edited by M. Flourens (Paris: P. Dumenil, 1835-1836), 642-7, cited by King, *The Philosophy of Medicine,* 174.

141 In addition to the works of Blackman, King, Park and Daston, and Rousseau already cited, Blondel and Turner also appear in the chapter entitled 'Rabbits and Quacks' of Harvey Graham's (pseud.), *Eternal Eve* (Altricham: William Heinemann, 1950), 345-6. Numerous midwifery texts of the nineteenth century also referred to the debate, see for example Michael Ryan, *Manual of Midwifery* (Burlington: Smith and Harrington, 1835), 64-73. In another context, see P.-G. Boucé's 'Imagination, Pregnant Women, and Monsters in Eighteenth Century England and France', in G.S. Rousseau and Roy Porter (eds), *Sexual Underworlds of the Enlightenment* (Manchester: Manchester University Press, 1988), esp. 89-94. Barbara Stafford discusses this debate in her chapter on 'Markings' in *Body Criticism,* 281-339. Finally, Ian Stevenson delivered a lecture entitled 'The Mother's Possible Influence in Birthmarks in cases of the Reincarnation Type' on 22 January 1989 at 'Parapsychology: A State-of-the-Art Conference' in New York. A more extensive account appears in Stevenson's *Reincarnation and Biology: A Contribution to the Etiology of Birthmarks and Birth Defects,* vol. 1 (London: Praeger Publishers, 1997), esp. 104-75.

142 See, for example, L.J.A. Lowenthal, 'Daniel Turner and "De Morbis Cutaneis"', 517-23, and R. J. Mann, 'Daniel Turner, the First British Dermatologist', 62-6. Even the more historically grounded writing of P.J. Hare perpetuated Turner's unfavourable reputation in his *Our Credulous Countryman.* One important exception is the short article by A. Lyell, 'Daniel Turner ... The Man Seen in the Pages of His Book of the Skin', 162-70. Here (168), Lyell explained Turner's

reliance upon authority more as a reverence for earlier works than as a blind acceptance of their word.

7

Exposing the 'Secret Disease': Recognizing and Treating Syphilis

Despite little demographic evidence, historians and sociologists have argued that syphilis or *lues venerea* (i.e., venereal plague or pestilence) was rife, apparently endemic in Enlightenment London.[1] Contemporaries linked its prevalence with 'whore mongering' or prostitution; a trade which, like the disease, was deemed 'epidemical and spreading'.[2] London prostitutes were found 'plying their trade' at all public shows, feasts, churches, plays, parks; the same types of places to which, contemporaries claimed, most cases of syphilis owed their origin.[3]

These conditions, however, were not peculiar to the eighteenth century. London prostitutes had been blamed for the spread of syphilis for several centuries. Sufferers in the 1700s, however, typically claimed to have acquired their disease through misfortune or accident, laying less emphasis on the sinful or Providential origins of this disease than their Puritanical forebears had done.[4]

Social campaigns to control venereal disease in Enlightenment London had not been implemented like those Edmund T. Burke, Paul McHugh, and Allan Brandt have described for later centuries.[5] The physician and satirist Bernard Mandeville's 1724 suggestion to curtail the spread of venereal disease by legalizing public prostitution and better regulating London's stews was never enacted.[6] Similarly, little action was taken upon Robert Poole's suggestion that by denying prostitutes the necessary medical treatments, they would become 'more cautious and circumspect in their Behaviour'.[7] And few contemporaries appear to have supported preventative measures such as the condom, which purportedly gained its introduction to London through Daniel Turner's writings.[8] Instead, many physicians and surgeons appear to have expressed more concern over determining whether syphilis originated as a 1492 'Columbian Exchange' or if documents proved it had existed in twelfth-century Southwark brothels.[9]

Contemporary sources suggest that one particular socially constructed view of venereal disease existed during this period: its secret nature. A 1730 London advertisement promoted both a lotion and an elixir for the 'Secret Disease', local parlance for venereal disease.[10] Sufferers and healers generally claimed syphilis was contracted through coupling the secret parts. If contracted through secret dalliances, the inflicted kept their predicament secret from their spouse, at least initially.[11] In fear of his reputation, one victim paid a quack twenty-five guineas for his complete treatment – ten for its 'cure', and fifteen for 'Secrecy'.[12] Some obtained their treatments through secret shop entrances, often during the night, and medicines were sent through 'utmost Privacy' to individuals, many of whom used 'Feigned Names'.[13] Some patients even wore masks to keep their identity secret when personally calling upon practitioners.[14] And numerous advertised medicines claimed their panacean power was derived from secret ingredients. Given this context, it is not surprising that venereal disease had, in common parlance, become known as the 'secret disease'.

As syphilis was among the most common disorders contemporary practitioners claim to have treated, it is of interest to uncover what they recognized as syphilis (i.e., determining an occupational construction of syphilis for this period). Thus, this chapter begins by examining the typical appearance of London's syphilitics as described in contemporary medical, surgical, and quack writings. Given the public concern over identifying the 'proper' type of practitioner to treat this disease, the relation between the presentation of syphilis and the selection of a practitioner is examined. As many syphilitics were purportedly 'cured' of their disease, contemporary descriptions of 'cure' are included. Finally, the techniques by which several contemporaries achieved their cures are discussed.

The contemporary literature on venereal disease was vast; scores of publications in the English vernacular alone were published during the first half of the eighteenth century (see Table 7.1). Few topics in medical history have attracted as much attention as syphilis.[15] Thus, for the historian, the need for selectivity arises. As this book focuses upon the surgical and medical careers of one contemporary London practitioner, Daniel Turner, this chapter emphasizes his writings, the patients he treated, the treatments he administered, and the criticisms raised against these treatments. Selecting Turner's writings over those of his contemporaries is somewhat justified as Turner was one of the most outspoken London authors on venereal disease. Still, to better contextualize my account of Turner, his arguments are studied in relation to those of his explicit allies and opponents. In particular, the views of his compatriots John Marten, William Cockburn, Thomas Dover and Joshua Ward as well

Turner's Works	Publication Date	Authors
	1670-90	Harvey, Wiseman, Ucay, Manwaringe
	1691-1700	Lister
	1701-5	
	1706-10	T.C., Spinke, Marten, Warren
	1711-15	Boulton, Cockburn, Harris
Syphilis	1716-20	Beckett, Cam, Wiseman, Nicholson
Modern Quack	1721-5	Chicoyneau, Dunn, de Sigogue, 'J.C'.
Discourse Concerning Gleets; *Letter to Mr. Fern*; (Hutten's) *De Morbo Gallico*	1726-30	Petit, Boerhaave, Cockburn, Garlick, Brown, Cam
Ancient Physician's Legacy … Survey'd; *Discourse on Quicksilver*; *Account of M. Belloste's Pill*; *Case of Barton Booth*; *Mr. Ward Consider'd*	1731-5	Sparrow, Belloste, Brest, Dover, Bradley, 'Country Physician', 'Mercurialist', 'Hydrargyrum', Knight, Atkins, Packe
(Luisinus) *Aphrodisiacus*; *Syphilis Part II*	1736-40	Clutton, Robinson, Douglas, Armstrong, Astruc, 'Country Physician', Desault, 'Philo-Chymicus'

Table 7.1
Vernacular English writings on venereal disease (1670–1740)

as French authorities on this disease, Jean Astruc, François Chicoyneau, Augustine Belloste, and Pierre Desault are compared with his own writings.

Recognizing the 'Clapped' and the 'Poxed'

Despite the appellation of the 'secret disease', contemporary texts, treatises, and lengthy advertisements frequently described various physical manifestations of syphilis. Indeed, the secret disease was among the most visible diseases of the early Enlightenment. Although its manifestation was not uniformly consistent, the accounts paint a verbal image of the physical afflictions from which syphilitics suffered.[16] Accounts typically concentrated upon how venereal diseases affected the most visible regions of the body, namely the head, hands and arms. Genital afflictions were also described.

The typical composite head-to-toe account which follows includes all of what Turner described as the 'Principal, univocal, pathognomonical, or ... demonstrative Signs' of syphilis.[17] Crusty scabs or pustules were found among the hairs of the head, often accompanied by deep-seated swellings or node-like protuberances from the cranium.[18] The nostrils, throat and palate were typically affected with ulcers and 'gummy Swellings' of the membranous parts, whereas the bony substructure of the nose and palate was often eaten away by the caries ensuing from long-standing syphilis. Some of Turner's patients grew concerned about the pox when they noticed that the food they ate or pipe smoke they inhaled came out through their nostrils; a sign which Turner interpreted as syphilis poisons having eaten through their palate. The 'venereal venom', Turner argued, made bodily humours so 'sharp and corrosive' that they ate into the cheeks, made 'sores [i.e., shankerous ulcers] in the Mouth, upon the Tongue and Lips ... and prey[ed] upon the Bone'.[19]

Reddish-brown scales formed along the insides of the fingers and the palm of the hands of syphilis victims. These scales and the 'Boils and Blotches' formed elsewhere over the body arose from syphilitic poisons in the blood which 'strive' to 'throw themselves out'.[20] The small joints of the hands were, like the bony facial structures, often affected with 'caries'. These joints, particularly in children, first appeared swollen and later erupted as the caries spread from inside out. Deep-seated swellings and node-like protuberances, according to Turner, had a propensity for developing along the ulna (i.e., the medial bone of the forearm). Glandular tumours commonly developed in the groin, and hard chancrous ulcers formed on, in, or around the genitalia. At times, purulent matter dripped from the urethra, and victims experienced excessive pain while urinating. One patient vividly described this excruciating pain in the following letter, dated 9 September 1710.

> Oh! Now I have a pressing to make water -----
> Oh! it scalds me to Pieces -----, 'tis like Fire ----
> Oh! Pocky Wh--re--, Thank God for a little
> Ease, – I have heard and read of p--ssing Pins and Needles,
> but never felt what it was till now---
>
> Occassion to P--ss again--Oh! what shall I do?--Oh!
> that this dribbling was over--it makes me Shudder--Scalding
> hot Water--just like Fire--as red almost as Blood---
>
> For God sake send me some Ease, I feel it coming again ...
> Pray be Plain in your Direction.[21]

Nodous protuberances similar to those growing from the ulna also affected the tibia of the lower leg. Similarly, the small joints of the ankle were affected like those in the hands. Swellings or gumata (i.e., strumous tumours filled with a 'gumous' substance) also arose from many muscle beds in diverse locations about the body; their size and painfulness were claimed to increase during the very early hours of the morning. These lesions accounted for the nocturnal pain which kept many syphilitics from bed rest until morning.

The signs of the 'infection' did not always appear all at once on everyone who became infected, and sometimes they did not appear at all.[22] Individuals without 'demonstrative' signs were not, however, necessarily free from infection. Most authors claimed that venereal disease existed in stages and that diagnostic signs of the disorder may not yet have become apparent. When this situation arose, Turner claimed it was not 'improper' to enquire whether the patient had formerly laboured under any 'Commemorative' symptoms of syphilis, to find out by what method they had been cured, and using this information, to determine the likelihood of whether any of that 'old Leaven' (i.e., from an earlier case of the pox) may still be 'mixed therewith'.[23]

Authors disagreed over distinctions between different stages or 'degrees' of venereal disease. John Marten, for example, described four stages of venereal disease, beginning with an infection confined to the genitals, progressing through stages of severity until, in the fourth stage, the patient's brain and bone marrow had become totally corrupted.[24] Others distinguished between inward and outward venereal diseases. One patient, for example, was told he suffered from an 'inward Pox', and that if it had been accompanied with 'Running or Blotches on the outside of his Body, the practitioner could have cur'd him for half the Money'.[25] Turner distinguished cases of venereal disease as either recent or confirmed. It was 'very necessary' to distinguish between these types, he argued, for each required 'very different' forms of treatment.[26] He identified a recent or first infection by a 'dripping' of purulent matter (i.e., pus) from the urethra, often accompanied by a genital chancre which, he claimed, produced much 'Pain and Smart' when making water. This infection, which Turner preferred to call *stillicidium purulentum*, was known among contemporaries as 'the dropper', 'the burning', 'gonorrhoea', 'gleets', or more colloquially, 'the clap'. If this infection was not 'dried up' whereby the 'venom' was not 'evacuated', Turner argued 'a Pox may happen to commence'.[27] The pox (i.e., syphilis or 'lues') was commonly regarded among practitioners as a late stage of venereal disease. For Turner, it represented the confirmed or second stage of the disease which was, he claimed, the 'usual Consequence' of an untreated, 'ill-treated', or 'empirically flubber'd over' clap.[28] Thinking of venereal diseases as being malignant or corruptible, and syphilis, in particular, as a more chronic, advanced consequence of untreated gonorrhoea is consistent with the contemporary idea of a 'metastatic translation' which, as Malcolm Nicholson has convincingly argued, was 'virtually [a] constant feature' of eighteenth-century disease theory.[29]

Some writers claimed venereal disease was difficult to distinguish from other similarly appearing distempers. Thomas Spooner, for instance, stated it was difficult to distinguish syphilis from 'the Itch'; a disorder apparently at least as common as the pox. Turner, however, argued that the Itch was contained or 'circumscrib'd' within the 'cuticular Compage' (i.e., the skin) whereas venereal disease, being of a more 'septic, arsenical, or caustic Quality', often 'corrupt[ed] not only the outward Teguments' but also 'devour[ed] ... Flesh and Bone'.[30]

Practitioners were apparently most concerned in their patients being able to distinguish between the gleeting (i.e., running) associated with gonorrhoea and the 'the whites' or *Fluor Albus*, a common female disorder described as the issue of a 'slimy yellowish matter' instead of a normal menstrual discharge.[31] Many women believed their 'Running' to be the whites, and let it 'run into the last Degree of a Pox, before they knew what their illness was, or looked for [a] proper Remedy'.[32]

Some practitioners distinguished syphilis from skin diseases more upon the patient's moral fibre than the outward manifestations. One

1721 account claimed that if a patient presented with 'Ulcers or running Sores, red, yellow, blue, or dark Spots, Pimples, or Blotches on the Face, Arms, Legs, or any other Part of the Body' and was deemed to be of 'sober discreet' character, he was diagnosed with scurvy. But if he was 'inclined to wantonness by reason of his Youth, or sly Countenance' then he was diagnosed with 'the Pox'.[33]

Unlike many of his contemporaries, Turner also distinguished between different individuals' susceptibilities to venereal disease. Men, for example, were claimed to be 'easier infected' and 'sooner cured' than women.[34] And it was not impossible, he argued, for patients with 'peculiar temperaments or constitutions' to be 'pox'd almost as soon as [they were] clap'd'.

Contemporary accounts suggest that patients and practitioners alike apparently shared the belief that venereal diseases could spread through the body in a malignant, sequential fashion. The public's concern about even a suspicion of having 'been clap't' prompted them to seek immediate care. The 'Women of the Town' (i.e., prostitutes), for example, took 'Alarm' as 'soon as their Water disturbs them', and immediately sought cures.[35] Similarly, most of Turner's patients 'applied themselves' to him within days of first noticing a 'scalding' upon making water or a continuous discharge from their genitals. As discussed in Chapter Three, Londoners commonly suffered disorders, particularly surgical disorders like ulcers, tumours, and hernias for many months, even years before seeking care. What, then, prompted people to seek immediate care if they believed themselves to be venereally infected?

For many, perhaps most, it was fear. 'Syphilophobes' loomed large in the anecdotal literature. And in reality, the quacks of Turner's day, as Roy Porter has shown, commonly traded upon the fears of potential patients.[36] Fear drove people to obtain any medicine advertised to effect an immediate cure, thereby preventing the consequences of a lingering pox. Some feared being 'found out' by their spouse. Others feared that the 'telling' signs of the disease would 'risque their Characters in the [business] World'.[37] This fear was particularly common, according to Turner, 'among the Tradesmen or Citizens' who worried that without rapid treatment, syphilitic throat infections would cost them their 'proper Tone of their Voice', and consequently, 'their Reputation'.[38]

Obtaining Cures

Scores of English vernacular publications from the first half of the eighteenth century indicate that a venereal patient's chief concern was obtaining a rapid cure. Selling a curative product largely depended upon effective advertising. London was filled with advertisements for 'curing' venereal disease. Francis Doherty has recently argued that 'Being in the venereal trade meant cashing in on anything that might be guaranteed to bring in the customers'.[39] The public was frequently inundated with potential cures through handbills passed their way or posted on signboards throughout the city, through practitioners hawking their cures on the streets, at booksellers or coffeehouses, and through many pages of advertisement in the rapidly expanding periodical press. Those who thought themselves venereally inflicted could shop for remedies as consumers shopped for goods.

Case study evidence indicates that many venereal sufferers first turned to the local, self-acclaimed healers whose advertisements had appeared most convincing. Others, particularly middle-class men who had not initially sought out street practitioners, often called upon the advice of their peers in coffeehouses or barbershops, those 'dens of male comradeship'.[40] Here, not only could they check their suspicions with the experience or knowledge of their comrades, they could actually select from a variety of curative remedies sold within. Although the ingredients of the remedies most barbershops offered were secret, the name brands were often the same as the products advertised on quackbills posted around the city. Thus, many of the same products appear to have been distributed to different classes of patients through different venues and, at times, for different prices. This exchange of commerce indicates that an intra-London drug trade was already well formed .

Medical historian, W.F. Bynum has cogently argued that the treatment of venereal disease actually became a special form of practice or speciality in eighteenth-century England.[41] I agree that some practitioners, both quack and professional, gained their reputation and amassed vast wealth as venerologists. However, most of this literature together with the surviving case history evidence from the first half of the century suggests that syphilis treatment remained in the domain of a surgeon's care. That is, surgeons were both publicly and occupationally recognized as caretakers of syphilis; at least of the stubborn, resilient, recurrent, or previously mismanaged cases of syphilis. I offer several reasons as to why this form of the disease primarily remained part of general surgical practice.

English surgeons were, at least as far back as the 1585 writing of William Clowes, traditionally provided with practical information about treating syphilis.[42] At this time, and in the early eighteenth century as well, orthodox surgeons were primarily treating externally manifest disorders whereas internal disorders were treated by physicians. As mentioned above, syphilis was recognized and diagnosed primarily upon its external appearance; therefore, its care, as many surgeons argued, fell among the surgical trade.

Turner, for one, claimed that 'if we consider many of the [Signs] and Symptoms' of syphilis, undertaking its 'Cure' was by 'right' the surgeon's province. For the cure, he expounded, often required 'manual Operation'. Treating syphilis implied having to apply caustics to 'lay open the Venereal Abscesses, to rub down the Verrucae, to extirpate Caruncles; ... to lay bear rotten Bones, or [to apply] Cauteries ... [upon bones] for Desquamation'. To meet these needs, Turner argued that a surgeon's knife and scissors were most appropriate. After presenting this scenario, Turner concluded, 'it must be granted, that the Surgeon is the most proper Person to be consulted' for treating syphilis.[43] Similar arguments appear in contemporary writings of surgeons John Marten, James Douglas, Edward Dunn, and physicians Richard Boulton, Richard Brown, John Freind, and Bernardino Ramazzini as well as in popular works such as Campbell's *London Tradesman* and newspapers such as *The Grub-Street Journal*.[44]

Identifying surgeons as caretakers of syphilis was also consistent with European models. By the early eighteenth century, European syphilis treatises of François Chicoyneau, Jean Louis Petit, Augustine Belloste, Vincent Brest, Pierre Desault, and Jean Astruc had been translated into the vernacular and were sold in London bookstalls. The manual treatments recommended in these works were often explicitly and favourably cited by English surgical authors, indicating an adoption of some foreign methods in treating this disease. These particular French writings appear to have held the most sway with English surgeons; what better way than to emulate French treatments of what the English so readily referred to as the 'French Disease' (or 'French Pox')?[45]

Surgeons also appear to have accepted their responsibility of manually administering long, labour-intensive treatments. A contemporary case book from St Thomas' Hospital, for example, indicates that surgeons William Cheselden, Josiah Paul, and James Ferne routinely attended and administered treatments for many 'foule' (i.e., venereally diseased) patients over standard 21- or 31-day courses of treatment.[46] John Douglas stated that patients outside the hospital often received treatments for one, often two months.[47] From what we know about contemporary medical practice, many London physicians, particularly those of the College, were less likely to embark upon such lengthy, time-consuming, manual, labour-intensive types of treatment.[48]

Surgeons' laborious efforts were likely, however, to have been driven by the lucre of treating syphilitics. Syphilis was present in all social classes, having completely cut through the traditional English barriers which demarcated stratifications between classes.[49] Physicians in London, particularly those of the College, are typically portrayed as primarily treating the moneyed or upper-class patients, whereas surgeons appear to have treated any who sought their care and were brought to their surgeries. To convince a potential patient to undergo a lengthy, extensive course of treatment, secluded in either the surgeon's home or other rented accommodations, surgeons contracted their services for set fees. Given that thousands of people appear to have been afflicted with some venereal disorder, securing syphilis treatment as part of the surgical trade offered surgeons a way to gain a more constant, predictable, steady business than did treating other types of accidents.

Finally, and perhaps most importantly, since patients continued to willingly seek surgeons to treat syphilis, at least the stubborn or recurrent types of syphilis, it must be considered that surgeons were able or at least were thought to be able to successfully 'cure' this disease. Evidence abounds that syphilis was curable.[50] For example, Samuel Palmer, admitting surgeon to the Lock Hospital in Southwark and correspondent of Turner's, reported that between January 1719/20 and January 1720/21, 108 of the 115 syphilitics he admitted were later 'cured and discharged'.[51] At St Thomas' Hospital, nearly all of the 34 'foule' patients treated for syphilis between 1 May and 1 September, 1726 were discharged as 'cur'd'. John Douglas, surgeon to Westminster Infirmary, claimed to never have sent one of his 'several hundreds' of venereally diseased patients away 'uncured'.[52] Edward Dunn and William Cockburn attested to similar curability in their public (i.e., non-hospital) practices. Before explaining how they achieved these cures, let us consider what contemporary surgeons considered as being 'cured'.

Syphilis Cured?

Twenty-six of the thirty patients Turner described in his 1717 *Syphilis. A Practical Dissertation of Venereal Disease* became 'cured' through his treatment. Four patients died, two of which Turner claimed died not from his hands, but from the intervention of a quack. Turner's depiction of a cured patient generally represents the accomplishment of one or more of ten therapeutic goals. Namely, cure involved 'eas[ing] the Smart' of making water, 'lessening the

Running' of the clap, 'mending the colour' of the urine, and 'drying up' scabs and pustules. In addition, he sought to 'resolve' the bubos, 'mundify' the chancrous ulcers, 'reduce' nodous protuberances, restore the ability to swallow with ease, preserve the voice, and 'relieve' the 'Great [nocturnal] Pain' in the head or legs.

To achieve these cures, Turner's patients often underwent months of therapy. For example, salivating a patient, a common procedure more fully described below, required, at least in theory, that a patient be 'laid down' (i.e., bed ridden) for a month. 'Strictly conform[ing] to the Rules prescribed, keeping [to one's] ... Chamber the whole time', Turner argued, greatly 'contribute[d] to the success of these Cures'.[53] Yet, he claimed that ''tis seldom' surgeons 'have such Opportunity' of this 'Convenience'.[54] Despite the shared public and occupational belief that an incompletely cured clap led to a confirmed pox,[55] Turner acknowledged that surgeons often compromised ideal syphilis treatments according to the patient's demands. One patient refused salivation on the grounds that his work 'Affairs ... [did] not favour ... such recess from [his] Business'.[56] Thus, Turner resolved to treat him by fumigation, a less confining form of treatment. Another gentleman also refused to be salivated because his 'concerns in merchandising being very Great' would 'by no means ... allow his getting out of the way' for the entire month which Turner's treatment required. Only when his condition was greatly exacerbated did he submit to salivation. Another patient discharged himself from Turner's full course of treatment having 'reckon[ed] himself well'.[57]

Turner described most of his patients as becoming completely cured, healed, or restored to 'a perfect State of Health'. One 'Sober and virtuous Gentlewoman' was, after weeks of treatment, reported to be 'in every Way improved'.[58] Turner described another patient's 'Appetite, Complexion, and Flesh' as being fully 'recruited' after ten weeks of therapy.[59] One gentleman was improved to a 'sound State' excepting that his swallowing and speech were not 'so readily performed as before'.[60] Only one patient reportedly received little benefit. Although this patient 'subsist[ed]', Turner claimed he did so 'very miserably'.[61]

Cure appears to have been the general state of a patient at the time he was 'dismis'd' from private care or 'discharg'd' from hospital. Few contemporaries reported what we would call patient follow-up. Turner, however, provided glimpses into the futures of five patients he claims to have 'cur'd'. One gentleman was described as 'fat and lusty' a year later, whereas the cure of another 'stood firm', so Turner was informed, some two years after treatment.[62] One gentleman married a year after treatment, but whether through his previous infirmity or his advanced age, the patient claimed to Turner that 'his [marital] Abilities' were 'not answerable to his Inclinations'.[63] Another patient Turner cured, being 'well tired with Venus's wars ... enter'd those of Mars' in which, he learned, he was 'not long after ... killed in an Engagement'.[64] But one of Turner's 'cured' patients was not entirely freed from his troubles. According to Turner, it was

> many Months, I may say Years, before he [i.e., the patient] would believe he was well, if he does yet: For [a] long Time after ... when he was hot with riding or walking in the Summer Time, ... [and] an Efflorescence [appeared on the] Parts of the skin next to [the earlier 'Stigmata' of syphilis], he would come to me as a Person affrightened, for fears of his Malady returning; and having read much of the Disease, especially the Quack Bills, ... he would apply every Symptom to himself: So that if his Head ached ever so little, as after a drinking Bout it did sometimes, or a Pimple appeared about him, nay if it was but a Flea-bite, ... it was sufficient to cast him into a Fit of Melancholy, and make him pass away whole Nights ... feeling of his Nose and Shin Bones.[65]

Finally, Turner argued that curing a patient required removing all of the 'venereal venom' that was lurking within. This point distinguishes Turner's meaning of cure from the 'Aim' of 'London Quacks'. The latter, it was argued, only sought to stop the urethral running and heal the outward sores, whereas they disregarded the possible consequence of a secondary infection or confirmed case of the pox.[66] London physician Edmund Packe cautioned against believing in this quackery as treatment and noted 'Nothing is more common, and indeed unavoidable, than a Return of Distempers (with their Symptoms) ... one Day after ... [a practitioner] believe[s] they are cur'd'.[67] To overcome this calamity, surgeon John Douglas urged orthodox practitioners to pursue a course of treatment 'untill the symptoms have all disappeared, and some little time after'.[68]

Relatedly, Turner discredited reports of patients being 'partially cured', a 'new Phrase' he claimed the French commonly used for 'palliating'.[69] One type of palliation for syphilis was described in a contemporary verse.

> When Noses drop, and Shins do scale,
> And Mercury and Aegypticum fail,

When Bubos, Pains, and Chancrous Sores in spight
Of Art the tottering Tenement hourly fright;
When Strength is wasted, Flesh become
Past help of China and Guaiacum,
Then Doctor cease, poor Patient must endure,
And be content with patching, where's no Cure.[70]

The principles of the French 'Partial' cures are discussed below. Suffice it to say here that Turner argued that 'Partially cured' patients were likely to retain their inward poison and consequently never become fully cured.

Treating Syphilis

The 'acceptable' forms of treating syphilis had changed by 1739, the date of Turner's last publication, from the standard therapies used thirty years earlier. Turner had not instigated this change; and in many ways he remained one of the old guard whom 1739 critics claimed were 'biggots to antiquity'.[71] Rather, his writings illuminate many contemporary concerns over administering effective but non-hazardous remedies. Additionally, they exemplify how being deemed a 'quack' or a 'guardian of orthodoxy' depended as much upon the way a practitioner administered treatments as upon his qualifications to practise.

No single universally accepted treatment existed to cure syphilis. Rather, exponents of a variety of therapies appeared in the contemporary surgico-medical literature. Many of the remedies promoted here as well as in quack handbills contained some form of mercury. Prince's Powder, for instance, a red precipitate of mercury, was one of the most common 'Chemical Quack Remedies' and was also prescribed in Quincy's *Pharmacopoeia*.[72] Mercury was also among the most common ingredients present in the remedies distributed gratis to charity patients, sold to commoners in local shops, and offered to the aristocracy, the nobility, and the royal household.

According to some contemporaries, mercury was a godsend; to others, the devil incarnate.

Mercury as us'd, the Body fills,
With wholesome Goods, or noxious Ills,
And quickly Cures, or quickly Kills.[73]

Like most London practitioners of the 1710s treating venereal disease, Turner was a mercurialist. He claimed mercury was the 'specifik' or 'antidote' for syphilis.[74] Indeed, he claimed, it was the 'only antisyphilitic Remedy ... we ... know of'.[75] Turner administered mercurials both externally and internally. Topically applied mercurials, he claimed, digested, deterged, and cicatrized the external ulcerations of syphilis. But some 'subtil Particles' of these external mercurial preparations would, he continued, also 'insinuate' themselves 'thro' the Pores [of the skin] into the Lymphatic Vessels' whereby they were 'instantly convey'd to the Glandules' to 'subdue' the venereal 'Poison lodg'd therein'.[76] For 'mild' forms of the pox, Turner frequently prescribed the use of calomel (i.e., mercurous chloride or *mercurius sublimatus dulcis*) to be 'given inwardly'.[77]

During the time, various forms of mercury were available for the use of surgeons, physicians, and quacks. White sublimate, calomel, red, white, yellow, and green precipitates (i.e., oxides of mercury), natural and artificial cinnabar (i.e., mercury and sulphur) as well as crude mercury or quicksilver could be obtained from apothecaries.[78] Mercurial products were administered internally by mouth, externally by frictions, fumigations, salivations, clysters, or as impregnated plaisters applied on the limbs, worn as girdles or as socks.

Numerous disputes ensued over selecting the precise form of treatment. Turner distinguished himself from other mercurialists by restricting his use to particular forms of administration. Indeed, he grew quite incensed over the panaceic use of crude or metallic mercury which he claimed many contemporaries used. Crude mercury, he argued, was quacked from London streets, and distributed by 'Plowmen, Farmers, [and] Swine-heard' who were 'destroying' local inhabitants as 'people do with Buckets of Water, to quench the Fire of another Nature'.[79] Turner claimed first-hand knowledge of its effects from his early surgical career.[80] But the hazardous consequences he observed in his and other surgeons' patients had prompted him to abandon its use, and he urged fellow London surgeons to stop using it, too.[81] Specifically, Turner suggested that practitioners reduce the amount of external mercury they applied and omit the use of orally administered crude mercury entirely.

Turner regarded mercury taken internally as inefficacious against the syphilis poisons in the body. It was 'doubtless the Case', he argued, that many 'thinking the [oral mercurial] Remedy is working Miracles in their Blood, might find it in their Breeches, or on the Ground, if they mist it in the Close-Stool'.[82] Anecdotal stories and experiments abounded in the literature recounting how orally administered mercury quickly passed through one's system. Many patients humorously described how their mercury often 'slip[ped] away with a Crepitus'.[83] Perhaps the most entertaining tale was that of a 'mercurial Lady' who,

> while Dancing at a publick Assembly, happened to let go some Particles of the Quicksilver she had taken in the Morning, which shinning on the Floor, in the midst of so great an Illumination, like so many Brilliants, ... [prompted] several [others to] stoop down to take them up; but finding themselves deceived, it afforded much Laughter among the Gentlemen, and Blushing among the Ladies, especially she that was most concerned.[84]

Turner also recalled how the surgeon Henry Bradley had administered pre-weighed daily doses of mercury totalling sixteen pounds over nine months. During which time, by 'Washing' the mercury from his 'Excrement, as it came from his Body', he reserved his collection 'in a Bottle'. Upon weighing it afterwards, he found 'there wanted only one Ounce and [a] half' of sixteen pounds. The discrepancy, he claimed, was 'lost in the washing'.[85]

Turner deemed the inefficacy of internally administered mercury was due to its minimal absorption. He argued that if little mercury was actually absorbed, then this explained why so many practitioners had administered increasing doses without achieving success. He concluded that the increasing doses actually produced an internal toxicity. Thus, increasing internally administered doses of mercury only quickened its toxicity, ultimately killing the patients, while leaving their syphilis unchecked.

To persuade readers of this point, he described an experiment which he had performed. Turner employed a young man to remove the 'stomach and Intestines of a Bitch', and then tie a 'firm Ligature around the Rectum'. He then poured a measured quantity of crude mercury through the oesophagus into the stomach, tied the upper end off, and 'shook it about till [the mercury] was past over the Pylorus [region of the stomach], and had entered the Intestines'. After waiting 'some Hours', he shook it again, let the mercury settle to a lower point in the intestine, and repeated this procedure until he 'perceived the whole Mass [had] fallen down upon the Ligature, at the lower end of the Rectum'. At this time, he noted that 'not one' of the globules of mercury had 'passed thro' the lining of either the 'smaller or larger Gut'. Only when pricking the lower bowel wall with a pin, after first compressing the mercury into that region, did any mercury spill out.[86] Turner argued that this experiment demonstrated that mercury was not absorbed from the stomach or intestines, regions where he deemed absorption would have occurred, on its passage through the animal guts. Thereby, he offered experimental 'proof' to prohibit readers from administering such an unabsorbable, and thereby inefficacious, treatment.

Turner did not completely reject the use of crude mercury, only its oral administration. Indeed, he favoured its use when applied 'in the way of Unction', literally rubbing it into the body. Mercurial unctions were commonly used in the 1710s and 1720s to bring forth the internal venereal poisons through the excessive production of spittle or saliva; a process labelled salivation or ptyalismus. Turner advocated this use of mercury, and described the two 'safest and most commodious' ways to salivate patients which were 'generally used by the surgeons of the Town'. Calomel was to be 'given inwardly' for the mild pox, whereas crude mercury was externally applied by 'way of unction' for the 'stubborn or rebellious' pox.[87] In this later procedure, mercury was rubbed upon a syphilitic's arms and legs in sufficient quantity to excite the noxious humours to induce the production of ample spittle.[88] The spittle was thought to contain the poisonous venom. Beginning with the ankles and slowly proceeding up to the thighs, the mercurial unguent was rubbed in so as to allow the mercurial 'Globules' to be 'leisurely ... blend[ed] ... with the Lymph', whereby they were then 'dispose[d]' to take 'the ready Road to the Fauces, and miss the Intestines'.[89]

Turner avoided treating the chest or belly this way in fear of harmful effects. The 'pores of the other parts' were, he claimed, 'sufficient to lett the Mercury into the Blood, which being once Admixt there with', it was 'less material by what particular Pores it had its first Admittance'.[90] With his patient's safety still in mind, he urged colleagues to stop using 'so much greasing or daubing' of mercury when a small amount will produce the same effect. Additionally, he warned surgeons that 'too sudden[ly] r[a]ising' a salivation and 'too long [of its] continuence' provoked 'Accidents' that often proved fatal.[91]

In 1736, Turner claimed that 'several hundred Persons' were salivated 'yearly, in the Cities and suburbs of London and Westminster'.[92] Earlier in the century, salivation had become the standard for treating 'foule' (i.e., venereally diseased) patients admitted to St Bartholomew's and St Thomas' hospitals, London's 'sacred sanctuaries for the sick'.[93] A hospital pupil at St Thomas' noted that these methods 'may safely be us'd according to Turner'.[94]

When a patient would not salivate, Turner recommended the use of a cinnabar fumigation.[95] Cinnabar was a mixture of mercury and sulphur. If the patient's whole body was to be fumigated, he or she was placed upon a seat that was 'perforated' somewhat 'like the close Stool'. A blanket was wrapped around the patient, entirely 'enclosing' the body and head, and was secured to a hook in the ceiling.[96] Cinnabar was sprinkled on a hot iron placed below the seat, and the fumes ascended through the chair, guided by an inverted funnel so that they would flow 'all round the Diseased Parts' (see Figure 7.1).[97] If fumigation was to be used primarily for treating stubborn syphilitic ulcers in the nose, mouth and throat, as Turner recommended, the blanket-enclosed patient was directed to hold the cinnabar in an earthen platter on his knees and to inhale the fumes repeatedly. Turner generally 'smoaked' or fumigated these patients in the 'Night and Morning ... for about a week'.[98] As in salivating, Turner urged practitioners to keep patients 'confined' to their houses 'During the Course' of treatment. Fumigation, however, offered the opportunity for those whose 'Business would not permit' confinement, to go 'about their Affairs as usual, only wearing a bit of Flannel under their chin, as a Muffler, to keep their Throat warm'.[99]

For patients whose temperaments or state of disease prevented these means from effecting a cure, Turner considered the use of Guaiac, also known as *Lignum vitae*, the 'pock wood' and the 'Indian cure' or 'Indian Decoction'.[100] Guaiac, a wood introduced into Spain and Portugal from the New World in the early sixteenth century, developed a mixed reputation in Europe over the following two centuries regarding its efficacy in curing syphilis. In 1728, the 'guaiacum vogue' was 'once again revived'.[101] 'Must the venereal Patient, who ... can receive no Help from Mercury, be forsaken as desperate?' 'No', claimed the respected medical sage and Turner's Continental contemporary, Herman Boerhaave. Just 'read [Ulrich von] Hutten's Treatise [*De Morbo Gallico*], and ... you shall find [that] the most intricate or deeply radicated Evils of this kind, may be scoured out or cleansed away by a strong Lixivium of Guaiacum'.[102]

Turner had read Hutten's *De Morbo Gallico* (1533) in the early years of his surgical practice (see Figure 7.2). Indeed, he was so intrigued with it at the time, claiming 'no Physician, has given us ... a better and more graphical Account of the Disease', that Turner made himself 'Master of the Old English Letter, the Orthography ... and many obsolete Words and Phrases' used in the old earlier printed version, and 'transcribe[d]' it into 'our modern Idiom'.[103] Turner later used this transcript to provide historical background about syphilis for his own work in order to add 'some account of the Rise and Progress of that Disease'.[104] He eventually republished Hutten's *De Morbo Gallico* in the 'modern' English vernacular together with a lengthy introduction in 1730.[105] In the introduction, Turner claimed that both Hutten and Boerhaave were 'endevouring to prove' that 'there is in this Decoction [of guaiac] something peculiar' which after being 'raised into Steams' and 'incorporated with the Blood ... unites more readily with the Morbific Particles' than did mercury, thereby easing their discharge in the 'Form of Dew or Vapour'.[106]

Despite publishing Hutten's and Boerhaave's use of guaiac, he and most of his London colleagues remained sceptical whether it would actually 'succeed where Mercury will not'. He mentioned having used it on only one patient, and few London colleagues offered any account of having used it either. He withheld further

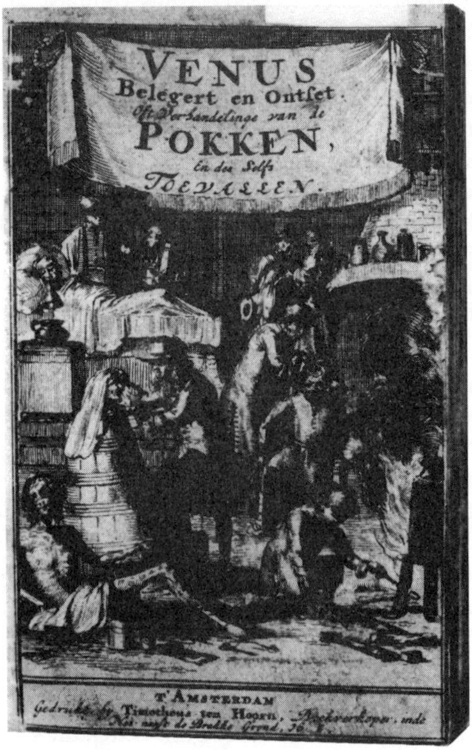

Figure 7.1

The scenario of various syphilis treatments, including fumigation and salivation. Frontispiece to Steven Blankaart's *Venus Belegert en Ontset* (1685, Wellcome Institute Library, London)

endorsement of guaiac until its efficacy could be 'more thoroughly' tested. To perform such 'experiments', Turner envisioned London hospital surgeons and physicians as the ideal experimenters.

Hospitals

By 1730 six hospitals existed in London.[107] St Bartholomew's, St Thomas' and the Westminster Infirmary were general hospitals, whereas Guy's, The Lock, and Kingsland hospitals also accepted patients deemed as 'Incurables'. Incurables were 'generally understood' to include individuals suffering 'loss of limbs, blindness, ... other natural or accidental deformities', specific distempers,

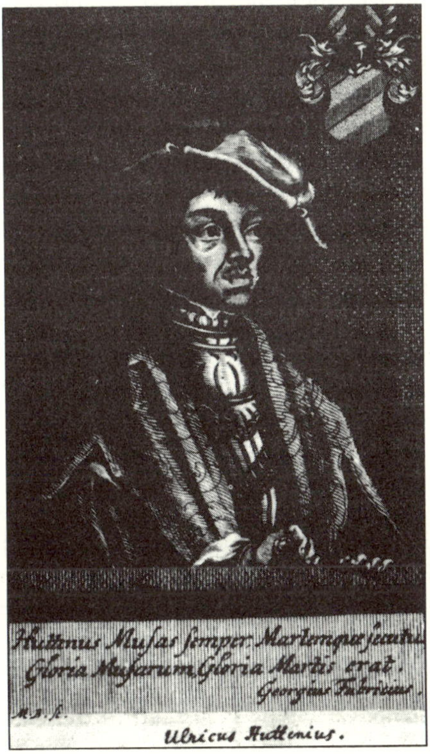

Figure 7.2
Ulrich von Hutten, 1488-1524
(M.B., Wellcome Institute Library, London)

including asthma, consumption, cancers and 'even old age itself'. Syphilitics who were unable to obtain 'cures' elsewhere often turned to these hospitals as their last resort for help.[108]

Turner recommended that guaiac's efficacy be tested on the syphilitics at one of London's 'hospitals of Incurables'. Although he treated such patients from his home-based surgery, he was aware of hospital practice through collaboration with Richard Blundell of St Bartholomew's, James Dansie of Kingsland, and Samuel Palmer and Peter St Hill of The Lock.[109] Through these contacts, Turner learned that syphilitics were present in large numbers at these hospitals. Moreover, these patients were obliged to obey the hospital orders read to them upon admission. Failing to do so put them upon 'perill of being excluded [from] the Hospital'.[110] This condition, Turner intimated, made them more willing to comply with any suggested 'experimental' treatment.[111]

Turner's depiction is consistent with John Bellar's 1714 proposal of using hospitals as places where the effects of new remedies might regularly be tested upon a large number of patients. Thus, if any benefit of guaiac was to be found, he claimed it would be more readily observed in a hospital with many experimental subjects. Hospitals had, in the early eighteenth century, begun to refine what Michel Foucault termed the practitioner's 'gaze'. Patients in these hospitals would, Turner claimed, be 'under the Care of Gentlemen [in] every Way qualified for making their observations, [and] having Opportunities beyond most others of singling out what Subjects they please to work on in this way'.[112]

Treating Syphilis: Who's a Quack?

In his 1718 *The Modern Quack*, Turner identified five types of quack: the 'Empirical Practitioner' or mountebank, the 'Libelling Quack' or 'practicing Pamphleteer', the 'Chyrurgick Barber', the 'Pretending Bonesetter', and the 'City Doctress'.[113] These characterizations primarily identified various types of the 'thousands of false Pretenders' which Turner claimed filled the streets of London.[114] In addition, Turner argued there were variously 'qualified' practitioners who practised some form of quackery as well. These quacks included anyone 'bred up to a Mechanic Employment ... [who falsely] setup for a Doctor or Surgeon'; one who after living only 'a Year, two or three, with one ... of the Profession ... endeavor[s] to screen himself' with an ecclesiastical license to practise; one 'legally bred up' in the profession, but who advertises particular universal remedies; or one trained in 'Physic, Pharmacy or Surgery who ... intermeddles in all three'.[115]

Turner regarded it as quackery for a surgical or medical author to 'conceal ... from the Reader' anything he knew that might be of help to patients.[116] In particular, he despised authors who promoted secret remedies. It was this fault, Turner claimed, that lay at the heart of a work entitled *The Symptoms, Nature, Cause and Cure of a Gonorrhea* (1713). He rebuked the author of this work, his contemporary and fellow licentiate of the London College of Physicians, William Cockburn, for keeping the ingredients of the curative remedy he promoted a secret.

In contrast to Cockburn's quackery, Dr Thomas Dover openly disclosed his remedy for venereal disease: orally administered quicksilver. Turner's opposition to this form of administration has been previously discussed. However, he expressed particular outrage at Dover for promoting his remedy not only for venereal disease, but as a 'panpharmicon' or panacea. Indeed, Dover recommended using large doses (i.e., several pounds) of mercury as a cure for disorders including hysteria, intestinal infestation and obstruction, scrofula, infertility, asthma, elephantiasis, scorbutic ulcers, and venereal disease.

Dover first propounded his panaceic claims of quicksilver in *The Ancient Physician's Legacy to his Country* (1732). In the following year, the surgeon, Henry Bradley and an anonymous 'Country Physician' were among the first to counter Dover's claims. But it was Daniel Turner who, in 1733, made what has been called the first 'serious examination' of Dover's writing, dissecting it piecemeal in his *The Ancient Physician's Legacy Impartially Survey'd*.[117]

A publishing war ensued, chiefly between Turner and Dover, but backed by respective allies as well. Within the following year, a number of anonymous authors, identifying themselves by such titles as 'The Mercurialist' and a 'Gentleman of Trinity College, Cambridge', upheld Dover's use of mercury.[118] Dover, too, republished his *Ancient Physician's Legacy*, defending his claims of quicksilver on grounds of both theory and practice. According to Dover, injuries resulting from any mercurial agent were due to the agent's shape or form. Hazardous agents, he argued, always appear marked with 'spiculae, points, and edges'. Thus, quicksilver, which always retained its 'globular form', was perfectly harmless.[119] Dover added further support of mercury's efficacy by publishing eight signed testimonials. In disapproval of those who dubbed him the 'Quicksilver Doctor' and 'Quicksilver a-la-mode', Dover defended his opponent's rebuff, arguing 'Pray do not you gentlemen, physicians, surgeons, and apothecaries prescribe it [i.e., mercury] almost every day of your lives? I avow you do; only you disguise it, and I give it in such an open honest manner that my patient cannot be deceived in taking it'.[120]

Dover's detractors, including Turner, provided much first- and second-hand case evidence that the large quantities of mercury Dover used had produced hazardous effects. They scorned him for returning to the practise of the 'Ancients', i.e., seventeenth-century practitioners who administered mercury in the much more unregulated fashion. Turner claimed he 'might forgive [Dover's] Quackery if [only] he would quack safely'.[121]

As in many contemporary medical disputes, no quick resolution over Dover's practice was reached.[122] Neither the College of Physicians nor the Society of Apothecaries made an official pronouncement regarding Dover's treatments. Rather, each side continued to gain adherents by publicly denigrating its specific opponent.

Turner entered into a similar dispute against the physician Augustine Belloste. Belloste had become renowned in France for his mercurial pill, reputedly effective in treating all forms of venereal disease. Turner initially vowed that Belloste had an 'Honest Intention of serving the Public'.[123] But his anger flared when Belloste, 'like most other Men, ... resolv'd to make the most he could of his Nostrum'. Turner claimed that as

> Soon as I found him making a Secret of what is known to the Whole World, i.e., valuing so common a Remedy at an extravagant Rate ... I was forced to alter my Opinion both of the Man and his Medicine; and can esteem the latter no other than a Piece of vile Empiricism.[124]

To resolve contemporary dilemmas over selecting the most efficacious and least harmful form of therapy, Turner proposed that a more open and accurate method of reporting case evidence was needed. His efforts to compile case studies are best exemplified by his tirade against Joshua Ward.

Ward, trained as a drysalter with no qualification in physic, surgery, or pharmacy, developed a reputation as a dispenser of his emetic 'Pill & Drop', a medicine that Marjorie Nicolson rightly claimed was 'one of the most notorious medicines of the XVIII Century'.[125] Ward had returned to London from France in the early 1730s, having 'supported himself chiefly by the sale' of the nostrum during sixteen years on the Continent.[126] He ascended the ladder of social recognition soon after his return by curing George II's dislocated thumb; a task the royal surgeons and physicians had been unable to achieve. From this newly derived social status, Ward began his practice, or more accurately his business, of dispensing his 'Pill & Drop' in London.

Principally, Ward advertised his 'Pill & Drop' as effective in treating numerous disorders, not the least of which was venereal disease. He claimed some twenty thousand individuals benefited from this remedy during his first nine months in London. But opposition to Ward's remedy, as well as his popish proclivity, quickly followed. He was first attacked on 28 November 1734 in the *Daily Courant*. The *Daily Journal*, the *Advertiser*, and *Gentleman's Magazine* soon joined the campaign against Ward's practice. His most relentless foe, however, was the *Grub-street Journal*.[127]

Turner, too, became one of Ward's 'most active critics'.[128] Indeed, Turner displayed more vehemence against Ward than upon any other single individual throughout all of his writings.[129] His argument combined elements of his disputes with Cockburn, Dover and Belloste. In addition, he explicitly opposed Ward 'trying Experiments with Remedies, so often hazardous' to 'Great Numbers of ... People, who, ... so readily come' to him, and 'promiscuously' taking his pill and drop in 'want of proper Information' of what they are actually taking.[130]

In order to demonstrate how Ward's claims ran contrary to what he represented as orthodox practice, Turner gathered much case evidence demonstrating the 'mischief' caused by Ward's 'Pill & Drop'. One 'poor Fellow', for instance, who had been Turner's patient 'for a Venereal Head-ach' produced 'between sixty and seventy Stools' and was in 'the most imminent Danger of his Life' after taking only 'One single Pill'.[131] Turner reprinted twelve similar incidents that had previously appeared in the *Grub-street Journal* and the *Gentleman's Magazine* for the 'Satisfaction of all those in whose Hands' the periodicals had 'not fallen'.[132] He was joined by many allies seeking to depose Ward by exposing the identity of the 'Pill & Drop'. By gathering testimonials as evidence of the previously untold miseries resulting from Ward's remedies, they hoped to convince the public to quit using his medicine.

The efforts to suppress Ward's claims offer insight into what contemporaries viewed as tests and proof of the effects of unknown remedies. Some, like 'Philo-Chymicus', and later, John Page, performed comparative assays between Ward's 'Pill & Drop' and known substances in order to ascertain the identity of any harmful ingredient in Ward's concoction.[133] Turner compared the colour and internal 'workings' of Ward's medicine with his general knowledge of other strong emetics, arsenicals and antimonials.[134]

In a pamphlet to James Jurin, one of the Censors of the College of Physicians, Turner explicitly adopted Robert Boyle's guidelines for experimentally testing Ward's remedies as a way of avoiding hazards. Specifically, Boyle had urged that any newly claimed remedy be put 'into the Hands of some learned and experienced Physician of his Acquaintance, to make ... Trials therewith, ... [that] might be done with Safety, and to report' the consequences back to him. If the remedy was found to be 'safe and beneficial', he 'encourage[d]' its use. But if it was in 'any ways detrimental', he argued that 'the Danger' be 'point[ed] out', and the remedy laid 'wholly aside'.[135]

Turner's actual plan to gather evidence against Ward's claims ran along somewhat different lines. Rather than promoting new trials of Ward's medicine in the hands of 'some learned and experienced Physician', Turner appealed to the public to 'send an Account of what they know ... from taking of these Medicines' (see Figure 7.3). He requested reports of both the 'Good and Bad Consequences', claiming that only in such gathering of information can 'equal Justice ... be done'. He specified that contributors provide 'Facts' which they had 'truly' observed, together with 'Patient's Names and Places of Residence'. Turner specifically urged parish clerks to 'lay the strictest Injunction' upon parishioners to 'make a true Report' of the incidents 'immediately ensuing' upon taking Ward's medicine. This information was to be left in a letter addressed to Turner at John Clarke's Bookshop under the

ADVERTISEMENT.

WHOEVER ſhall think fit, to ſend an Account of what they know, of the Good or Bad Conſequences (that equal Juſtice may be done the ſame,) from the taking of theſe Medicines; by a Letter directed for the AUTHOR, to be left at Mr. JOHN CLARKE's, Bookſeller, under the *Royal Exchange*, the Favour will be acknowledged; and provided the Facts are truly ſtated, with the Patients Names, and Places of Reſidence, at leaſt private Allowance for any diffident Perſon to ſatisfy themſelves of the Truth of ſuch Facts; the Perſons Name who ſends ſuch Information, ſhall be made no other Uſe of, than he himſelf gives free Permiſſion.

Figure 7.3

Daniel Turner's public appeal for first-hand testimonials regarding the efficacy of Joshua Ward's 'Pill & Drop'. From D. Turner, *The Drop and Pill of Mr Ward Consider'd* (1735, Wellcome Institute Library, London)

Royal Exchange. Turner swore to keep the informer's name confidential if so desired.[136] Thus, the public would compile the data of which Turner viewed himself the ultimate arbiter.

Whatever responses Turner may have received remain unknown. But all the publicity drawn to Ward's remedies appears to have actually supported his business. Ward established three privately run infirmaries in London for charity patients, for whom he took direct charge. This business captured the attention of some of Turner's professional colleagues. Dr Packe, for example, supported Ward's claims for his 'Pill & Drop' after seeing first-hand how Ward was treating his patients. He wrote an invective against Turner's 'injurious Treatment of Mr Ward' and encouraged Collegiate physicians to follow the 'God-like' example he claimed Ward exemplified by dispensing such 'extraordinary' medicines to the poor.[137] This dispute over Ward's claims illustrates the diversity and discordance over ideas about medicines and medical practice that existed among Collegiate physicians during this period.

Having thoroughly elucidated the role of external and internal medicine in his 1714 *De Morbis Cutaneis*, Turner also regarded it as quackery to treat only the outward or visible manifestations of a disease without considering whether the patient may also be suffering internally. An example of this type of quackery is seen in Turner's attack of the treatment described in a 1729 *Treatise on the Venereal Disease*. The author of this work, the renowned Leiden physician, Herman Boerhaave, described that venereal patients should be treated until all visible symptoms and signs of the disease had vanished.[138] If, 'after a strict Enquiry', no such signs were found, Boerhaave recommended that the external parts be washed, bathed, and covered with a mucilage or medicated emplaister.[139]

Turner argued that 'if the Absence of Symptoms ... [was to] be your Guide' for treating venereal patients, or even those suspected of being venereally infected, one had a 'sorry Chance' of curing a patient. For often, he claimed, individuals come to practitioners in fear after mingling with a 'foule' partner before any signs of the disease were 'to be expected'.[140] He further claimed that a consequential pox could develop if the practitioner only treated the visible clap instead of entirely expelling the venereal venom. Thus, Boerhaave's therapeutic aim of healing only the outward signs of venereal disease was, to Turner, quackery.

Turner expressed further concern over Boerhaave's implication that these patients should be treated with only external medicine. Treating a patient only with 'Lotions and cataplasms' and omitting the 'proper Alexipharms, internally administer'd' was, he argued, not 'much wiser' than expecting one 'bit by a mad Dog or Viper ... to be cur'd by [only] an outward Salve or Ointment'.[141] Rather, Turner claimed, one must 'evacuate the Malignity' of the 'Poison' first by 'Proper [internal] Purgatives', and then work to 'heal the Ulceration by Agglutinants or Balsamics'.[142]

Salivation, Friction or Purges?

Not all of Turner's contemporaries accepted salivation as a sure cure for syphilis. More adamantly, many denounced Turner's use of salivation as an 'ineffectual & pernicious' form of treatment. Some, like Montpellier physician, François Chicoyneau, proposed instead using small doses of 'Quicksilver Ointment' applied by 'friction'. His popularization of this treatment gained acclaim on the Continent where, as later in England, it became advertised as the 'Montpellier Method'.[143]

Turner openly opposed Chicoyneau's argument. Separately replying to each of Chicoyneau's points, Turner claimed experience had taught him to the contrary. Salivation had, he argued, annually cured 'Hundreds' of London patients, many of whom had 'fruitlesly' undergone previous treatments only with frictions.[144]

Another French physician, Pierre Desault of Bordeaux, claimed that the 'whole Secret' of curing syphilis derived from 'keeping the Patient's Body open by Clysters'.[145] Thereby, in modifying the 'Montpellier Method', Desault recommended that syphilitics be treated primarily by purging, accompanied by mild frictions. Turner opposed Desault's method, and resorted to his standard reply of never having 'seen or known' anyone with an inveterate pox to be cured without submitting to salivation.[146]

Desault met Turner's objections through correspondence, but their differences were aired to a wider audience through the intervention of London surgeon, John Douglas. Douglas claimed to have treated 'several hundreds' of venereal patients by friction and gentle purgation without ever sending 'one away uncured'.[147] In 1739, Douglas published an 'Answer' to Turner's 'bitter Invectives, false Insinuations and Gross Misrepresentations' of Desault's method of cure. Can 'T——r and company' not see, he argued, the difference between

> spitting four, five, or six pints a-day, for a month, sometimes two, while suffering with all of the parts of the mouth inflammed, ulcerated, tumified, and excessive[ly] painful, the

> face puffed up, the voice suppressed and inarticulate, and such a difficulty in swallowing that it is seldom possible to get the smallest quantity of liquids down, ... and taking two or three gentle purges a-week, and eating heartily all the while?[148]

Douglas identified four surgeons and six physicians in London who also favoured frictions without salivation, and claimed he was working to have all the local hospitals 'fitted up' to use purges and only mild frictions.[149] He also insinuated that Turner retained the practice of salivation primarily because it was more 'profitable' than short-term frictions.[150] Jean Astruc, France's most authoritative venerologist, also argued that 'all Degrees' of venereal disease could be removed by 'mercurial Remedies without [bringing the patient to] a Salivation'.[151]

Comparing Douglas' writing from 1737 to 1739 with that of Turner's over the preceding twenty years offers important insight into the change of accepted orthodox syphilis treatment. By the late 1730s, Douglas was promoting the use of only small amounts of mercury through frictions, certainly not enough to bring on the salivation that he despised. Support for frictions as opposed to salivation had begun gaining strength some ten years earlier. It was also at this time that guaiac, Dover's mercurial remedy, and eventually Ward's 'Pill & Drop' began to gain public and professional support as well. Thus, it appears there was a general, though gradual, movement towards finding alternatives to salivation as a method for treating syphilitics. Why was this so, and what does this say about Turner?

Neither the College of Physicians nor the Barber-Surgeons' Company formally urged practitioners to quit salivating patients in favour of other methods. Indeed, a constituency of both physicians and surgeons may be found among the supporters of each alternative therapy as well as among the old guard of 'sworn salivators'. Thus, promoting an alternative to salivation was not, at this time, so clearly divided along surgeon-physician lines as some historical accounts have suggested.[152] Although salivating hospital patients does not appear to have declined, salivations by public (i.e., non hospital) surgeons under whom patients had more say about their treatment distinctly lost the level of support it boasted of some ten years earlier. Several new alternatives were available whereby patients had more time to go about their day-to-day business, without having to be 'laid down' for a month. Only brief contact with practitioners was required, whether the practitioner was qualified or quack.

As Turner had argued, quackery was more inclusive than the

practice of qualified mountebanks. Indeed, any supporter of an unpopular remedy was considered by some members of the orthodoxy to be a quack. By 1739, salivation was no longer considered an orthodox form of treating syphilis by many qualified London practitioners. What then of Turner? If Douglas be our guide, and he is the only contemporary guide to this issue we have, he insinuates that by his 'bigottry' to 'antiquity', by his adherence to 'old' outmoded 'notions' and practices rather than adopting the less hazardous 'modern' forms of treatment, and by retaining 'old forms' of treatment merely 'because they are profitable', Turner was nothing better than a quack. 'Rail T[urner] rail! Your Craft's in danger, if the truth prevail'.[153]

Having led London's crusade against quackery from 1695 through 1739, Turner's practice was ultimately designated as quackery by a similarly aged, similarly trained surgical colleague. What an ironic turn for Turner, the physician most keenly attuned to abolishing quackery in all London. Turner's situation, at least from Douglas' view, exemplifies W.F. Bynum's dictum that 'quack is as quack does'.[154]

Notes

1 R.P.T. Davenport-Hines, *Sex, Death and Punishment: Attitudes to sex and sexuality in Britain since the Renaissance* (London: Collins, 1990), esp. 34-40; W.F. Bynum, 'Treating the Wages of Sin: Venereal Disease and Specialism in Eighteenth-Century Britain', in W.F. Bynum and Roy Porter (eds), *Medical Fringe & Medical Orthodoxy 1750-1850* (London: Croom Helm, 1987), 5-28; and Fernando Henriques, *Prostitution in Europe and the New World* (London: Macgibbon & Kee, 1963), 171. The contemporary French scene is described in F. Buret, *Syphilis in the Middle Ages and in Modern Times*, vols II and III (Philadelphia: F.A. Davis), 247-64, Claude Quetel, *Le Mal de Naples: historie de la Syphilis* (Paris: Seghers, 1986), translated by J. Braddock and B. Pike as *History of Syphilis* (Cambridge: Polity Press, 1990), 73-105, and Kathryn Norberg, 'From Courtesan to Prostitute: Mercenary Sex and Venereal Disease, 1730-1802', in Linda E. Merians (ed.), *The Secret Malady: Venereal Disease in Eighteenth-Century Britain and France* (Lexington, Kentucky: The University Press of Kentucky, 1996), 34-50.

2 Daniel Turner, *Syphilis. A Practical dissertation on the Venereal Disease* (London: J. Walthoe, 1717), 72. Unless otherwise noted, future references to *Syphilis* are taken from the 4th edition, 1732. See also R.P.T. Davenport-Hines, *Sex, Death, and Punishment*, 17-54.

3 Vern Bullough and Bonnie Bullough, *Women & Prostitution: A Social History*, (Buffalo, New York: Prometheus Books, 1987), 173. The sexual promiscuity in these areas filled contemporary ballads like those in *The London-Bawd; with her Character and Life*, 4th ed (London: for John Gwillin, 1711). See also 'The Playhouse is their place of traffic', chapter 14 of E.J. Burford's *The Orrible Synne: A Look at London Lechery from Roman to Cromwellian Times* (London: Calder & Boyers, 1973), 178-88. For a postmodern view of prostitution, see Shannon Bell, *Reading, Writing and Rewriting the Prostitute Body* (Bloomington, Indiana: Indiana University Press, 1994).

4 R.P.T. Davenport-Hines, *Sex, Death, and Punishment*, 38-39. For a discussion of the previous Providential views of venereal disease, see P. Quetel, *History of Syphilis*, 73-5 and John Addy's *Sin and Society in the Seventeenth Century* (London: Routledge, 1989), 145-7.

5 Edmund T. Burke, *The Venereal Problem; a description of the venereal diseases, their history, their prevalence in Great Britain, their effect upon the national life, the factors causing their propagation and spread, and a discussion of methods for their control and eradication* (London: H. Kimpton, 1919); Paul McHugh, *Prostitution and Victorian Social Reform* (London: Croom Helm, 1980); and Allan M. Brandt, *No Magic Bullet: A Social History of Venereal Disease in the United States Since 1880* (New York: Oxford University Press, 1985). For a modern re-reading of syphilis and prostitution, see also Mary Spongberg, *Feminizing Venereal Disease: The Body of the Prostitute in Nineteenth-Century Medical Discourse* (New York: New York University Press, 1997).

6 Phil-Porney [pseud. of Bernard Mandeville or Charles Ogle], *A Modern Defense of Publick Stews: or, An Essay upon Whoring, as it is now Practis'd in these Kingdoms* (London: A. Moore, 1724), later published under the title *The Natural History of Both Sexes*. Vern Bullough discussed Mandeville's attempts at reform in 'Prostitution and Reform in Eighteenth-Century England', *Eighteenth-Century Life*, ix, n.s. 3 (1985): 61-74.

7 R. Poole, *Physical Vade Mecum*, Dedication, xi.

8 D. Turner, *Syphilis*, 107. For a full account of the search for the origins of this prophylactic, see William E. Kruck, *Looking for Dr. Condom*, American Dialectic Society publication no. 66, (University, Alabama: University Alabama Press, 1981).

9 Daniel Turner, for example, placed the 'Geneology' of syphilis before the reign of Henry VI (1421-71) based on documents shown to him by Mr Grainger of the East India House, a 'Great Admirer of Antiquities', *Syphilis*, 12-13. St Thomas' Hospital

surgeon and enthusiastic antiquarian, William Beckett proposed similar arguments in three papers published in the *Philosophical Transactions of the Royal Society*. See his 'An Attempt to Prove the Antiquity of the Venereal Disease, long before the Discovery of the West Indies', *Philosophical Transactions of the Royal Society*, xxx (1717-19), 839-47; 'A Letter concerning the Antiquity of the Venereal Disease', *Philosophical Transactions of the Royal Society*, xxxi (1720-1), 47-65; 'A Letter to Dr. Halley ... in answer to Some Objections made to the History of the Antiquity of the Venereal Disease', *Philosophical Transactions of the Royal Society*, xxxi (1720-1), 108-12. Physician John Freind, however, placed the origin of the Neapolitan disease in the late fifteenth century in his *History of Physick*, 2nd edn, vol. 2 (London: J. Walthoe, 1727), 351, 356-8. Alfred Crosby's *The Columbian Exchange: Biological and Cultural Consequences of 1492* (Westport, Connecticut: Greenwood Publ. Co., 1972) remains a reputable historical account of the socio-demographic consequences of this exchange. For a recent investigative examination of pre-Columbian accounts, see Jon Arrizabalaga, John Henderson and Roger French, *Before Syphilis: The French Disease in Renaissance Europe* (New Haven, Connecticut: Yale University Press, 1996).

10 *The Practical Scheme of the Secret Disease* (London: H. Parker, 1730). R.P.T. Davenport-Hines labeled the chapter of his historical look into venereal disease as 'The Secret Disease' in *Sex, Death and Punishment,* 16-54, and James Cleugh depicted syphilis in the title of his *Secret Enemy: The Story of a Disease* (London: Thames and Hudson, 1954).

11 For a view into this delicate matter, see Mary Margaret Stewart, '"And blights with plagues the Marriage hearse": Syphilis and Wives', in Linda E. Merians (ed.), *The Secret Malady: Venereal Disease in Eighteenth-Century Britain and France* (Lexington, Kentucky: The University Press of Kentucky, 1996), 103-13.

12 Daniel Turner, *The Modern Quack*, as cited by W.F. Bynum, 'Treating the Wages of Sin', 20.

13 *The Practical Scheme of the Secret Disease*, 5.

14 D.Turner, *Syphilis*, 319.

15 J.K.Proksch's monumental bibliography remain the most comprehensive to date. See his *Die Litteratur uber die venerischen Krankheiten*, 3 vols in 5 (Bonn: Hanstein, 1889-1900). See also J.K. Proksch, *Die Geschichte der venerischen Krankheiten*, 2 pts (Bonn, Hanstein, 1895). Ludwig Fleck's *Genesis and Development of a Scientific Fact* (Chicago: University of Chicago Press, 1979);

D.B. Perett's 'Ethics and Error: The Dispute between Ricord and Auzias-Turenne over Syphilization, 1845-70', (Ph.D. thesis, Stanford University, 1977); and J.H. Jones' *Bad Blood. The Tuskegee Syphilis Experiment* (New York: Free Press, 1981) provide more recent histories of this disease. See also the Stanislav Andreski's Weberian analysis of *Syphilis, Puritanism and Witch Hunts. Historical Explanations in the Light of Medicine and Psychoanalysis with a Forecast about Aids* (Basingstoke, Hampshire: MacMillan, 1989).

16 This verbal imagery compensates for the paucity of contemporary artistic renderings of syphilis. R.S. Morton provided an artistic overview of 'Syphilis in Art' in a series of articles published in *Genitourinary Medicine*. For discussion of the art in the seventeenth and eighteenth centuries, see Part 3 of this series in lxvi (1990), 208-21. Two chapters in Linda E. Merians (ed.), *The Secret Malady: Venereal Disease in Eighteenth-Century Britain and France* (Lexington, Kentucky: The University Press of Kentucky, 1996), are also devoted to art. Namely, N. F. Lowe, 'The Meaning of Venereal Disease in Hogarth's Graphic Art', 168-82, and Rose A. Zimbardo, 'Satiric Representation of Venereal Disease: The Restoration versus the Eighteenth-Century Model', 183-95. Robert Wilkins provides several graphic representations of syphilitics in Chapter 11. 'Pox and Clap: The Great Unmentionables' in his *The Fireside Book of Deadly Diseases* (London: Robert Hale, 1994), 197-229.

17 D. Turner, *Syphilis*, 1739, 85.

18 Afflictions of the scalp were, at least among certain classes of men, quite noticeable as their heads were generally kept shaved beneath their wigs. For example, in order to show Turner the scabs on his scalp, one patient was described as first 'lifting up his wig, and taking off the Rags he had put on [the scalp] to prevent the[ir] Adhesion' to the wig. See Turner's *Syphilis*, 1727, 253.

19 D. Turner, *Syphilis Part II*, 187.

20 D. Turner, *Syphilis*, 28. Such arguments also appeared in contemporary literature accounting for the sores on plague victims.

21 John Marten, *A Treatise of the Venereal Disease*, 7th edn (London: for the Author, 1711), 456-7.

22 D. Turner, *Syphilis*, 1717, 26.

23 D. Turner, *Syphilis Part II*, 93-94.

24 Roy Porter provides a most useful overview of Marten's perspective of venereal disease in '"Laying Aside Any Private Advantage", John Marten and Venereal Disease', in Linda E. Merians (ed.), *The Secret*

Malady: Venereal Disease in Eighteenth-Century Britain and France (Lexington, Kentucky: The University Press of Kentucky, 1996), 51-67.

25 D. Turner, *Syphilis*, 124.

26 D. Turner, *Syphilis*, 1717, 17.

27 *Ibid.*, 24-5.

28 *Ibid.*, 81.

29 Malcolm Nicholson, 'The Metastatic Theory of Pathogenesis and the Professional Interests of the Eighteenth-Century Physician', *Medical History*, xxxii (1988): 281.

30 In Daniel Turner's lengthy preface to his translation of Aloysius Luisinus' *Aphrodisiacus, Containing a Summary of the Ancient Writers on the Venereal Disease* (London: John Clarke, 1736), ix-x. E.L. Zimmerman has more fully discussed this work in 'Early Collections of Syphilogic Works. Aloysius Luisinus and His Influence on Syphilology', *Bulletin of the History of Medicine*, iv (1936): 582-99.

31 John Quincy, *Lexicon Physico-Medicum; or, A New Physical Dictionary* (London: A. Bell, 1719), 157. According to John Quincy, the whites was a 'Distemper common to the Female Sex' arising from a 'Laxness of the Glands of the Uterus, and a cold pituitous Blood'.

32 D. Turner, *Syphilis*, 1717, 27. Turner mentioned a 'great Dispute among ... modern Writers' over distinguishing these diseases, but appears to have explicitly accepted Walter Charleton's distinction based upon the quantity of fluid and whether it flowed throughout the month (*ibid.*, 30-2).

33 *Medicina Flagellata: or, The doctor Scarify'd* (London: J. Bateman & J. Nicks, 1721), 18.

34 D. Turner, *Syphilis*, 1717, 34-5. Contemporary accounts also describe that a man's susceptibility to syphilis depended upon whether he was circumcised and whether the whores with whom he dallianced were frigid. For, as the physician Gideon Harvey had proposed in his *Great Venus Unmask'd*, frigid whores were 'less contagious' than those who openly enjoyed their pleasures.

35 D. Turner, *Syphilis*, 27.

36 R. Porter, *Health for Sale*, 135-9.

37 D. Turner, *Syphilis*, case 9, 362.

38 *Ibid.*, case 9.

39 F. Doherty, 'Anodyne Necklace', 281.

40 R.P.T. Davenport-Hines, *Sex, Death and Punishment*, 41.

41 W.F. Bynum, 'Treating the Wages of Sin' esp. 22-5.

42 William Clowes, *A Briefe and Necessarie Treatise, Touching the Cure of the Disease called Morbus Gallicus* (London: Flesher, 1587).

43 D. Turner, *Syphilis*, 1717, preface. Turner also described special medical preparations applied to candles which were passed up the genital openings to detect venereal caruncles, 61-2.

44 R. Campbell, *London Tradesman*, 52-3; and J.T. Hillhouse *The Grub Street Journal* (New York: Benjamin Blom, 1967 reissue), 263.

45 Jeremy Black noted the English gentry's preference for French surgeons in treating venereal disease in his *The British and the Grand Tour*, (London: Croom Helm, 1985), 111.

46 The Medical Library, St Thomas's Campus, UMDS, 'Charles Oxley Notebook, Case notes of surgical patients admitted to St Thomas's Hospital, 1725-26', MS. S2.a.6., final section 'Observationes and Ptyalismum pertinented'. See also P.K. Wilson, 'Sacred Sanctuaries for the Sick', 53-54.

47 John Douglas, *A Dissertation on the Venereal Disease*, Part III, 27.

48 Roy Porter noted that many London physicians spent their days in coffeeshops writing prescriptions and never actually saw most of their 'patients'. Yet, physicians of the early eighteenth century appear to have been more sympathetic to treat venereally diseased patients than the European physicians Ulrich von Hutten described two centuries earlier. Hutten described that physicians typically 'fled from the presence of syphilitics'. Hutten, *De Morbo Gallico*, 1730, as cited by R. Davenport-Hines, *Sex, Death and Punishment*, 25.

49 D. Turner dedicated the second section of his *Syphilis. Part II* to two surgeons. One of these, Mr James Dansie, surgeon to the Hospital at Kingsland, had, according to Turner, treated many syphilitics 'of high Rank and Condition'. The poor were also not deprived of syphilis. Stanley Dana Nash argued they, too, had their share of infected prostitutes. See Nash's 'Social Attitudes towards Prostitutes in London from 1752-1829' (Ph.D. thesis, New York University, 1980), 9.

50 James J. Walsh provides an interesting psychological explanation of historical cures in his *Cures. The Story of Cures that Fail* (New York: D. Appleton, 1923), esp. vii-ix, and 1-12.

51 D. Turner, *Syphilis*, 377-78. Similar reports for 1731-37 appear in D. Turner's *Syphilis. Part II*, 233. Linda E. Merians discusses The Lock as a speciality hospital for the treatment of syphilis in 'The London Lock Hospital and the Lock Asylum for Women', in Linda E. Merians (ed.), *The Secret Malady: Venereal Disease in Eighteenth-Century Britain and France* (Lexington, Kentucky: The University

Press of Kentucky, 1996), 128-45.

52 John Douglas, *Dissertation on Venereal Disease* Part III (London: For the Author, 1739), 53.

53 D. Turner, *Syphilis*, 1717, 147.

54 *Idem.*

55 *Ibid.*, 32.

56 D. Turner, *Syphilis*, 1727, 255-6.

57 *Ibid.*, 211.

58 *Ibid.*, 240.

59 *Ibid.*, 261.

60 *Ibid.*, 235.

61 *Ibid.*, 292.

62 *Ibid.*, 271, 300.

63 *Ibid.*, 208.

64 *Ibid.*, 275.

65 *Ibid.*, 224.

66 D. Turner, *Syphilis*, 1717, 36.

67 Edmund Packe, *An Answer to Dr. Turner's Letter to Dr. Jurin* (London: J. Roberts, 1735), 20.

68 J. Douglas, *Dissertation on Venereal Disease*, Part II, 37.

69 D. Turner, *Syphilis*, post case 30.

70 J. Marten, *Treatise of Venereal Disease*, 515.

71 J. Douglas, *Dissertation on Venereal Disease,* Part III, 153.

72 Turner noted the quack's common distribution of the Prince's Powder in *Syphilis,* 1717, 66. This same remedy was recommended in Quincy's *Pharmacopoeia Officianalis & Extemporanea; or, A Complete English Dispensatory* (London: A. Bell, 1719), 663, as cited in Leonard J. Goldwater's *Mercury. A History of Quicksilver* (Baltimore, Maryland: York Press, 1972), 239.

73 J. Marten, *Treatise of Venereal Disease*, 651.

74 D. Turner, *Syphilis*, 147, 154.

75 *Ibid.*, 370.

76 D. Turner, *Syphilis. Part II*, 41.

77 D. Turner, *Syphilis*, 1717, 106. George Urdang constructed a historical survey of the preparations and uses of calomel in his 'The Early Chemical and Pharmaceutical History of Calomel' in Tenney L Davis (ed.), *Chymia. Annual Studies in the History of Chemistry*, vol.1 (Philadelphia: University of Pennsylvania Press, 1948), 93-108.

78 Quincy's *Pharmacopoeia* (1719), listed sixteen forms of mercurials including crude quicksilver, Arcanum Joviale, Mercurius Sublimatus, Calomel, Mercurius Resuscitatus, Mercurius Praecipitatus ruber, albus, and viridus, The Prince's Powder, Panacae Mercurii rubra and

alba, Turpethum Minerale, Arcanum Corollinum, Aethips Mineral, and Cinnabar Nativum and Factitium. J. Marten's *Treatise of Venereal Disease* includes even more preparations of mercury, see 663.

79 D. Turner, *Syphilis*, 151.

80 *Ibid.*, 100-107.

81 Among the harmful consequences of crude mercury treatment Turner described were haemorrhages from the 'Lungs by the Mouth, and from the Brain by the Nose', blood vessels of the adnata 'burst[ing] open', and the loss of vast quantities of blood in the stool. See D. Turner, 'A Discourse on Quicksilver', in idem, *The Ancient Physician's Legacy Impartially Survey'd* (London: J. Clarke, 1733), 'By Way of Postscript', 131-80. John Marten, among many others, also noted that 'Ill prepared' and 'untimely Administration' of mercury often led to 'Tremors, Spasms, Pains, Weaknesses, Lamenesses, Impediment of Speech, loss of hearing, Tasting, Smelling, [and] decay of Sight. See Marten's *Treatise of Venereal Disease*, 651.

82 D. Turner, *Discourse on Quicksilver*, 144.

83 *Idem.*

84 *Ibid.*, 144-5

85 *Ibid.*, 143-4.

86 *Ibid.*, 136-8. Several contemporary experiments with crude mercury were reported in the Royal Society's *Philosophical Transactions*. Investigations somewhat similar to Turner's are to be found in Dr Madden's 'Account of what was Observed upon Opening the Corpse of a person who had Taken Several Ounces of Crude Mercury Internally', xxxix (1735-6), 291-4, and Dr Cantwell's 'Pernicious Effects of Crude Mercury given Internally', xl (1737-8), 139-42.

87 D.Turner, *Syphilis*, 1717, 106. Turner, however, like his contemporary Henry Bradley, was not opposed to using other mercurials internally. Bradley was primarily opposed to Thomas Dover's claims of the panaceic powers of crude mercury. See Bradley's *Physical and Philosophical Remarks on Dr. Dover's late pamphlet, entitled, The Ancient Physician's Legacy* (London: C. Rivington, 1733).

88 Turner specified that mercury's transport through the skin was aided by mixing it with terebinthe (turpentine) or Axungia (hog's lard). He disagreed with Gideon Harvey's widely reputed *Great Venus Unmask'd*, 2nd edn (B.G. for N. Brook, 1672), which advocated the use of many pots of Quicksilver (*ibid.*, 190-1). Additionally, he argued that patients would receive added benefit if allowed to rub in the mercurial unguent with their own hands. Bernardino Ramazzini

also described this as one way of avoiding this disease of surgical tradesmen. See his *Treatise of the Diseases of Tradesmen* (London: for Andrew Bell, Ralph Smith, Daniel Midwinter, Will. Hawes, Will. Davis, Geo. Straughan, Bern. Linot, Ja. Round, and Jeff Wale, 1705), 25.

89 D. Turner, *Syphilis*, 1732, 275.

90 D. Turner, *Syphilis*, 189-90.

91 *Ibid.*, 205. Among the 'accidents' Turner listed were diarrhoea, dysentery, sickness and vomiting, sore mouth, haemorrhages, over-costiveness, dropsy and palsy (title page).

92 D. Turner, *Aphrodisiacus*, xxxv.

93 Turner's phrase for the two hospitals as used in his *Apologia Chyrurgica. A Vindication of the Noble Art of Surgery* (London: 1695), 115. I previously described St Thomas' practice of treating venereal disease in 'Sacred Sanctuaries for the Sick', 40-1.

94 In 'Observations and Ptyalismum pertinented', in Charles Oxley Notebook.

95 D. Turner, *Syphilis*, 84, 217.

96 D. Turner, *Syphilis*, 1727, 173.

97 D. Turner, *Syphilis*, 1717, 51.

98 D. Turner, *Syphilis*, 1727, 62-3.

99 *Ibid.*, 173.

100 D. Turner's 'Prefatory Account of Professor Boerhaave's New Comments on the Venereal Disease; and some Animadversions thereon', prefaced to Turner's *A Discourse Concerning Gleets* (London: John Clarke, 1729), xlii. Robert S. Munger discussed the origin and uses of Guaiacum in 'Guaiacum, the Holy Wood from the New World', *Journal of the History of Medicine*, iv (1949), 196-229. B. Ramazzini suggests that quaiacum and mercury were not mutually exclusive remedies. Specifically, he found guaiacum useful to 'correct' the disorders 'occasion'd by the Mercury'. Ramazzini, *Diseases of Tradesmen*, 25.

101 R.S. Munger, 'Guaiacum', 218.

102 [D. Turner], *De Morbo Gallico*, by Ulrich von Hutten, translated by T. Paynell, revised by Daniel Turner (London: J. Clarke, 1730), Preface to the Reader. For a survery of Hutten's influence, see Thomas G. Benedek, 'The Influence of Ulrich von Hutten's Medical Descriptions and Metaphorical Use of Medicine', *Bulletin of the History of Medicine*, lxvi (1992), 355-375.

103 *Ibid.*

104 *Ibid.* Turner was probably also drawn to Hutten's explicit 'Reproof' of the action of the 'Secret-mongers' of quack medicines and those

'Learned Triflers' who, according to Hutten, 'thought nothing could be done but from certain physical Axioms ... [or according to] their "Canons" of theory', from which 'there was no deviating'. Rather, Hutten 'valued and esteemed' men not 'pinn'd ... down to these Rules ... but [who] practis[ed]' only by a 'simple Method, [which was] confirmed to them by Observation, and justified by Experience'. D. Turner, *De Morbo Gallico*, 1730, preface. Turner reiterated similar sentiments in his own writings some two centuries later.

105 Sufficient contemporary interest existed among some London physicians to introduce a 'new Impression' of classical medical works in the English vernacular, for example T. Dale's translation of Jodocus Lommius' *A Treatise of Continual Fevers* (London: T. Brotherton, 1732). Others turned their interest to compiling histories of particular diseases, such as John Armstrong's *Synopsis of the History and Cure of Venereal Diseases* (London: A. Millar, 1737).

106 D. Turner, *De Morbo Gallico*, Preface to the Reader.

107 St Bartholomew's, St Thomas', The Westminster Infirmary, Guy's, The Lock, and Kingsland hospitals.

108 Samuel Wilks and G.T. Bettany, *A Biographical History of Guy's Hospital* (London: Ward, Lock, Bowden & Co., 1892), 83.

109 Turner appears to have accepted the Barber-Surgeons' Company's 1695 denouncement of hospitals as 'breeding' grounds for 'Illiterate and Unskillful pretenders' of surgery. J.F. South, *Memorials of the Craft of Surgery*, 246-7.

110 Item 46 of the 1707 St Thomas' Hospital Orders, reprinted in R. Poole's *Physical Vade Mecum; or, Fifth Gift of Theophilus Philanthropos* (London: E. Duncomb, 1741), preface, lii. Poole also desired for these rules to be 'set up in each Ward, in publick View'.

111 In the hospital, a patient's ability to select their practitioners and their type of therapy was drastically curtailed from what N.D. Jewson, R. Porter and L. Beier have described for the contemporary city marketplace medical practice. N.D. Jewson, 'Medical Knowledge and the Patronage System', 369-85; R. Porter, *Health for Sale*, 2-59; and L. Beier, *Sufferers & Healers*, 8-50. For a contemporary view of syphilis treatment in French hospitals, see Joan Sherwood, 'Treating Syphilis: The Wetnurse as Technology in an Eighteenth-Century Parisian Hospital', *Journal of the History of Medicine and Allied Sciences*, l (1995), 315-39.

112 D. Turner, *De Morbo Gallico*, Preface to the Reader.

113 D. Turner, *Modern Quack*, To the Reader, 2-4.

114 D. Turner, *Apologia Chyrurgica*, 131.

115 *Ibid.*, postscript, 151-3.

116 D. Turner, *Syphilis*, 1717, close of preface.

117 L.A.G. Strong has previously recounted part of Turner's disagreement with Dover in his *Dr. Quicksilver 1660-1745. The Life and Times of Thomas Dover, MD* (London: Andrew Melrose, 1955), 163-6. Kenneth Dewhurst provided a more accurate account in his *The Quicksilver Doctor. The Life and Times of Thomas Dover Physician and Adventurer* (Bristol: John Wright, 1957), esp. 141-73. See also D.N. Phear, 'Thomas Dover 1662-1742, Physician, Privateering Captain, and Inventor of Dover's Powder', *Journal of the History of Medicine and Allied Sciences*, ix (1954), 139-56, and R.S. Morton, 'Dr Thomas ("Quicksilver") Dover, 1660-1742', *British Journal of Venereal Disease*, xxxxiv (1968), 342-6.

118 Dover scholars concur that the 'Gentleman of Trinity College, Cambridge' was Dover himself. Dover had received his M.B. from Cambridge in 1687; however, he had been admitted as a 'pensioner to the Scholar's table' at Caius College.

119 K. Dewhurst, *Quicksilver Doctor*, 155.

120 Thomas Dover, *The Ancient Physician's Legacy*, 6th edn (1742), 75, as cited by Dewhurst, 153.

121 D. Turner, *Ancient Physician's Legacy ... Survey'd*, 59.

122 Dover's work continued through at least eight editions, the last printed in 1771. And after both Dover and Turner were dead, respected authorities like George Cheyne continued to laud mercury as the 'only true Panacea, and Universal Antidote'. See Cheyne's *The Natural Method of Cureing [sic] the Diseases of the Body and the Disorders of the Mind* (London: G. Strahan and J. and P. Knapton, 1742), 119. D. Harley discussed similar outcomes of disputes in his 'Honour and Property', 138-64.

123 D. Turner, as cited by [T. Dover], *Enconium Argenti Vivi: a Treatise upon the Use and Properties of Quicksilver* (London: for Stephen Austin, sold by J. Roberts, [1733]), 61-4.

124 *Ibid.*, 62.

125 Marjorie H. Nicolson, 'Ward's "Pill and Drop" and Men of Letters', *Journal of the History of Ideas*, xxix (1968), 177. For other accounts on Ward, his reputation, and his medicines see H. Selfe Bennett, 'Joshua Ward, 1685-1761', *Proceedings of the Royal Society of Medicine. Section of the History of Medicine*, ix (1916), 100-12; W.A. Campbell, 'Portrait of a Quack: Joshua Ward (1685-1761)', *University of Newcastle Medical Gazette*, (June 1964), 118-22.

126 M. Nicolson, 'Ward's 'Pill and Drop', 177-8. Both the pill and drop primarily acted as emetics.

127 The campaign lasted several years, and according to a historian of

periodical publication, Ward's 'Pill & Drop' was given more space in the 'Grub-Street Journal' than any other subject in the paper's history. J. Hillhouse, *Grub-Street Journal*, 272.

128 Eric Jameson, *The Natural History of Quackery* (London: Michael Joseph, 1971), 45.

129 Given Turner's disputatious nature as evidenced by his more well-known dispute with his colleague James Blondel, the enormity of his opposition against Ward is even more significant.

130 D. Turner, *The Drop and Pill of Mr. Ward Consider'd* (London: J. Clarke, 1735), 28.

131 *Ibid.*, 15.

132 *Ibid.*, 29-32.

133 Philo-Chymicus, *Pillulae Wardearae Dissectio & Examinatio: or Ward's Pill Dissected and Examined ... Discover'd* (London: Osborne's, 1736), and John Page, *Receipts for Preparing and Compounding the Principal Medicines Made use of by the late Mr. Ward* (London: Henry Whitridge, 1763).

134 One London physician, Edmund Packe, opposed Turner's attempts to identify the composition of Ward's medicine by 'Analogy'. However, he did not describe any more rigorous chemical testing. Instead, he merely generalized that the effects of harsh emetics were not comparable to the benefits derived from Ward's 'Pill & Drop'. E. Packe, *Answer to Dr Turner's Letter*, title page. Packe attacked Turner piecemeal throughout the work.

135 E. Packe, *Answer to Dr. Turner's Letter*, 9.

136 D. Turner, *Ward's Drop and Pill ... Consider'd*, 38.

137 E. Packe, *Answer to Dr. Turner's Letter*, 34.

138 D. Turner, *Essay on Gleets*, xxix.

139 *Ibid.*, xx.

140 *Ibid.*, xxix.

141 *Ibid.*, xxii-xxiii. Elsewhere, Turner presented a similar argument against Cockburn's claim that only 'pocky Chancres' required 'Internals', for the rest were completely 'removed' by 'Topicks'. See Turner's *Syphilis*, 1732, 84.

142 D. Turner, *Discourse on Gleets*, xxii-xxiii. Turner avoided mercurials in treating a simple clap, for calomel, he claimed, was too strong of a purgative, and crude mercury lacked 'those Agglutinating Particles' (*ibid.*, 31, 51-2).

143 For a description of this method, see F. Chicoyneau, *The Practice of Salivating shewn to be of no Use or Efficacy in the Cure of the Venereal Disease*, translated by C. Willoughby (London: J. Roberts, 1723) and R. Brown, *A Letter from a Physician in London ... giving an Account of*

the Montpellier Practice, (London: J. Roberts, 1730).

144 D. Turner, *Syphilis*, 1727, 352.

145 D. Turner, *Syphilis. Part II*, 164.

146 Turner published correspondence from Desault's countryman, Monsieur Perochon of Bordeaux in favour of salivation in which Perochon claimed Desault's method was 'entirely exploded' such that he knew no one still following this practice in Bordeaux. D. Turner, *Syphilis Part II*, 245-6. It is noteworthy that this is the only contemporary Frenchman whose writing or practice Turner explicitly favoured. More often, Turner reflects the National tradition of remaining what Jeremy Black describes as 'Natural and Necessary Enemies' against France. See Black's *Natural and Necessary Enemies. Anglo-French relations in the eighteenth century* (London: Duckworth, 1986).

147 J. Douglas, *Dissertation on Venereal Disease*, Part III, 53. Interestingly, he claimed that although they were 'well cured' without the 'least visible sign of the distemper remaining', 'two or three ... still pretended to have pains here and there' due to the 'fear of paying' for their treatment.

148 *Ibid.*, 27.

149 *Ibid.*, 154-5. 'What say ye to this?' he added, 'Is not the milch cow [his depreciating term for Turner] in danger of going dry?' Douglas identified physicians Mead, West, Douglas, Sanders, Nisbett, Owen, and Wodrow in support of friction as well as surgeons Paisely, Deverell, Glen, and Horton.

150 *Ibid.*, 153.

151 J. Astruc, *Treatise on Venereal Disease*, as cited by D. Turner in *Aphrodisiacus.* Astruc held little regard for Turner's writing style, claiming it was 'not so methodically delivered ... nor placed in that order as might have ... afforded a fuller Insight into the Nature of this Distemper' as cited by Turner, *Syphilis. Part II*, viii. Turner, too, disapproved of Astruc's writing agenda to compile an encyclopaedic account of all known varieties and complications of venereal disease in a manner that obliterated the common presentation of the disease instead of concentrating on the practical means of cure. (Turner, *Syphilis. Part II*, 53-61).

152 C. Willoughby anticipated that opposition to salivation would generate a similar response from both physicians and surgeons as that over proposed safer and gentler methods of treating smallpox. See the introduction of his translation of François Chicoyneau's *The Practice of Salivating Shewn to be of no Use or Efficacy in the Cure of the Venereal Disease* (London: J. Roberts, 1723), iii.

153 J. Douglas, *Dissertation on Venereal Disease*, Part III, 153.
154 W.F. Bynum, 'Treating the Wages of Sin', 12.

8

Self-Styled Gentleman in London's Middle Class

As A.S. Byatt reminded readers interested in the biographical process,

> There are things which happen and leave no discernible trace, are not spoken of, though it would be very wrong to say that subsequent events go on indifferently, all the same, as though such things had never been.[1]

Indeed, much of Turner's life escapes present-day description as many details were unrecorded. Yet, agreeing with Byatt, it is 'wrong' for biographers to explain subsequent events of a person's lifetime without considering probable ways through which the subject's life has been affected. Daniel Turner, from at least the early 1690s, styled himself as a gentleman. Throughout his life, increasingly, he displayed the trappings associated with gentility. This concluding chapter chronologically reviews his attempts to attain a genteel standing. However, reminiscent of Byatt's above remarks, many of the details of his social climb from tradesman to gentleman were unrecorded.

Gentlemen

Turner's contemporary, Daniel Defoe, characterized a gentleman as 'A Person Born ...of some known or ancient Family; whose Ancestors have ... for some time been Rais'd above the class of mechanicks'. 'Heaven has given [the gentleman] ... his money, ... 'tis below him to get money, [but rather] his business to spend it.'[2] Thus, according to Defoe, the status of a gentleman in Enlightenment England was, to a large extent, fixed by his birthright.

Turner, however, had more humble beginnings than members of the genteel class which Defoe described. Born between the ranks of landed gentry and the artisans of the 'working' class, Turner was a member of what contemporaries identified as London's 'middlin' class. This 'middle rank of people', however, was not a distinct class. Rather, it was comprised of a 'number of differentiated ranks, orders, or degrees' of people.[3] Turner shared many of the 'genteel pretensions' representative of this class. In particular, Turner ambitiously strove to separate himself from the common lot, but had neither the birth right nor the wherewithal allowing him to be too upwardly mobile.[4]

Having been raised in a family of tradesmen, Turner had witnessed the need for many people to earn their living by working with their hands. During his early childhood, Daniel's brother, John Turner, the younger, like his father, John Turner, the elder, worked as a tallow chandler in their own home. This 'nauseous greasy Business' was hardly a gentleman's pursuit.[5]

Daniel also learned from an early age that profits could be gained from a trade. His brother, Samuel Turner, had acquired enough money through the taylor trade to 'raise' several estates.[6] John Turner the elder also became prosperous through his handicraft. At the time of his death in 1697, he bequeathed considerable sums to his family. Daniel's substantial £500 inheritance offered him a financial boost at precisely the time his own life's work was beginning.[7] This boost may indeed have provided him the wherewithal from which he sought to improve himself above the status of a common tradesman.

Following his father, Turner also became financially successful in his chosen trade. As a surgeon, he earned fees of up to £50 per year per patient.[8] Additionally, he maintained a townhouse and surgery in London's affluent Devonshire Square (see Figure 8.1).[9] If we believe his own account, patients came to desire his services over other practitioners, and colleagues recognized him as a valued consultant as well. Thus, Turner's practice was successful in several ways.

Turner's success as a surgeon appears to have been the direct result of a strong work ethic. This ethic was in no small way related to his 'duty' to serve as a useful 'hand-servant' to God. His religious living was also part of his pursuit of leading a virtuous life. Being in 'constant pursuit of Virtue' was, according to Turner's contemporary John Littleton-Costeker, how one

> Daily arrives at superior Degrees of Excellency; and 'tis from such Examples a Person is encouraged to become a good Christian: since he that is once so happy aspires to no less Things than to please and glorify God, to promote the general Good of Mankind, to be a Protection to the Virtuous in Distress, and to improve, as far as is possible, his personal Excellences in this Life, and to secure himself hereafter a most glorious and happy State in the World to come.[10]

Equally important, virtuous living was also considered the 'most important qualification of true gentility'.[11] Turner's constant pursuit of virtue may be seen not only as living according to strict religious convictions, but also as a visible display of genteel status. Indeed,

Turner exemplifies what D.C. Coleman has described as typical of many individuals of this period who 'possessed' enough 'ambition' to play the 'great game of life' of 'cross[ing] that divide' which distinguished the gentility from the common people.[12]

Turner and the Royal Society

Turner began his social climb early in his surgical career. Unlike many other surgeons or even the tradesmen in his own family, Turner never took an apprentice. It was quite unusual for a man like Turner, whom contemporaries regarded as a capable and masterful surgeon, never to have served as master to a young apprentice. Such a tutelage would have enhanced Turner's income – and acquiring wealth, after all, was necessary to acquire the trappings of gentility.[13] However, taking an apprentice would also have emphasized Turner's status as a tradesman. According to his contemporary, John Chamberlayne, 'All are accounted gentlemen in England who maintain themselves without manual labour'.[14] Turner's eventual turn to medical practice reinforced his desire to distinguish himself from the 'mechanick part of mankind'.

Turner's ambitions to elevate himself above the typical surgeon are also seen in his submission of a series of case reports to the Royal

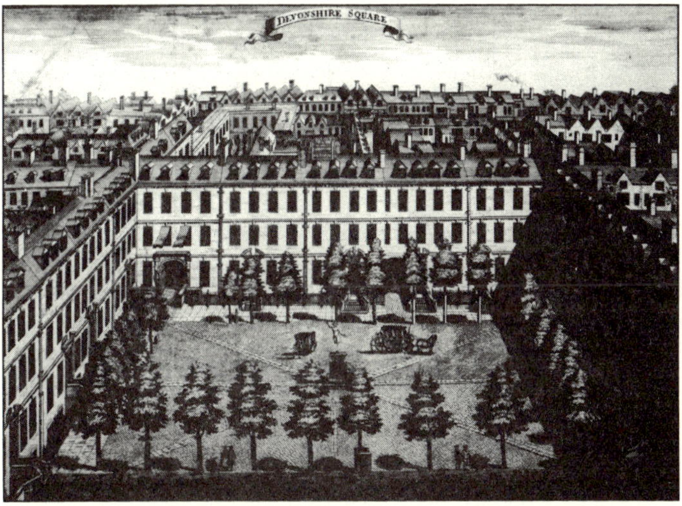

Figure 8.1
Devonshire Square, Bishopsgate Ward, London (Plate 39, *London Described*, 1731; Guildhall Library, London)

Society.[15] At this time, it was quite unusual for a surgeon to prepare any written reports, let alone reports before one of London's most august gatherings of gentlemen and scholars. Moreover, most of the reports presented before this Society were written by men who shared similar University education to the natural philosophers, physicians, and antiquaries who comprised the Society's fellowship.

In order to submit these reports, Turner had first gained the patronage of Edward Tyson, a gentleman by birth, Oxford graduate of medicine, leading London physician, lecturer at Barber-Surgeons' Hall, and anatomical procurator for the Royal Society.[16] Tyson had urged Turner to prepare reports for the Society about several autopsies which they had performed together. Submitting this series of consecutive reports before the Royal Society on Tyson's recommendation suggests that Turner was perhaps being 'groomed' for eventual election into the Society's fellowship. Tyson had proposed seven successful candidates to the Society's electorate before 1700.[17] As a Fellow of the Royal Society (F.R.S.), Turner would certainly have been placed among the leading scholars and gentlemen in London. But alas, this goal was never attained.[18]

We can only speculate as to why Turner was not admitted to the Royal Society. As mentioned in Chapter Five, Tyson himself had, by the mid-1690s, lost the favour of many Collegiate physicians in the Royal Society due to his opposition to the attempts of the 'ancient fellows" to control London marketplace medical practice. Thus, Turner's allegiance to Tyson may have actually diminished his chances of gaining Royal Society fellowship. Turner may not have been well known to Fellows other than Tyson. His trade practice of surgery was unlikely to have brought him into contact or consultation with many Society Fellows. Additionally, Turner was not a freemason, and thus he missed another opportunity to become known to the many masons in the Society.[19] In the Royal Society, men required an 'informal network of influence and dependency' like the masons to assure fellowship.[20] Historian Michael Hunter has argued that the better known the candidates were to the Fellows, the greater the likelihood of their gaining admission.[21] Who you knew was also important in gaining Fellowship as no 'specific procedures of certification and promotion' existed.[22] This was particularly true for surgeons as electing members of the Society viewed them, with very few exceptions, as unworthy of fellowship. Only six surgeons were admitted as Fellows between 1667 and 1700.[23] Most of these had Royal patronage or the backing of Hans Sloane, the influential Secretary of the Society.

One surgeon, William Cowper, who had also gained Tyson's patronage was elected a Fellow of the Royal Society. What, then, did Cowper have in his favour which Turner did not? Both Turner and Cowper completed their surgical apprenticeships in 1691, and both had their first papers on anatomy presented before the Royal Society two years later. Cowper, however, had proceeded to more elaborate writings on anatomical experimentation. He compiled a major opus, *The Anatomy of Humane Bodies*, in 1698. The anatomical descriptions in this work were based upon his extensive observations and experimentation, ideals upon which the Royal Society was founded.[24] Moreover, Cowper's contribution helped distinguish him as a scholar. As sociologist Steven Shapin has demonstrated, scholars were one of the 'special sort[s] of person[s]' the Royal Society brought into their fellowship.[25]

Without having been a gentleman from birth, not having acquired a University education, and not having become a published scholar in the same sense as Cowper, Royal Society Fellows appear to have given Turner little notice. Although he later offered one additional case study to the Society[26] and regularly kept abreast of the Society's *Philosophical Transactions*, one door to his desired elevation to a higher genteel status was closed.

Given this situation, it might at first appear unwarranted to search for further possible associations between Turner and the Royal Society. However, finding the motto of the Royal Society, 'Nullius in Verba' (on the word or authority of no one), beneath an engraved portrait of Turner (ca. 1714) prompted further investigation (see Figure 8.2).[27] Why would Turner, not a Fellow of this Society, publicly associate himself with their motto? Michael Hunter has interpreted Turner's use of the motto as suggestive of the 'growing kudos of the Society'.[28] Displaying the motto of this well-known Society of gentlemen and scholars suggests that Turner may have used it as both decorum and as an outward display that he held many ideals and, perhaps at least in his mind, the status that outsiders associated with the Fellows of this Society. Contemporaries in London and on the Continent who saw this widely published portrait may have, as one historian has done, assumed Turner had ascended to F.R.S. standing.[29]

In the late seventeenth century, this motto represented the Society's 'determination to withstand the domination of authority and to trust all statements by appeal to the facts'.[30] Like the Society, Turner claimed to have refused accepting any word or individual as an authority whose claims opposed the observations he found in his own practice. In this sense, there is no discrepancy between the message in his writings and the motto found beneath the frontispiece portrait he included in many of his publications.

A 'Professional' in Early Enlightenment London

Finding few surgeons turning to medicine suggests that physicians discouraged this occupational shift. Indeed, part of the idea of a 'profession' represented having the right to exclude individuals whom fellow professionals deemed as unqualified. Many members of the College scorned the 'sort of men not of academical but mechanic education' as unfit to practise physic.[31] Although Turner had proved himself knowledgeably competent in the medical art, and had enjoyed long-standing working relationships with several London physicians, he likely received considerable rebuff from the Collegiate physicians who abhorred this entrée into medicine.

Before I examine the consequences of Turner's move into the

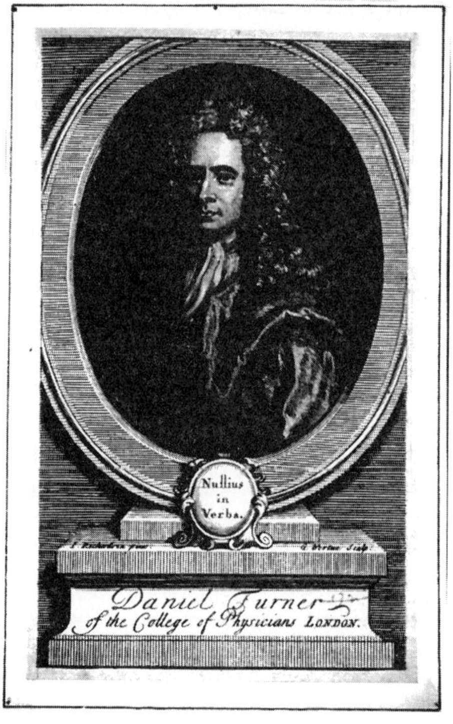

Figure 8.2

Daniel Turner and motto. (G. Vertue engraving after J. Richardson, ca.1712-14; Wellcome Institute Library, London) 'profession' of physic, it is necessary to explain the historical construct of 'profession' and 'professional'. 'Controversy exists as to what constitutes a profession and, indeed, whether any universal definition is possible.'[32] Toby Gelfand's words of 1980 remain potent nearly two decades later. As he showed in his exemplary study of the eighteenth-century emergence and restructuring of the French surgical 'profession', surgeons exhibited the qualities which, at different periods over the century, likened their organizational structure to that of physicians – a learned 'profession' in the traditional sense.

Identifying what specifically constituted professions in early modern England remains an active area of investigation. Gelfand argued that, for the French, few would 'dispute medicine's claim' to professional status.[33] However, Margaret Pelling has offered a series of examples and future questions to consider around her argument that the 'professionalism' of medicine in England existed more as a goal than a reality.[34] Harold Cook has demonstrated that the standards by which physicians gained authority as professionals had shifted by the early eighteenth century.[35] Geoffrey Holmes, concentrating upon Augustan England, considers that in addition to clerics, lawyers, and physicians, many 'nascent professional occupations' existed during this period.[36] By 'nascent professional occupations', Holmes meant all of the 'organizational structures' which upheld three basic characteristics: providing a vocation for the whole of a man's working life, undergoing a long and carefully regulated course of training in that vocation, and working in a vocation through which men offered services to their community.[37] Among these 'nascent professions', Holmes included architects, school masters, writers, and surgeons among others.

Building upon Holmes' work, Wilfrid Prest has challenged scholars to examine two new lines of research in order to better understand the socio-cultural formulation and acceptance of nascent professions. First, he proposed that future investigation should focus upon less eminent, more common 'professionals' in order to ascertain more typical information about who was actually involved in these careers and the variety of ways these individuals gained this 'professional' status. Second, Prest claimed that both the 'social identity' of these 'professionals' and the nature of work they performed must be explained.[38]

Turner's career move offers a study of a less eminent practitioner who described both the social differences between surgeons and physicians as well as the different types of work he performed as a surgeon and physician. Therefore, examining Turner's career change in light of Prest's challenge allows us to develop a better understanding of how one individual who became part of a 'profession' presented himself to and was received by other members of society.

General historical accounts lead us to believe that most physicians during the early eighteenth century distinguished their types of practice from the more manual practice of surgery. Surgery was literally a handicraft, whereas physic was, at least in the traditional sense, a 'profession'. Paula Backscheider has described that holding the status of a 'professional' in Defoe's London 'told' contemporaries that one was 'a person with some power' and that one did not have to earn a living by working with his hands.[39] In this sense, it may be accepted that turning to the practise of physic from the practice of surgery would have 'told' Turner's contemporaries that he was no longer exclusively practising the manual trade of surgery. Also, by casting away a literal handicraft image, Turner was possibly improving his social standing.

As a surgeon, Turner effected little change in reforming surgical training and practice. However, his persistence in proposing ways to improve the surgical art after he became a physician suggests he envisioned his new position as influential towards the acceptance of his proposals. For at this time, physicians of the College maintained a stronghold over the practice of surgery, dictating what treatments surgeons could and could not perform. Thus, by offering instruction to young surgeons and becoming established as an authority in this field, Turner appears to have believed himself more able to effectively reform the surgical art as a physician author than as a practising surgeon.

Turner also used his status as a physician to inform fellow physicians about what he perceived to be their erroneous conceptions of surgical practice. For example, Turner explicitly defended surgeons against the 'Charges' raised in fellow physician, Walter Harris' *Dissertationes Medicae & Chirurgicae*. Turner offered multiple cases as evidence to dissuade readers of Harris' 'very gross (and surely undeserved)' claims that surgeons were 'ignorant', 'cruel and hard-hearted', and prone, whether for 'Lucre' or 'to save [themselves] the Trouble of looking longer after' patients, to a 'Wicked' and hurried malpractice.[40]

Successful Upward Mobility

Having cast away his handicraft image as a surgeon, Turner, the physician, acquired a professional status which greatly affected his life. In December 1711, Turner quit surgical practice and became a licensed physician. Within a month of gaining this professional standing, he married Elizabeth Altham.[41] The timing of Turner's change in professional and marital status suggests that they were not unrelated.

Elizabeth was a daughter of James Altham, a member of the English landed gentry with an estate, Mark Hall, in Latton, Essex.[42] Several of her brothers and brothers-in-law were university-educated clergymen and attorneys.[43] Allowing Elizabeth to marry a 'professional' such as a physician would have been more acceptable to the genteel Althams than her marrying a tradesman surgeon. To further ensure the Althams of his worthiness, Turner drew up a pre-nuptial agreement with his 'intended', guaranteeing her £1000 if she survived him.[44] Through this marriage, Elizabeth gained financial security and Turner, by marrying into landed gentry, gained upward mobility.

Turner lived during a period when social prestige and influence were integrated with an 'economic gradation' in the 'pyramid' of wealth.[45] His decision to become a physician better enabled him to amass considerable wealth. Contemporary physician Richard Mead averaged an annual income of £5,000 to £6,000 from his practise of physic.[46] Others enhanced their professional income through investments. David Hamilton, for instance, purchased £10,000 in Bank of London stock. John Radcliffe placed £35,000 in a new annuity loan, and Caleb Coatesworth, who like Turner had turned from surgeon to physician, invested £25,000 in the East India stock in 1723-4.[47]

Turner displayed his prosperity in part through the acquisition of land. As early as 1727, he invested in several estates around the home counties. These transactions involved approximately 136 acres of land in the parishes of Datchworth and Aston in Hertfordshire. In succeeding years, he acquired five other estates in Hertfordshire, Essex, and Middlesex, together with two freehold houses, one ground rent and one freehold estate around the city of London.[48] It was 'quite usual', F. Bastion has claimed, for a prosperous man to 'invest some of his profits in land, ... as a first step towards establishing a family of landed gentry'.[49] Moreover, displaying wealth through land holdings represented another way in which Turner put forth a genteel image.

Turner also displayed his wealth in an impressive retinue of attendants maintained at his London townhouse (see Figure 8.1). Having the attendance of servants, maids, coach and coachmen showed that Turner was a prosperous man.[50] But then, this was a typical retinue for Turner's Devonshire Square neighbours including

Richard Craddock and George Finch, Governors of St Bartholomew's Hospital, and the Levant merchant, Edward Radcliffe. The Duke of Devonshire also maintained an elaborate residence on the square.[51] Turner informed his readers of his affluent surroundings by identifying his residence at the close of the preface in each of his major writings.

As early as 1714, Turner displayed a coat of arms beneath one of his engraved portraits (see Figure 8.3).[52] Publicly displaying these arms was one of Turner's most visible attempts to define himself as a gentleman. However, the arms Turner displayed were not his by 'right' of descendance. Rather, they had originally been granted to John Turner of Bletchingley (Surrey) in 1604.[53] In Daniel Turner's lifetime, these Turner arms were held by Thomas Turner, of St Dunstan's-in-the-West until 1715, and by his son John, of Helden, until 1747.[54]

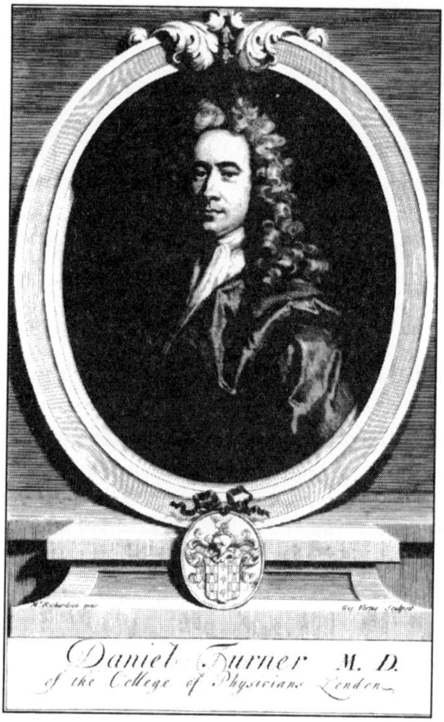

Figure 8.3
Daniel Turner and coat of arms. G. Vertue engraving after J. Richardson, ca.1712-14 (Wellcome Institute Library, London)

T.D. Mathew, Windsor Herald of the College of Arms, supports my research findings that Daniel Turner had no 'demonstrable right' to these arms by descent.[55] Turner may, however, have purchased the right to display this coat of arms from London's Painter-Stainer's Company which, early in the eighteenth century, carried out 'legitimate searches' for heraldry rights.[56] Nevertheless, by emblazoning these arms beneath his portrait, Turner created an image of his descendance from a distinguished family. As Defoe claimed, 'We live in a general Disguise, and like the Masquerades, every Man dresses himself up in a particular Habit'.[57] Knowing, however, that Turner's arms were probably purchased, and certainly not his by descendance, provides further evidence that Turner intentionally 'dressed' himself in the 'Habit' of recognizable genteel status.

Turner's 'social consciousness', to use Harold Perkin's phrase, became formally displayed through a 'stylized behaviour'. Displaying the appearances of success and gentility were crucial aspects of the 'Character' which Turner deemed medical as well as surgical practitioners should uphold. 'It will behove' a practitioner, Turner argued, to 'appear always neat in his Attire, avoiding the Extremes of the Fop and the Sloven'. As William Hogarth claimed, 'we know the very minds of the people by their dress'.[58] Daniel, too, may have learned through his brother Samuel, a taylor, about the powerful use of clothing as a means of displaying status. Many considered that their taylor 'not only makes their Dress, but, in some measure, may be said to make themselves'.[59] Additionally, Turner claimed it was important to 'have such a competent Estate, as may support a handsome Figure in Life' in order to be 'taken Notice of in the World'.[60]

Each of these displays served at least two purposes for Turner. First, they fulfilled his own criteria of the 'Character' or 'Properties' required of a physician. And second, they were consistent with Turner's attempts to display himself as a gentleman. As Perkin argued, there are many 'outward signs' which 'proclaim[ed]' a person's self-perceived status. For Turner, his manner, speech, deportment, dress, liveried equipage, size of house and household, and, most probably, even the kind of food he ate were adopted as a form of displaying a particular position in society.[61] Not only did he use these trappings to acquire patients, but he appears to have been ever conscious of using them to style himself as a gentleman.

Turner as Author and Authority

Turner claimed that after twenty years of practice, he found surgery a most 'toilsome' way to earn a living.[62] As a physician, Turner

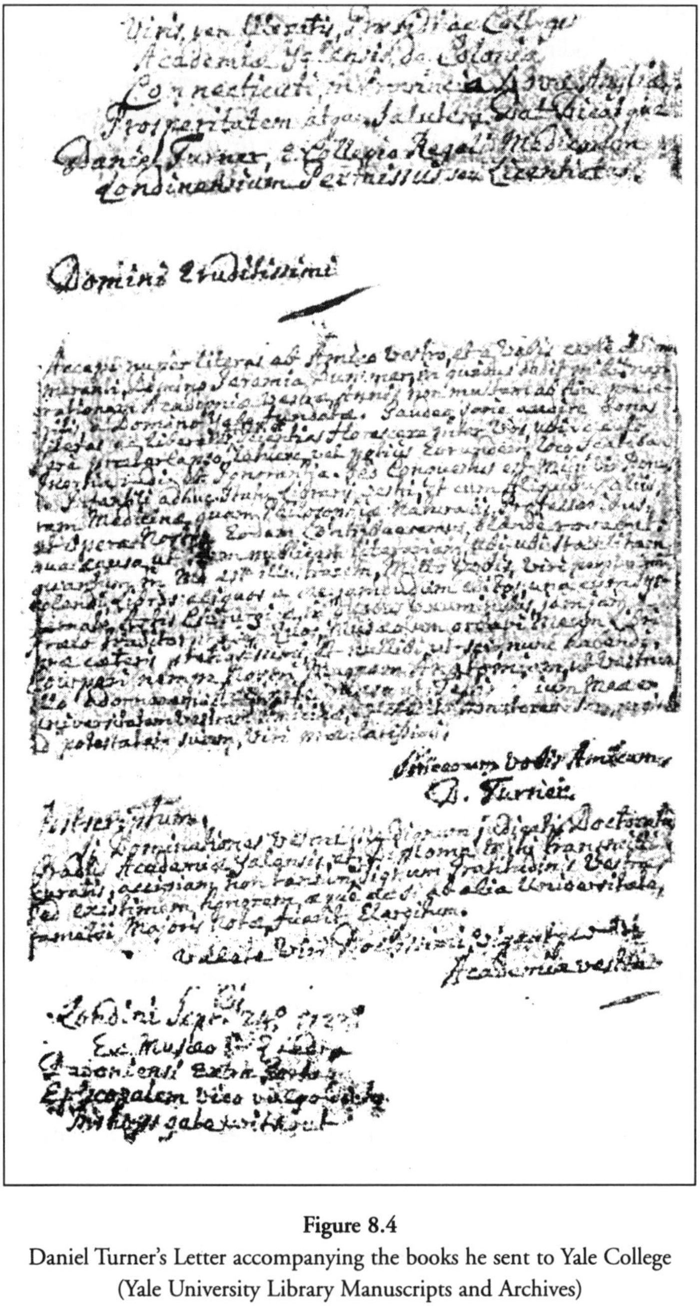

Figure 8.4
Daniel Turner's Letter accompanying the books he sent to Yale College
(Yale University Library Manuscripts and Archives)

described himself as much more at 'leisure'.[63] Leisure, as Perkin reminds us, was not synonymous with idleness. Rather, it strictly meant having the 'freedom to pursue any interest, taste or pleasure consonant with the honour of a gentleman', without 'further need to demean oneself by earning a living'.[64]

Turner used his newly acquired leisure time to read and to write. 'He who is not at leisure to survey the Labours of others', Turner argued, 'is scarcely likely to oblige us with any of his own.'[65] Turner, indeed, 'obliged' us with many of his own works. He published six major texts between 1714 and 1739. Seven relatively shorter treatises and revisions of two 'ancient' works also appeared over the same period. Compared with his contemporary physicians, Turner's writing represents a major literary output. The extent of this output suggests that Turner was ambitious to become known through the quill and the press.

What did Turner hope to gain from authorship? His prolific writings suggest that he was driven to become recognized as an authority: specifically, an authority in surgery. This focus stems in part from his familiarity with this field. During his twenty years of surgical practice, he had collected many 'loose Pages' of extensive notes on the patients he treated.[66] In their 'undigested' state, Turner viewed them to be of little use to anyone. But by converting them into a book which would serve as instructive guidelines for 'junior' surgeons, he could secure their usefulness and become a published author. For Turner, this accomplishment appears to have implied gaining some sense of authority as well.

The multiple, up to six editions of seven of his surgical writings suggest that he became well known in his field.[67] His publishers and booksellers offered testimonials that there was 'no need to say any thing to recommend [Turner's *Art of Surgery*]' as it had already been 'so well approved by the most noticed Practitioners of the same Art'.[68] Thus, relying upon these accounts and the author's own claims, Turner appears to have become established as an author, and thereby, an authority in his field.

Turner turned to publishing, in part, to gain the acceptance of his university-trained medical colleagues. Most physicians had a common educational background, but Turner was, in many ways, an outsider and a self-made physician with only a self-education in physic. Writing, therefore, offered Turner an opportunity to display his knowledge in an attempt to convince his critical colleagues of his worthiness to be recognized as a physician.[69]

Additionally, he used writing to address the immorality of

quackery. Like the efforts taken by the Society for the Promotion of Christian Knowledge, the Society for the Encouragement of Learning, and the whole Reformation of Manners campaign, Turner addressed the literate public with a religious zeal, cautioning them about the dangers they faced, and promoting ways through which they could escape these dangers.

Turner appears to have had another motive as well: to preserve the memories of the dead. His reliance upon the descriptions of 'ancient' writers exemplifies his appreciation for their authoritative wisdom. In a manner similar to the humanists, Turner used the 'ancients' to 'present examples to the living'.[70] Most explicitly, his case studies represented histories 'by way of example', teaching readers how to virtuously pursue their art.[71] Of course, a display of 'classical' knowledge was also a sign of gentility.

Finally, Turner also wrote for financial gain and as a means of demonstrating virtuous living. In a meritorious manner, he sought 'honest profit' for his work. For some authors, the 'want of money' was the 'only motive to writing'.[72] But for Turner, it was also his 'Duty' to share the knowledge and abilities he viewed himself as holding – a duty both to the public and to God. As discussed in Chapter Five, Turner's religion was central to his lifework. Thus his writing, in part, fulfilled his earthly worthiness and proved himself reverent to God.

Turner Buys a Medical Degree

In her popular *Restoration London*, Liza Picard argues that surgeons were not commonly viewed as gentlemen, although 'some of them confused the issue by qualifying as physicians as well'.[73] Turner

> 1723 Mr. *Daniel Turner* of *London* ſent to the Library ſundry Volumes of his own Works, on Phyſick and Chirurgery; and a Collection of other valuable Books, principally on the ſame Subject; and particularly the large Volume of *Cowper's Anatomy*. Whereupon the Truſtees ſent him a *Diploma*, creating him *Doctor of Phyſick*.

Figure 8.5

Description of Turner's gift to Yale as recorded in Thomas Clap's *The Annals or History of Yale College* (1766, Beinecke Rare Book and Manuscript Library, Yale University Library) contributed to this confusion for historians. In September 1722, Turner forwarded a letter to the 'President and College of the Academy of Yale' in the 'Colony of New Haven'. The letter accompanied a collection of twenty-five books he 'robbed' from his own library (see Figures 8.4 and 8.5).[74] This contribution was, in part, a response to the Academy's efforts to build up their library. As early as 1707, potential London book donors were being solicited for contributions. 'Chiefly through the efforts of Jeremiah Dummer', Connecticut's 'agent' in London, more than seven hundred volumes had been collected by 1714, and six hundred more were added during the following four years.[75] Dummer had solicited books from luminaries including Richard Steele, Richard Bentley, William Whiston, Dean (later Bishop) Kennet, John Davie, Isaac Watts, Joseph Thompson, Richard Blackmore, Edmund Andes, William Bates, Richard Horsey, Mr Goodchild, and Elihu Yale. Additionally, natural philosophers, physicians, and surgeons including John Woodward, Thomas Burnet, Edmond Halley, John Allen, John Atkins, John Colbatch, Richard Mead, Hans Sloane, and Isaac Newton contributed copies of their own writings to Yale's library.[76] Yale librarian, Andrew Keogh later claimed that 'practically all of the current books of importance' were included in Dummer's shipments.[77]

Turner was not one of the most 'Liberal Benefactors' or 'Generous Gentlemen' through whom, according to the Trustees, the 'Influence of Heaven ... cast a smiling aspect' upon the 'Nursery' of Yale College.[78] Sir John Davie donated 168 works, primarily theological. Elihu Yale gave 32 books in 1714 and another 437 in 1718, many of which were medical writings. Far above all other benefactors, Bishop George Berkeley donated 'some nine hundred volumes' in 1733. Still, Turner's contribution, some twenty-five titles in thirty-two volumes, was considerably more substantial than the donations from other medical or surgical men.[79] His contribution included eight works of biblical commentary, seven of British history, topography, and trade, one work on ethics, four works by other medical authors and five volumes of his own writings.[80] (The specific titles he contributed are listed in Appendix 3.)

Turner explicitly intended his donation to help 'good literature and the liberal arts and sciences ... flourish' in a land where, he claimed, only 'crude indifference and ignorance' had previously 'reigned'.[81] It is difficult to ascertain what these particular works signify about Turner or how they may have influenced his own life. For example, it is unknown whether most of these works came into Turner's hands through inheritance, through purchase, or as gifts;

thus, speculations about the importance any individual book may have had to Turner are inconclusive.[82] However, the entire donation distinctly altered his life.

In the postscriptum of the letter accompanying this contribution, Turner noted that in return for these books, he would be most grateful to receive a doctoral degree from the Yale College.[83] Jeremiah Dummer supported this plea, endorsing Turner as a 'very Learned Physician and worthy Gentleman', and encouraged the Academy authorities that they would 'do [them]selves great honour' by conferring the desired degree.[84] On the following commencement day at Yale College, 11 September 1723, Timothy Woodbridge, rector, *pro tempore*, honoured this request, and granted Turner an honorary Doctor of Medicine degree, the first medical degree issued from Colonial America.[85] A diploma signifying this degree was forwarded to Turner.[86]

Dummer claimed he 'took ... pains' to get the censors of the College of Physicians to 'honour & ratify' this diploma, but his efforts 'prov'd in vain'. That College, he claimed, was presently 'enrag'd' at how easily English 'physicians' could purchase medical diplomas from Glasgow for only 'small sums' without ever being examined by the College. And in an attempt to 'discourage every thing of that kind', the College continued to show 'no Countenance but to Graduates at Oxford & Cambridge'.[87]

It is somewhat ironic that Turner himself had previously denounced those who secured 'surreptitious' degrees from diploma mills like Glasgow.[88] Yet he regarded his Yale degree as quite distinct from a purchased degree. He respectfully accepted this doctorate as a symbol of his erudition of medical knowledge, his recognition as an accomplished author, and his affluence to contribute to a learned institution's growing 'Republic of Letters'. Thereafter, he openly signed himself 'Daniel Turner, M.D., of the College of Physicians in London'. Contemporaries, too, acknowledged Turner's doctoral status, although some jested that his M.D. more truthfully represented a *multum donavit* than a learned title.[89]

Other Gentlemanly Endeavours in Publishing

Turner held high regard for books and book publishing. He had acquired a large library, from which he made the previously mentioned donation to Yale College. Compiling such a library was another effort to display himself as a man of wealth and erudition, and as a gentleman.[90]

Turner also gained personal notice through book subscription. Subscribers were the financial underwriters who paid the author's or bookseller's costs in advance in order to put a particular work into print. After publication, the subscribers received a copy or copies of the completed work. The books most often subscribed to tended to be large or elaborate works which were financed by 'the more affluent members of society'.[91] Thus, subscribing to book publication often signified belonging to a genteel class. 'Every person of quality', claimed historian Leslie Stephens, 'felt himself bound to promote' authors by subscription.

Turner subscribed to the production of two works: John Hughes' *A Complete History of England* (1706) and Henry Pemberton's *A View of Sir Isaac Newton's Philosophy* (1728).[92] Hughes was a poet of relatively little note in 1706, gaining more fame and affluence through his later works.[93] Some nine hundred subscribers supported Hughes' *History*. Finding that Samuel Turner of Fryday-Street and John Turner of Tottenham also subscribed to this work suggests that Daniel Turner's subscription may have been part of a family financial venture. Alternatively, Hughes may have been a family friend.

Unlike many Newtonians who subscribed to Pemberton's *View*, Turner's help in financing this work stemmed from non-natural philosophy matters. Pemberton had previously achieved renown for 'superintend[ing]' the publication of Newton's *Principia*; a work many contemporaries claimed was destined for posterity. This previous successful venture gained its major financial backing from moneyed Whig subscribers.[94] Turner, a staunch Tory and explicit opponent of Pemberton's medical theorising, was unlikely to support any publication which espoused Newtonian theory. However, he probably envisioned that subscribing to Pemberton's *View* was a sure way to generate wealth, public notice, and to establish an enduring display of being a financially able supporter of this tribute to Newton. However, unfortunately for Turner, Pemberton's work was 'not remunerative to himself, and [the work] was regarded as disappointing'.[95]

Turner also interacted with other parties of the London book trade: book congers. As book publishing was quite expensive, booksellers often pooled their resources to purchase the copyrights of individual manuscripts from authors, forming what was called a conger. The congers controlled much of the trade of books between booksellers and helped protect copyright holdings under the 1709 law.[96]

Turner published his works through members of congers including Charles Rivington, J. Lacy, and John Clarke. Early on, Turner may not have made significant sums for the sale of his copyrights. But as he became better known, his later works commanded higher fees as booksellers were likely to make more money from their sales. 'Known authors' who, like Turner, saw their works carried into a number of printings were able to sell their copyright for several hundred pounds.[97] Turner's later writings and the reprinting of his earlier works were primarily acquired and published through the same member of a local conger: John Clarke.[98] Disappointingly, records of his transactions with Clarke have not survived.[99]

Turner in the Popular Press

In addition to gaining renown as a prolific author of surgical writings, Turner also became known to readers of the *Grub-street Journal*. This weekly newspaper was published by a consortium of booksellers from 8 January 1730 to 29 December 1737. One historian claims it was the 'liveliest, wittiest, and most original' periodical of the 1730s.[100] This pro-Pope, anti-Walpole paper 'descended with ... gusto into the mirky cockpit of personal controversy' for its 'daily food', while satire and irony served as its 'breath of life'.[101] Topics related to medicine and surgery in this journal included the repeated attacks on medical quackery, the censoring of a randomly compiled anatomy text, the existence of microscopic animalcules, the ethics of performing operations on criminals, and discussions of various remedies claimed to cure the bite of a mad dog and venereal disease.[102]

In the 26 February 1730 number of the *Journal*, 'Ephriam Quibus, M.D.', alias botanist John Martyn, denounced various styles of writing used by contemporary medical authors. Among the writings he disapproved of were those composed in what he called the 'digressive' style. This style, he argued, was exemplified by those passages which were designed to 'agreeably amuse ... us, and call us off from the uneasy attention, in which the relation of a melancholy case is apt to ingage [sic] us'.[103] The 'gentleman' whom Martyn claimed 'excell[ed] most in this is the learned Dr. DANIEL TURNER'.[104] He denounced Turner for using this style, particularly for the 'swelling epithets' which he claimed filled Turner's *Art of Surgery*, the 'greatest Master-Piece' of the digressive style Martyn claimed he 'ever saw'.[105]

In later years, Turner himself used the *Grub-street Journal* as his major organ in a campaign against the 'quack', Joshua Ward. Turner's specific disagreements with Ward, as discussed in Chapter Seven, were consistent with the *Journal's* scorn for anything new or which varied from established principles. Additionally, it met the publication's chief aim of combating unorthodox, irregular forms of practice.[106] By publishing in the *Journal*, Turner not only enhanced

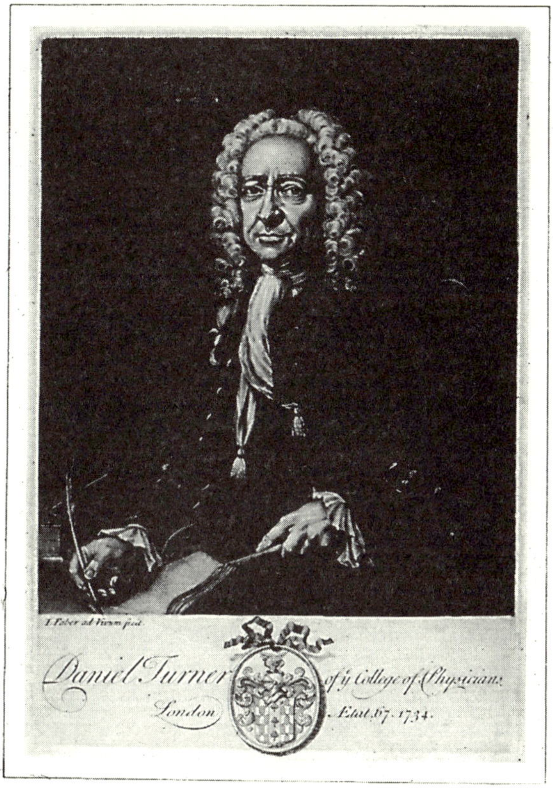
Daniel Turner
of ye College of Physicians
London
Ætat.67. 1734.

Figure 8.6
Daniel Turner. (Johan Faber mezzotint, taken from life, 1734; Yale University Library)

his reputation as an authority, but he also became known to a larger, public reading audience.

Portrait of a Man of Letters

Turner's display of his reverence of books and writings is perhaps best shown in a mezzotint which he had produced in 1734 (see Figure 8.6). In this portrait, Turner is seated at a writing desk surrounded by shelves filled with large leather-bound books. The artist, Johan Faber the younger, captured Turner in the act of writing, quill in hand.[107] His delicate right hand grips a quill similar to how he previously held his scalpel. Veins stand out on his well-aged left hand which is holding the bound volume in which he was writing. In this image, we are unmistakenly introduced to Turner as a writer or man of letters.

Related to his display of arms and his personal motto, Turner's regular use of engraved portraits in his published writings indicates a further adoption of the signs of genteel status. 'There is no passion so universal', Richard Steele claimed in an opening number of *The Guardian*, as the 'vanity of being known to the rest of mankind, and communicating a man's parts, virtues, or qualifications to the world'.[108] One common contemporary way of making oneself, as well as one's work, known was by taking 'care to affix his own image opposite to the title-page of his learned treatise'.[109]

Turner's regular use of portraits offers information about his self-image: first, by employing prominent London portraitist Jonathan Richardson and engraver George Vertue, and second, by the clothing and demeanour in these engravings. The first engravings of Turner (Figures 8.2 and 8.3) appeared in 1714. The engraver, George Vertue, created this work from a portrait painted by Jonathan Richardson.[110] Richardson, an intimate of Hogarth, earned a 'respectable following' in early eighteenth-century London as a 'faithful painter of faces'.[111] In addition to gaining success in portraiture for sitters including Alexander Pope and Dr Richard Mead, he also became widely recognized for his writings on painting.

Although all accounts lead me to believe his portrait of Turner was faithfully accurate in every detail, Richardson's writings provide more instruction into 'reading' what he was actually attempting to portray about Turner. 'A Portrait', Richardson claimed, 'is a sort of General History of the Life of the Person it represents.'[112] To sit for one's portrait was to have 'an Abstract of one's Life written and published, and ourselves consign'd over to Honour, or Infamy'.[113] Indeed, for Richardson, painting was 'another sort of Writing'.[114] He claimed that a portraitist represented his subject's life 'more expressly, and particularly' than a biographer would ever be able to formulate.[115] For in 'making a Portrait', although the 'Complexion and each particular Feature may have been Carefully Observ'd and Imitated ... what is Most Important remains; the Air, the Mind, the Grace, the Dignity, the Capacity, the Vertue, Goodness, &c.'[116]

Turner had himself represented in the portrait wearing a collegiate gown and a fashionable full-bottom wig. Although not exclusively symbolic of the medical profession, it was popularly construed that 'a physician can no more prescribe without a full wig, than without a fee'.[117] The pictorial elevation of Turner, surrounded by a finely ornamental oval frame upon a romanesque pedestal, presumably signifies Richardson's attempt to represent Turner's demand to be portrayed as someone of importance. Turner's self-perception is further proclaimed by the display of either a coat of arms or the *Nullius in Verba* motto.

Turner's stiffly characterized, youthful face represents an assuming, self-knowing look like that typically found in contemporary British portraiture.[118] Turner would have appeared to contemporaries as intellectual and dignified, well-set and fully filling the qualities represented by the collegiate gown enwrapping him. His pale face, gentle and smooth in complexion, conveys a like impression of his moral fibre. Turner's forthright posture indicates he is a man of virtue. There is every semblance of Turner's confidence and capability of fulfilling his professional role.

Turner's image between 1714 and 1734 had metamorphosed. No longer was he wearing the satin robe of his professional calling. Instead, he was dressed in a more rugged, but fashionable gentleman's coat, matching waistcoat, and a Steinkirk cravat loosely knotted under his chin, with one end passing through a buttonhole in his coat.[119] That clothes were important to Turner is not surprising, given the comment of physician and satirist Bernard Mandeville that 'People ... are generally honour'd according to their clothes ... [and] from the richness of them we judge their wealth'.[120] In keeping to 1730s fashion, Turner's wig was cut shorter than those featured in previous engravings.[121] No longer is 'M.D.' emblazoned after his name, but rather his coat of arms is embellished and more prominent. Contemporaries must have recognized the sitter as a man of letters and, by his dress, an accomplished man of letters at that.

Turner's face in this mezzotint by Johan Faber is that of an aged 67-year-old man. The gaunt, smooth, and handsome face of his youth has become filled with the wrinkles and bulges of ageing. The earlier face, noting an air of self-assurance, now appears more streaked with a seriousness or sternness fitting that of a wise and learned man. The books, ever powerful in Turner's life, symbolize his having amassed a vast knowledge from a long life of reading and attest to his accomplishments as an author. This mezzotint illustrates the 'Gentleman of great Erudition: in whose Books the Reader will find abundant Pleasure and Information', the appellation that surgeon James Handley verbally conveyed about Turner to readers of his *Colloquia Chirurgica*.[122] Overall, this engraving, taken from life, presents Turner in the act of what, I believe, he regarded as his most important accomplishment: becoming a man of letters.

1741

In 1741, England's governmental power was still in the grips of the

Whig statesman, Sir Robert Walpole. Although the nation was at peace, surgeons continued to fight with barbers in their combined Company. The number of Fellows in the College of Physicians had greatly dwindled from its 1700 level, and licentiates comprised a considerable proportion of the medics practising in London.[123] Quacks, however, still predominated in London's medical marketplace.

In 1741, Daniel Turner had lived three-quarters of a century, an age most of his contemporaries never reached.[124] Thirty years had passed since the winter he 'quit' the practice of surgery,[125] yet he had remained a faithful campaigner towards improving the surgical art. He claimed to have expended the 'utmost of [his] Power' to compose *The Art of Surgery*, the work he apparently regarded as his single most significant contribution to this cause, hoping it would 'serve, not only the present, but the succeeding Generation'.[126] Witnessing its sixth reprinting in 1741, Turner had seen it in constant demand for nineteen years. By this time, Turner was also known both in London and on the European Continent for his writings on the power of the maternal imagination and on syphilis.

Through his practice as a surgeon, Turner attended many Londoners on their deathbeds, but he claimed to have 'rarely' contemplated his own mortality. 'It is surely One of the greatest Oversights of Life, that in our healthful state, we too seldom entertain our Minds about the State of Sickness, and more rarely think on that of Death.'[127] With 'shame', Turner confessed that 'amidst the Hurry of this busy World', he 'carelessly' disregarded his own 'transitory Nature', neglecting to pay attention to the 'Emblems' of the human skull in his study and over his bedstead.[128] As he claimed of his colleagues, 'one would think' that with the physicians' 'continual dealings with Mortality', death 'should take up all their Thoughts'.[129] Instead, Turner claimed they were 'the least of all concern'd' with dying except their sorrow 'for want of More Employment'.[130]

Death appears to have approached Turner in 1707 and 1725. In the later case, he claimed that too much 'Study and Attendance upon the Sick' had 'impair'd' his 'weakly Constitution', leaving him in such a state that he concluded he 'shall write no more'.[131] This forecast proved false, but it was typical of many contemporary writers' expressions of their impending doom.

Turner's devotional confessions indicate that he came to face death with an assurance of the hereafter. In standard will and testament language, he resigned his soul to his Creator, 'wishing for Salvation'.[132] Turner appeared to have followed the advice he had previously offered surgical readers in 1725:

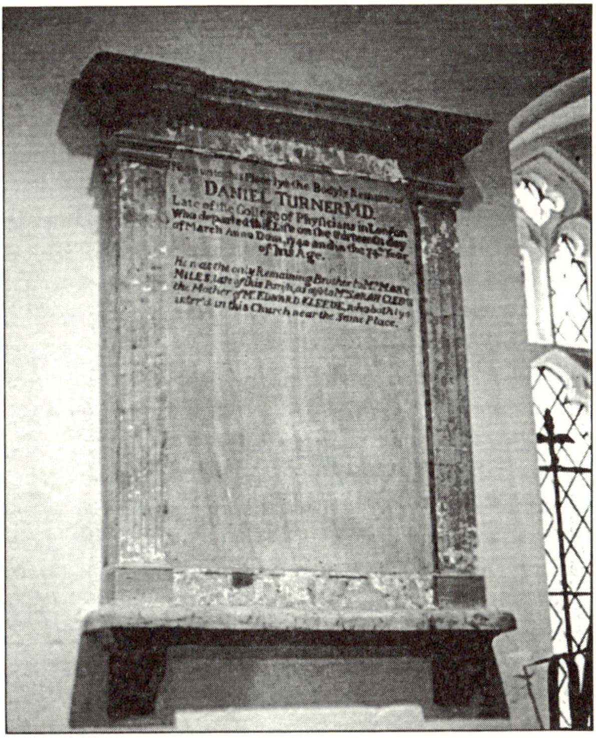

Figure 8.7
Daniel Turner's commemorative tablet, St Mary and St Andrew Church, Watton-at-Stone, Hertfordshire (Author's own photograph)

> Let them wait their appointed Time, and die like men; Let them rejoice that they are shortly going to meet those brave Men [who have gone before].[133]

Turner's 'appointed Time' came on 13 March 1740–41. The winter was one of the coldest in London's recorded history.[134] He may have been with the family of his sister, Mary Miles, in Hertfordshire at the time, for he was interred seven days later in the graveyard of the Watton-at-Stone parish church near the Miles' home, 'Watton Hall alias Watkins Hall'.[135]

Turner provided for his family through his 'Last Will and Testament' drawn up in his own hand on 10 July 1740. From this will, we learn that Turner had amassed real estate in London, Hertfordshire, and Essex, and had invested £1,000 in a South Sea

Corporation annuity. His wife, Elizabeth, received her £1,000 from Daniel's personal estate according to 'certain Articles of Agreement' drawn up before their marriage. His two daughters, particularly Mary, his unmarried youngest daughter, received most of his real estate. As was customary among men of means who were not in debt, Turner also allocated money 'for mourning' to be distributed to family members.[136] He also left money to his executors, an 'old Acquaintance', the Antiquary John Murray, and, according to custom, to each of his coachmen, footmen and maid servants living with him at the time of his decease.

The precise whereabouts of Turner's final resting spot remains unknown. His sister, Mary Miles, was probably the one who donated money for the tablet commemorating Daniel which hangs on the south wall of the Watton-at-Stone church (see Figure 8.7).[137]

This stone is unusual in that two-thirds of the tablet has been left blank. Neither Turner's wife nor his children appear to have followed him to rest in Watton-at-Stone. Paradoxically, the design of this 'incomplete' tablet of death is consistent with much of the way Turner lived. The romanesque features resemble the ostentatious markings found on the commemorative tablets of gentlemen. The style of the lettering and the composition of Turner's tablet, however, are of a markedly inferior quality. But this quality is only noticeable through careful scrutiny. More superficially, the display on Turner's tablet stands well above the quality of the common gravestone.

An 'Imaginary Epitaph' for Dr. Turner
Good Dr. Turner is deprived of breath,
And turn'd into another world by death:
'Twas a good turn for some, that gave him birth;
And having had his turn, he's turn'd to earth.[138]

Notes

1 A. S. Byatt, *Possession* (London: Vintage, 1991), 508.

2 *Daniel Defoe, The Compleat English Gentleman*, Karl D. Bulbring (ed.), (London: David Nutt, 1890), 13, 65.

3 Joseph Butler, 1740, as cited by J. W. Saunders, *The Profession of English Letters* (London: Routledge and Kegan Paul, 1964), 119.

4 P. Earle, *The Making of the English Middle Class*, 3-4.

5 According to R. Campbell's *London Tradesman*, a tallow chandler was much less 'genteel' than the related craft of a wax chandler, 271.

6 Land Deed (1688), Hertfordshire County Record Office, D/EAS 3131.

7 John Turner's will, written on 4 August 1691, stipulated that Daniel received £250 during his apprenticeship, and, as an incentive to learn his chosen trade, another £250 upon its completion. Daniel, however, had completed his apprenticeship before his father's death in 1697. Public Record Office, Chancery Lane, Prob.11/440.

8 Little, however, is known about the fee arrangements Turner made with most of his patients.

9 Ralph Davis discussed the environment around Devonshire Square in his *Aleppo and Devonshire Square: English Traders in the Levant in the Eighteenth Century* (London: Macmillan, 1967), esp. 2-3. See also Anonymous, *London Described, or, The Most Noted Regular Buildings Both Publick and Private with the Views of Several Squares in the Liberties of London & Westminster* (London: Thos & John Bowles, 1731), plate 39, and John Stow, *A Survey of the Cities of London and Westminster*, John Strype (ed.), (London: A. Churchill, J. Knapton, R. Knaplock, J. Walthoe, E. Horne, B. Tooke, D. Midwinter, B. Crowse, R. Robinson, and T. Ward, 1720, 1st edn 1593), vol. 1, Bk 2, Ch. 6, Bishopsgate Ward, 90-3, with a plate of Bishopsgate-Street Ward.

10 John Littleton Costeker, *The Fine Gentleman; or, The Compleat Education of a Young Nobleman* (London: J. Roberts, 1731), 49-50.

11 G.C. Brauer, *The Education of a Gentleman*, 13.

12 D.C. Coleman, 'Gentlemen and Players', *Economic History Review*, 2nd series, xxvi (1973), 96.

13 Geoffrey Holmes discussed surgical apprentice fees in *Augustan England*, 213-15. See also J.L. Axtell, 'Education and Status in Stuart England: The London Physician', *History of Education Quarterly*, x (1970), 147, and P. Earle *The Making of the English Middle Class*, 93-5.

14 Edward Chamberlayne, *Magnae Britanniae Notitia; or, The Present State of Great Britain*, 38th edn. (London: S. Birt, 1755), 179.

15 See Daniel Turner's 'Remarks, taken upon Dissecting … a Maid ... who dyed of an Ascites', *Philosophical Transactions of the Royal Society of London,* xviii (1693-94), 15-20, 'Of a Stone found in the Gall-Bladder of a Woman', *Philosophical Transactions of the Royal Society of London,* xviii (1694), 111-112, 'Woman hydropical in the ... uterus', *Philosophical Transactions of the Royal Society of London,* xviii (1693-94), 20-3, and 'Observations on a Child bit by Mad Dog', *Philosophical Transactions of the Royal Society of London,* xviii (1693-94), 24-5.

16 For a detailed biographical account, M.F. Ashley Montagu provided a detailed biography of Tyson entitled *Edward Tyson, M.D., F.R.S. 1650-1708, and the Rise of Human and Comparative Anatomy in England* (Philadelphia: American Philosophical Society, 1943).

17 Tyson, elected into Royal Society fellowship in 1676, proposed the following successful candidates into the Society: Henry Eve (1681), William Payne (1681), Richard Robinson (1681), James Monson (1684), Jean-Nicolas Pechlin (1688), Raymond Viessens (1688), and William Cowper (1699).

18 Turner never appears on any list of candidates in the Minute Books of the Royal Society. Records of elections around 1700 often mention only the successful candidates.

19 Turner is not listed on the freemasons' lists of surgeons or physicians presented in J.R.Clarke's 'The Medical Profession and Early Freemasonry', *Ars Quatuor Coronatorum,* lxxxv (1972), 298-311. Much more investigation and opening of presently closed files is needed before our understanding of the contemporary importance of masonic activity is expanded. Margaret C. Jacob's *Living the Enlightenment: Free-masonry and Politics in Eighteenth-Century Europe* (Oxford: Oxford University Press, 1992) is a most useful beginning.

20 Tony Davies, 'The Ark in the Flames: Science, Language and Education in Seventeenth-Century England', in A.E. Benjamin, G.N. Cantor, and J.R.R. Christie (eds), *The Figural and the Literal: Problems of Language in the History of Science and Philosophy, 1630-1800* (Manchester: Manchester University Press, 1987), 94.

21 Michael Hunter, *Establishing the New Science: The Experience of the Early Royal Society* (Woodbridge: Boydell Press, 1989), 344-5.

22 J.R. Clarke, 'The Royal Society and early Grand Lodge Freemasonry', *Ars Quatuor Coronatorum,* lxxx (1967), 110-19, and Margaret C. Jacob's *The Radical Enlightenment: Pantheists, Freemasons and Republicans* (London: George Allen & Unwin, 1981), 112.

23 James du Moulin, Master of Surgery to Charles II and James II (1667); John Beaumont, Somerset surgeon and naturalist (1685);

Charles Bernard, later Sergeant Surgeon to Queen Anne (1696); William Cowper, (1699); Paul Buissiere, Huguenot surgeon (1699); and James Cunningham, surgeon to the East India Company (1699). Michael Hunter provided information about all Fellows elected prior to 1700 in his *The Royal Society and its Fellows 1660-1700* (Buckinghamshire: British Society for the History of Science, 1982).

24 Robert F. Buckman and J.William Futrell briefly discussed Cowper's background in their 'William Cowper', *Surgery,* ic (1986), 582-90. I alluded to Cowper's Fellowship in the Royal Society in 'William Cowper's Anatomy of Human Skin', 2-3.

25 Steven Shapin, '"A Scholar and a Gentleman": The Problematic Identity of the Scientific Practitioner in Early Modern England', *History of Science,* xxix (1991), esp 295-9. Questions remain regarding the extent to which Cowper, who plagiarized the plates and some of the text from the anatomist, Govard Bidloo, was actually viewed as a scholar by his contemporaries.

26 The only further publication of Turner in the *Philosophical Transactions* was a brief letter he wrote to James Jurin in 1725 regarding 'Insects voided by the Urinary Passages', *Philosophical Transactions of the Royal Society of London*, xxxiii (1725), 410-11. The brevity and context of this letter do not suggest that Turner believed he was offering major new insights.

27 This use of this motto or other symbolic representations of the Society by non-Fellows, however, appears to have been quite rare. Besides Turner, I have found only one other non-F.R.S. who created such an association with the Society. The instrument maker John Marshall displayed 'Royal Society' in his advertisement. But since he made instruments for the Society, it can be argued that he was using their 'appellation' as a form of advertising the status of people for whom he worked. An illustration of Marshall's advertisement is found in R. T. Gunther, *Early Science in Oxford* (Oxford: for the author, 1935), v.10, xxxii. Roy Porter has claimed (personal communication) that Turner's contemporary, Benjamin Martin, identified himself as 'F.R.S.' on the title pages of several of his books although he never attained such a position. For a more complete account on Martin, see John R. Millburn, 'Benjamin Martin and the Royal Society', *Notes and Records of the Royal Society of London*, xxviii (1973), 15-23.

28 M. Hunter, personal communication.

29 Edwin Oviatt mistakenly identified Turner as 'FRS' in his *The Beginnings of Yale (1701-1726)* (New Haven: Yale University Press, 1916), 422.

30 Henry Lyons, *The Royal Society 1660-1940. A History of its*

Administration and its Charters (Cambridge: Cambridge University Press, 1944), 39.

31 Charles Goodall, *The Royal College of Physicians in London* (London: M. Flesher for W. Kettilby, 1684), as cited by G. Holmes, *Augustan England*, 17.

32 T. Gelfand, *Professionalizing Modern Medicine*, Preface, xi.

33 *Idem.*

34 M. Pelling, 'Medical Practice in Early Modern England', 90-128.

35 Harold J. Cook, 'Good Advice and Little Medicine: The Professional Authority of Early Modern English Physicians', *Journal of British Studies*, xxxiii (1994), 1-31.

36 Geoffrey Holmes' 'The Professions and Social Change in England, 1680-1730' *Proceedings of the British Academy*, lxv (1979), 313-54 was followed by his wider analysis of the professions in *Augustan England.*

37 G. Holmes, *Augustan England*, 7-8.

38 Wilfrid Prest, 'Introduction: The Professions and Society in Early Modern England', in W. Prest (ed.), *The Professions in Early Modern England* (London: Croom Helm, 1987), 6-7.

39 P. R. Backscheider, *Daniel Defoe*, 527.

40 D. Turner, 'Some modest ANIMADVERSIONS on Dr. HARRIS', 555-70.

41 They were married by Mr Samuel Eastwicke in the London parish church of St Helen's, Bishopsgate on 6 January 1712. W. Bruce Bannerman, *The Register of St Helen's, Bishopsgate, London* (London: Harleian Society, 1904), 176.

42 Information on the Altham family is anonymously provided in 'Some Althams of Mark Hall in the 17th Century', *The Essex Review*, xvii (1908), 74-89, 134-46 and xviii (1909), 91-100; W. R. Powell (ed.), *Victoria History of the Counties of England. A History of Essex*, vol. 8 (Oxford: Oxford University Press for the Institute of Historical Research, 1983), esp. 189-90; Essex Record Office MSS D/P 344/1/1-4, T/P 195/16 and T/B 93; and Jonathan Edwards, *A History of Latton* (Ware: Herts Display Co. for The Church of St Mary-at-Latton, 1980).

43 Her brother James Altham (d.1766) was Rector of Latton, and later Woodford, and Vicar of St Olave, Old Jewry. Turner's brother-in-law, Roger Altham, D.D., once Rector of Latton, served from 1701-1729 as Rector of St Botolph without Bishopsgate, the parish in which Turner resided.

44 'Of the Articles of Agreement before Marriage, that part relating to Dower and Thirds', 10 December 1712, Hertfordshire County

Record Office, MS. D/EAS 1612 (867). According to Lloyd Bonfield, it was not unusual during this period for prospective bride's families to draw up pre-nuptial contracts stipulating particular agreements in order to protect the bride's future financial security. *Marriage Settlements, 1601-1740: The Development of the Strict Settlement* (Cambridge: Cambridge University Press, 1983).

45 Pat Rogers (ed.), *The Eighteenth Century* (Cambridge: Cambridge University Press, 1978), 35.

46 Arnold Zuckermann, 'Dr. Richard Mead (1673-1754). A Biographical Study' (Ph.D. thesis, University of Illinois, 1965), 219-20.

47 G. Holmes, *Augustan England*, 220-1.

48 Daniel Turner, Probated will (16 April 1741), Public Record Office, Chancery Lane, Prob.11/709.

49 F. Bastion, *Defoe's Early Life*, 145. For a more complete argument relating the acquisition of property to one's place in society, see H. Perkin's *Origins of Modern English Society*, esp. 38-56.

50 Additionally, Turner mentioned occasionally employing nurses and attendants to help him care for patients.

51 See, for instance, R. Davis, *Aleppo and Devonshire Square*, 16, and *The Names of the Governors of St Bartholomew's Hospital* ([London]: s.n., n.d.), 1, 4.

52 From a portrait in the Iconographic Collection, Wellcome Institute for the History of Medicine Library, London. *Burgess Portrait Catalogue*, No. 2998.1.

53 George J. Armytage (ed.), *A Visitation of the County of Surrey*, 15.

54 As seen in the illustrated Turner pedigree in William Berry, *Pedigree of the Families in the County of Kent* (London: Sherwood, Gilbert, and Piper, 1830), 274. I am grateful to Vivian Dickinson for this reference.

55 T. D. Mathew, personal communication.

56 Anthony Wagner, *Heralds of England: A History of the Office and College of Arms* (London: HMSO, 1967), 120, 167, 237, 365.

57 Daniel Defoe, *System of Magick* (London: J. Clarke, 1729), 336.

58 William Hogarth, *Analysis of Beauty*, as cited by Aileen Ribeiro, 'Fashion and Fantasy: The Use of Costume in Eighteenth-Century British Portraiture' in *The British Face: A View of Portraiture 1625-1850* (London: P. & D. Colnaghi, 1986), 22.

59 R. Campbell, *The London Tradesman*, 191.

60 Turner listed these qualities as the sixth and seventh parts of his representation of the 'Character of a good Physician' in *Discourse on Fevers* (1739), 333. The other qualities identified were to be of 'solid

Erudition' and 'sound Judgement'; 'strict Probity and Fidelity'; 'Great Honour ... Gravity and Modesty'; 'Courteous'; and not to be 'Loquacious or Proud' (331-4).

61 H. Perkin, *Origins of Modern English Society*, 24-5.

62 D. Turner, *Art of Surgery*, Preface, 6.

63 *Idem.*

64 H. Perkin, *Origins of Modern English Society*, 55.

65 D. Turner, *Art of Surgery*, vol. 1 (1725), preface.

66 D. Turner, *Art of Surgery*, Preface, 6.

67 David Foxon warns historians that second, third, fourth, etc. editions of books often indicate the bookseller's attempts to boost poor sales. See his *Pope and the Early Eighteenth-Century Book Trade*, revised by James McLaverty (Oxford: Clarendon Press, 1991), 31. Turner's booksellers, on the other hand, informed readers that Turner's books enjoyed 'wide sales'. D. Turner, *Art of Surgery*, vol. 1 (1725), The Book Sellers to the Reader.

68 D. Turner, *Art of Surgery*, vol. 1 (1725), The Book Sellers to the Reader.

69 For example, *De Morbis Cutaneis*, his first work published as a physician, was designed to 'convince' his professional colleagues that they had bestowed the 'privilege' to practice medicine upon 'no idle ... useless person'. (1714, Epistle Dedicatory).

70 Vivian Nutton more fully discussed this aspect of humanism in 'Humanist Surgery', 80-2.

71 D. Turner, *Art of Surgery*, vol. 2 (1722), 28. G.C. Brauer described a similar use of history as exemplifying virtue in more general contemporary education in his *Education of a Gentleman*, 76-7.

72 Samuel Johnson, *Works*, John Hawkins (ed.), (London: J. Buckland, 1787), 362.

73 Liza Picard, *Restoration London* (London: Weidenfeld & Nicolson, 1997), 87-8.

74 John E. Lane reprinted this letter and an English translation in his 'Daniel Turner and the First Degree of Doctor of Medicine', 372-4.

75 Andrew Keogh, 'The Growth of the University Library', *Yale University Library Gazette*, v (1931), esp. 129-31.

76 Anne Stokely Pratt, 'The Books sent from England by Jeremiah Dummer to Yale College', in *Papers in Honor of Andrew Keogh* (New Haven: Yale University Press, 1938), 15-16, 35; Franklin Bowditch Dexter, *Biographical Sketches of the Graduates of Yale College with Annals of the College History October, 1701 – May, 1745* (New York: Henry Holt & Co., 1885), 142; Thomas Clap, *The Annals or History of Yale-College* (New Haven: John Hotchkiss and B. Mecom, 1766),

15; and John E. Lane 'The Medical Books in the 1742 Yale College Library', *Yale University Library Gazette,* vi (1936), 85.

77 A. Keogh, 'Growth of the University Library', especially 129-31.

78 Anne S. Pratt and Andrew Keogh, 'The Yale Library of 1742', *Yale University Library Gazette,* xv (1940), 30.

79 Overall, between 1712 and 1729, 180 donors contributed 705 volumes to Yale's library.

80 T. Clap, President of Yale 'College', recorded the value of Turner's contribution in his *Annals or History of Yale-College,* 96. Bishop Berkeley gave Yale a 4th edition (1731) copy of Turner's *Art of Surgery* as part of his 1733 donation of 'some nine hundred volumes'. Andrew Keogh, 'Bishop Berkeley's Gift of Books in 1733', *The Yale University Library Gazette,* viii (1934), 16.

81 J. Lane, 'Daniel Turner and the first degree of Doctor of Medicine', 372.

82 I previously speculated upon what these books may have meant to Turner in my 'Reading A Man Through His Gifts: Daniel Turner's 1722 Book Donation to Yale College', *Yale University Library Gazette,* lxix (1995), 129-48.

83 *Postscriptum. Si Dominationes vestrae me dignum judicatis Doctoratus Gradus Acadmiae Yalensis, et Diploma mihi transmitti curatis, accipiam non tantum ut signum Gratitudinis Vestrae, sed existmam honorem, aeque ac si ab alia Universitate, tamesti Majoris Notae, fuerit elargitum. valete Viri Doctissimi vigaetque Academia vestra.*

84 J. Dummer, letter to the Academy, 10 September 1723, as printed by J.E. Lane, 'Daniel Turner and the first degree of Doctor of Medicine', 374.

85 J. Dummer letter to the Academy, 10 September 1723, as printed by J.E. Lane, 'Daniel Turner and the first degree of Doctor of Medicine', 374-5. William J. Prendergast, 'The first honorary degree of Doctor of Medicine was granted in New Haven in 1723', *Sunday Pictorial,* 13 November 1966. Yale had previously conferred an honorary bachelor's degree (1705), and five honorary master's degrees (1702 and 1719). The next honorary medical degree Yale conferred upon John Bartlett in 1779, and their first official MD was awarded in 1814. *Catalogue of the Officers and Graduates of Yale University in New Haven Connecticut 1701-1924* (New Haven: Yale University Press, 1924), 571, 574, and 486.

86 Letter from Jeremiah Dummer to Timothy Woodbridge, 25 February 1725, reprinted in Franklin Bowditch Dexter (ed.), *Documentary History of Yale University under the original charter of the*

Collegiate School of Connecticut 1701-1745 (New Haven: Yale University Press, 1916), 256-7. Dummer described this diploma as being 'set in fine hand', 'drawn up in a true Roman diction ... exceeding anything I ever ... saw from Harvard', and 'hansomly [sic] ornamented with flourishes'. Unfortunately, the whereabouts of this diploma remain unknown.

87 In 1721, the College of Physicians complained that Oxford too liberally issued honorary medical degrees. *Annals*, Royal College of Physicians MS, vol. 8, f.197a, 22 December 1721. Similar reprimand was issued against Cambridge on 1 March 1721/22 (*Annals*, vol. 9, f.1a).

88 D. Turner, *Modern Quack*, Dedication.

89 Joseph M. Toner, *Contributions to the Annals of Medicine and Medical Education in the United States before and during the War of Independence* (Washington, D.C.: Government Printing Office, 1874), 66.

90 J.W. Saunders claimed acquiring such a library was a common pursuit of every gentleman, *Profession of English Letters*, 120.

91 W.A. Speck argued that only a 'tiny percentage' of works published during this period were financed by subscription, in his 'Politicians, Peers, and Publication by Subscription 1700-50', in Isabel Rivers (ed.), *Books and Their Readers in Eighteenth-Century England* (Leicester: Leicester University Press, 1982), 50.

92 P.J. Wallis and R.V. Wallis, *Eighteenth-Century Medics* (Newcastle upon Tyne: Project for Historical Bibliography, 1988), 606. He was also probably the 'Mr Turner' who subscribed to the posthumous publication of Roger Altham's (his brother-in-law's) *Sermons Preached on Several Occasions* (1732).

93 Samuel Johnson, *Lives of the English Poets*, 2 vols, vol. 1 (London: J. M. Dent & Sons, Everyman's Library Edition, 1925), 369-72.

94 Nearly two thousand subscribers are listed on the sixteen pages between the contents and the introduction of this work. W.A. Speck discussed the motives underlying the subscriptions to Pemberton's *View* in 'Politicians, Peers, and Publication by Subscription', 60, 63-4.

95 Leslie Stephen and Sidney Lee (eds), *Dictionary of National Biography*, vol. 15 (London: Smith, Elder, & Co., 1909), 726.

96 Terry Belanger, '"Booksellers" Trade Sales, 1718-1768', *Library*, 5th ser., xxx (1975), 281-302.

97 J.W. Saunders, *The Profession of English Letters*, 121-2.

98 Clarke had previously been in a conger with Charles Rivington and J. Lacy, but after the mid-1720s, he took up the selling of all of Turner's writings on his own. H.R. Plomer claimed Clarke dealt

'almost entirely' in theological literature in *A Dictionary of the Printers and Booksellers Who Were at Work in England, Scotland, and Ireland, from 1668-1725* (Oxford: for the Bibliographical Society, Oxford University Press, 1922), 72.

99 Few booksellers' records from early eighteenth-century London have survived. Exemplary historical accounts from the surviving reords are found in Foxon's *Pope and the Early Eighteenth-Century Book Trade* and J.D. Alsop, 'The Publication of Benjamin Gooch's Surgical Works, 1765-74' *Publishing History*, xxv (1989) 13-26.

100 Bertrand A. Goldgar, 'The Grub-street Journal' in Alvin Sullivan (ed.), *British Literary Magazines. Vol. 1: The Augustan Age and the Age of Johnson, 1698-1788* (Westport, Connecticut: Greenwood Press, 1983), 147.

101 James T. Hillhouse, *The Grub-street Journal* (Durham, North Carolina: Duke University Press, 1928; New York: Benjamin Blom, 1967 reissue), 9, 37.

102 Hillhouse devoted a chapter in his *The Grub-street Journal* to the 'Law, Theology, and Medicine' controversies in the journal, *ibid.*, 226-94. Raymond Williamson discussed several of the medical controversies in more depth in his 'John Martyn and the Grub-street Journal, with Particular Reference to his Attacks on Richard Bentley, Richard Bradley and William Cheselden', *Medical History*, v (1961), 361-74.

103 *Memoirs of the Society of Grubstreet*, vol. 1 (London: J. Wilford, 1737), 36.

104 *Idem.*

105 This reputation of Turner filled many later biographical sketches including M. Noble (ed.), *Biographical History of England*, vol. 3, 284. Noble makes some erroneous speculations about Turner's descendants.

106 J. Hillhouse, *Grub-street Journal*, 249, 260.

107 Johan Faber the younger, it has been claimed, was 'esteemed the ablest artist of his time' in mezzotints, excepting John Smith. G. C. Williamson, *Bryan's Dictionary of Printers and Engravers*, vol. 2 (1903), 138-9.

108 *Guardian*, No.1, 12 March 1713.

109 *Idem.* For a general discussion of the social usefulness of contemporary portraiture, see Shearer West, 'Patronage and Power: the Role of the Portrait in Eighteenth-Century England', in: J. Black and J. Gregory (eds), *Culture, Politics and Society in Britain, 1660-1800* (Manchester and New York: Manchester University Press, 1991), 131-53. See also Marcia Pointon, *Hanging the Head.*

Portraiture and Social Formation in Eighteenth-Century England (New Haven: Yale University Press, 1993).

110 George Vertue, who created an engraving of Turner from Richardson's portrait, began work as a member of Sir Godfrey Kneller's Academy in 1711. His work, though of 'no great artistic merit', according to George C. Williamson, forms a 'valuable historical record, and his antiquarian researches and writings were of higher importance'. His large note book, purchased by Horace Walpole, forms the basis of Walpole's *Anecdotes of Painting in England.* George C. Williamson (ed.), *Bryan's Dictionary of Painters and Engravers,* vol.5 (London: George Bell and Sons, 1915), 294.

111 Richard Wendorf, *The Elements of Life: Biography and Portrait-Painting in Stuart and Georgian London* (Oxford: Clarendon Press, 1990), 136. Horace Walpole in his *Anecdotes of Painting* (Strawberry Hill: for Thos Farmer, 1762-71) claimed Richardson 'drew nothing well below the head' (vol.3, 413), and John Kerslake supported this claim in commenting on Richardson's portrait of Dr. Richard Mead in *Early Georgian Portraits* (London: National Portrait Gallery, HMSO, 1977), plates 528-38.

112 Jonathan Richardson, *The Connoisseur: An Essay on the Whole Art of Criticism, as it relates to Painting,* in J. Richardson, *Two Discourses* (London: W. Churchill, 1719), 45.

113 Jonathan Richardson, *An Essay on the Theory of Painting,* 2nd edn (Menston, Yorkshire: Scholar Press, 1971, 1725), 13-14.

114 Jonathan Richardson, *A Discourse on the Dignity, Certainty, Pleasure and Advantage, of the Science of a Connoisseur,* in J. Richardson, *Two Discourses* (London: W. Churchill, 1719), 17.

115 J. Richardson, *Essay on the Theory of Painting,* 13-14. Richardson fully appreciated the task of biography and discussed the peculiar relationship it held with portraiture. See Richard Wendorf's 'Ut Pictura Biographia: Biography and Portrait Painting as Sister Arts', in R. Wendorf (ed.), *Articulate Images: The Sister Arts from Hogarth to Tennyson* (Minneapolis: University of Minnesota Press, 1983), 98-124.

116 R. Wendorf, *The Elements of Life,* 144.

117 Gregory in Molière's *The Mock Doctor* (1732).

118 Desmond Shaw-Taylor, *The Georgians: Eighteenth-Century Portraiture & Society* (London: Barrie & Jenkins, 1990), 83.

119 Aileen Ribeiro and Valerie Cumming, *The Visual History of Costume* (London: B. T. Batsford Ltd, 1989), 122-41. See also Phillis Cunningham and Catherine Lucas, *Occupational Costume in England from the Eleventh Century to 1914* (London: Adam & Charles Black,

1967), 315.

120 Bernard Mandeville, *Fable of Bees*, as cited in Neil McKendrick, John Brewer, and J.H. Plumb, *The Birth of a Consumer Society: The Commercialization of Eighteenth-Century England* (London: Europa Publications Ltd, 1982), 52.

121 In addition to the pre-1714 engraving of Turner, a similar engraving, with only the change of a new, fuller face of a middle aged man appeared as early as 1732. In this later engraving, Turner's previous full-length wig had been replaced with a 'physical wig', the long bob style which replaced the full-bottom or physicians' dress bob. See. J. Stevens Cox, *An Illustrated Dictionary of Hairdressing & Wigmaking* (London: Batsford Academic and Educational, 1984), 118. John Woodforde claimed the full-bottom wig began to decline from fashion around 1720 in his *The Strange Story of False Hair* (London: Routledge & Kegan Paul, 1971), 27.

122 J. Handley, *Colloquia Chyrurgica*, 4th edn (1733), vii.

123 R.J.J. Martin, 'Explaining John Freind's *History of Physick*', 405.

124 E.A. Wrigley and R.S. Schofield have estimated that only 8.11% of England's population during this period ever reached the age of sixty. And for this time, they have calculated that average life expectancy was 39.5 years. See *The Population History of England, 1541-1871* (Cambridge: Cambridge University Press, 1989), 252.

125 D. Turner, *De Morbis Cutaneis*, 1723, 310.

126 D. Turner, *Art of Surgery*, vol. 1, preface.

127 D. Turner, 'Religio Medici Reformata', Praemonition, f. 35.

128 *Ibid.*, f. 36.

129 In the present era, surgeon Sherwin B. Nuland addressed the issue of how physicians and surgeons cope with patient's deaths in his popular *How We Die: Reflections on Life's Final Chapter* (New York: Knopf, 1993), especially 242-69.

130 D. Turner, 'Religio Medici Reformata', Praemonition, f. 35v.

131 D. Turner, *Art of Surgery*, vol. 1, Preface to the Reader.

132 Daniel Turner, Probated will.

133 D. Turner, 'Some modest animadversions of Dr. Harris' *Dissertationes Medicae*', 563.

134 P. Rogers, *The Eighteenth Century*, 32.

135 Parish Register, Watton Parish, Hertfordshire County Record Office, 20 March 1740/41. Turner's obituary in *Gentleman's Magazine*, xi (1741), 164 described him as an 'eminent Physician, and Author of several learned Treatises in Physic'.

136 C. Gittings, *Death, Burial and the Individual in Early Modern England* (London: Croom Helm, 1984), 54, 97, 206-10.

137 The tablet reads 'Nigh unto this place, lys the bodyly remains of Daniel Turner, M.D. Late of the College of Physicians in London Who departed this Life on the thirteenth day of March Anno Dom. 1740[/41] and in the 74th Year of his Age. He was the only Remaining Brother to Mrs Mary Miles, late of this Parish, as also to Mrs Sarah Cleeve the mother of Mr Edmund Cleeve, who both lye inter'd in this Church near the Same Place'. Robert Clutterbuck, *The History and Antiquities of the County of Hertfordshire,* vol. 2 (London: John Nichols & Son, 1821), 488. It was erected after Mary Miles' death in 1751.

138 [William Wadd], *Nugae Conorae: or Epitaphian Momentoes* (London: J.B. Nichols, 1827), 20.

9

Aftermath

Throughout this work, I have presented Daniel Turner's career as being both typical and atypical. Like many of his contemporaries, Turner gained his initial surgical training through apprenticeship, and he encountered patients who suffered from disorders that were comparable to those treated by his colleagues. His remedies and operations were consistent with those of many other orthodox surgeons in his day. Thus Turner's surgical career was, in many ways, typical for that of an early eighteenth-century London surgeon.

However, Turner distinguished himself from his surgical colleagues in several respects. Foremost, his devotion to writing established him as the most prolific author of surgical works in early eighteenth-century London. Through these works he endeavoured to improve the art of surgery and advance the status of surgeons by liberalizing them from what many saw as a mere mechanical handicraft. Although Turner never engaged a single apprentice, in one sense he aspired to become the master of all young surgical practitioners. The *Art of Surgery* was, according to Turner, the 'most instructive' surgical guide in the English tongue.[1]

Many of Turner's expressed viewpoints also distinguished him from his colleagues. His ardent opposition to theoretical medicine, particularly iatromechanical-based medicine, in favour of 'quasi-vitalist' beliefs was unusual among the surgico-medical authors in Newtonian London. His use of the skin as a rhetorical device to dismantle the barriers between surgery and physic was unique. His appeal to the public to judge for themselves whether the power of the mother's imagination existed or whether Ward's 'Pill & Drop' was efficacious also distinguished him.

Turner's actions may, in part, be explained in terms of an inner drive or duty. Eradicating London's mechanical theorists and quacks would fulfil both a practical 'duty' to improve London for future generations and a moral 'duty' to his Creator. The traditional restraint upon surgeons to administer only external medications contradicted what Turner argued was a surgeon's moral or ethical 'duty' to provide his patients complete cures. To meet this need, he diligently campaigned to change physicians' view of the body such that surgeons as well as physicians could legally treat the whole patient. He also perceived it as a duty to provide surgeons a new resource, the *Art of Surgery*, which specified the correct, ethical, and orthodox practice as a guide to deter them from adopting questionable, quack-like practices.

In addition to fulfilling any perceived duties, Turner also used his writings to enhance his social position. Early in his career, he displayed his abilities before the Royal Society. Gaining the Society's favour and ultimately being invited into its Fellowship would certainly have furthered Turner's contemporary reputation as a scholar. But Turner's quest for recognition by this Society was in vain. Still, Turner envisioned his own talents and abilities to be broader than one occupation could satisfy. He ambitiously sought to further his local recognition by turning from the practice of surgery to the practice of physic. As a physician, Turner was able to marry into a landed family, obtain the leisure through which he could turn his attention to writing, and eventually acquire land holdings of his own. To let his new status be known in London and in colonial America, Turner went to unusual lengths to obtain an M.D. He also envisioned that as a physician, his prescriptive writings to fellow practitioners would be more stringently followed.

Turner as Reformer

Turner's persistent campaign to reform surgical practice was not realized in his lifetime. Soon after the time of Turner's death, however, surgeons' accusations against barbers 'pretending' to practice surgery soon became passé. The barber-surgeon mould of Turner's generation was recast after the establishment of a Company of Surgeons independent from the Company of Barbers in 1745. Consistent with Turner's aim to elevate the status of surgeons, the establishment of this Company and, in 1800, the foundation of a College of Surgeons of London, did succeed in further 'advancing' surgeons' professional standing.

Reform, like revolution, is not a term that is coterminous with success. Reformers often initiate ideas which future generations use and refine in their own successive stages of reform. Indeed, the totality of a reformer's contribution may not be realized until many generations after his death.

It is in this sense that Turner, too, was a reformer. His ideas were not the explicit ones which initiated a paradigm shift in surgical thinking, but they do represent ideas which were incorporated into the surgeons' successful separation from the barbers. Turner's surgical prowess involved not only his demonstrable adeptness with the hand tools of his trade but also his skill at employing rhetoric as a tool to advance surgical reform. Additionally, Turner never relinquished his role as London's chief crusader against quackery. Beginning with his detailed description of the abuses his surgical colleagues faced in his 1695 *Apologia Chyrurgica*, through the warnings of quackery against the medical profession in his 1718 *Modern Quack*, as well as in his syphilis writings of the 1720s and 1730s, Turner persisted in exposing his professional enemies in order to improve the health care delivery and the reputation of surgeons and physicians in London.

Turner's Legacy as an Authority on the Surgical Art

It was recently claimed that Turner, as an author, 'used words to paint what he saw in strong colors not for the sake of using strong words, but in order to make a clear picture'. His case histories, the reviewer continued, 'take the place of pictures in a modern book'.[2] In a manner similar to that of his contemporary Daniel Defoe, Turner brilliantly depicted 'realistic domestic scenes and innocent recreations'.[3] As has been shown, Turner's case studies revealed detailed information and imagery of surgery, surgeons, and patients of early eighteenth-century London. How was Turner's composite of surgery viewed by its author and received by his contemporaries?

According to Turner's own account, he endeavoured, in the *Art of Surgery*, to save readers 'much Pains and Labour, as well as Expense' having brought 'every Thing curious' about the surgical art under their 'View at once'.[4] Herein lies the heart of Turner's belief that his writings formed a complete body of instruction. As such, Turner viewed this as his single most important publication. He compared this work with Richard Wiseman's *Chirurgical Treatises*, the work Turner 'believe[d]' was previously the 'best ... ever set forth in the English Tongue'. His frequent citations of Wiseman's ideas and procedures of surgical practice further support the reverence that he held for this surgical mentor.[5] Turner had claimed that Wiseman's work would 'be had in good Esteem, 'till some Gentleman of the Fraternity (of more Judgement, and the same Industry) shall supply his Defects'.[6] In short, Turner viewed his *Art of Surgery* as supplanting Wiseman's treatises. What did the future hold for Turner's greatest self-perceived contribution?

Despite Turner's forecast that his work would replace Wiseman's, the latter's text remained a classic of surgical writing. Chambers

Cyclopaedia (1738) claimed that Wiseman's work 'has been the foundation of most *Chirurgical* treatises since its publication'.[7] Later in the century, Samuel Johnson continued to rely upon Wiseman's treatises for examples of the surgical terms he defined in his *Dictionary*.[8] Leading surgeons like John Justamond acknowledged Wiseman as the 'Ambrose Parey of the English', and claimed that his 'System of Surgery' was 'not unworthy even of ... [the] more enlightened age' late in the century.[9]

Thus, Turner's work did not succeed in replacing Wiseman's; nevertheless, it gained considerable renown. Although 'one worthy surgeon' had predicted the *Art of Surgery*'s 'Fate' would be, like that of a painting, 'better esteemed ... [after] there was no more to be had from the same Hand' (i.e., after Turner's death), Turner assured his readers that this prediction had proved false. In fact, it appears to have been quite well received in England at the time of its publication. He claimed he 'lived to see' this work, in but 'little Time, taken into the studies, not only of those in the middle Form of Practice, but of the greatest Masters of the same Art'.[10] Furthermore, it was this grand reception which, Turner claimed, prompted his reissue of the work.

Historians frequently judge a work's success, in part, by examining the number of revised or reprinted editions. The *Art of Surgery*, first published in 1722, was expanded, chiefly by the addition of thirty-six case studies, in 1725.[11] This edition was reprinted in 1729, 1732, 1736, and once after Turner's death, 1741-42. By this measure, his work was more successful than most surgical and medical writings of his day.

Although 'The Booksellers' claimed Turner's *Art of Surgery* was 'under' translation, I have not found any indication that it ever appeared in a foreign language. Overall, there appears to have been little interest in translating English-authored general surgeries for a Continental European audience. Instead, surgeons and chirurgic-physicians in France, Germany, the Netherlands, and Italy boasted many of their own surgical writings. Indeed, many of these foreign works were translated into the vernacular English. This may reflect strong nationalist images that Continental surgery was superior during this period.

The lack of translation into another language does not, however, suggest that English works, like Turner's *Art of Surgery*, were not read or were not influential abroad. According to Turner's own account, his surgical text was received 'as well at Home as Abroad'.[12] This claim is supported by a favourable review of his work in *Acta*

Eruditorum, Leipzig, the German equivalent of London's *Philosophical Transactions*.[13] Its spread beyond England is also evinced by finding many copies of this work in long-established national and private libraries throughout Europe today.

Turner's opinion of the success his *Art of Surgery* achieved is corroborated by other eighteenth-century surgical authors. Percival Pott, a celebrated London surgeon of the later eighteenth century, claimed Turner's work was 'at that time generally looked upon as a true representation of the London practice', and that it was 'universally dispersed, and read all over the Kingdom'.[14] The influential German physico-chirurgus, Lorenz Heister, included Turner in the ranks of Wiseman, Douglas, Cheselden, Garengeot, Marinus, Morand, and Le Dran as helping advance surgery in modern times.[15] Particular surgical techniques or remedies were also praised by St Thomas Hospital surgeons, Royal Naval surgical author John Atkins, and the author of the popular *Domestic Medicine*, William Buchan. Readers could, James Handley claimed, find 'abundant Pleasure and Information' in Turner's work.[16]

The historical recognition of this work as a text remains somewhat precarious. Few, if any, besides its author, have regarded the *Art of Surgery* as a classic. Rather, Turner's work exemplifies the pattern of many works which enjoy a brief popularity, but become replaced in succeeding generations by writings more 'modern' to their own time. The *Art of Surgery* remains, it seems, conspicuously absent both from standard historical accounts of British surgery and from listings of principal surgical writings. This absence begs further consideration.

Hitherto, histories of surgery, with a few noted exceptions, have concentrated upon the discoverers of new techniques or anatomical parts. These histories, primarily authored by surgeons, have documented surgery's 'advancement' or 'progression'. For eighteenth-century English surgery, names like William Cheselden, William and John Hunter, Percival Pott, and John Abernethy usually appear. Other works have usually concentrated upon either the 'advancements' of surgery through hospital teaching and practice or the 'gains' of surgery through experiences and experiments performed during times of war. Civilian, city surgical practice has been overshadowed, and, with one notable exception, little interest has been shown towards examining the theory or rationale underlying the operative practice of surgery.[17]

Turner appears not to have discovered any new anatomical organ or pathway, nor gained renown for any novel operative techniques.

He did not commission engraved plates of instruments or anatomy – ways in which other surgeons gained renown. Despite a number of self-serving statements, Turner did not self-publicize in ways similar to Cheselden, Heister, and Hunter. These 'limitations' have, it seems, accounted in part for Turner's 'art' of surgery being overlooked. Additionally, like many Enlightenment London authors who met critical comment and satire of their work, Turner was no exception. One critic claimed Turner 'sinned ... most egregiously' by publishing 'cases of little consequence, and still more by mentioning them in terms indelicate and improper'.[18]

Turner's *Art of Surgery* received mixed responses from his own and from succeeding generations. T. Aubrey dedicated his *The Sea Surgeon, or Guinea Man's Vade Mecum* to Turner, as 'a Testimony of Respect'.[19] Other surgeons cited Turner's writings as faithful representations of their age. Eighteenth-century encyclopaedists of surgical writings dutifully recorded Turner's contributions.[20] But by 1800, Turner's image as an authority in surgery had lost its lustre. Turner had been eclipsed by British surgical authors including Percival Pott, William Hunter, and John Abernethy. These authors' works were relatively deplete of the sort of detailed, instructive, 'digressive' case histories Turner had used. For, rather than emphasizing the importance of treating the whole patient and using remedies and procedures gathered from ancient authorities as Turner had done, later eighteenth-century surgical authors highlighted the 'advancements' they said could be made in surgery by 'improving' surgical technique. Thus, once the surgeons were separated from the barbers, the surgical art which Turner sought to liberalize into a patient-oriented practice never successfully developed. Rather, eighteenth-century surgery remained a mechanical, instrument-oriented practice.

A Mixed Reputation

Although Turner's writings were widely read, not all of them met with approval. James Blondel's vehement verbal attacks against Turner's views over the power of the mother's imagination attracted other criticisms. Turner's writings on syphilis treatments prompted the tirade of his surgical colleague, John Douglas, who represented Turner as a quack. The popular press also denounced Turner. Specifically, they opposed his 'digressive' writing style.[21] Douglas identified Turner's method of contriving passages in his opponents works in order to satisfy his own objections as Turner's own invention; a rhetorical device Douglas labelled a 'Turnerism'.[22]

Despite the slanders, Turner's name and campaigns were advertised through the pamphlet wars, thereby promoting his public reputation during his lifetime.

By the early nineteenth century, most medico-surgical writers dismissed Turner altogether. Thomas Bateman, in his widely reputed *A Practical Synopsis of Cutaneous Diseases,* pointed out many passages in which he claimed Turner 'confounded' the study of skin disease. For this, he deemed Turner 'our credulous countryman'.[23] However, by 1850, a century after Turner's death, chroniclers of skin disease endorsed Turner's 'pioneering' contributions to dermatology. After that time, his enduring legacy, chiefly among dermatologists, is evinced by the use of 'Turner's cerate' well into the twentieth century.[24] Later in the twentieth century, some three hundred years after his birth, London physicians and surgeons paid tribute to Turner in their establishment of the Daniel Turner Dermatology Clinic.[25]

Synopsis

Examining Turner's career provides insight into the hierarchy of physicians and surgeons in the so-called 'marketplace' of practice in early eighteenth-century London. Turner identified the skin as the border between the two practices. Despite his multiple attempts to persuade physicians of the surgeons' need to penetrate this border in order to treat the whole patient, the skin remained a rigid barrier distinguishing physicians' and surgeons' official realms of practice. The only area of care in which their practices regularly overlapped this border was in the treatment of venereal disease. Here, perhaps the want of lucre overpowered the need of occupational identity.

Turner repeatedly represented 'quacks' as his greatest occupational threat. Unorthodox practitioners continued to treat many, perhaps the majority of 'patients' throughout the Enlightenment. Despite the outcries from practitioners like Turner, quacks and orthodox practitioners continued to coexist in London. 'Progress' for surgeons became less directed at restraining quack surgical practitioners, and more focussed upon the promotion of book learning as a way of liberalizing surgery from a mechanical trade.

Turner's writings also illuminate a surgical practitioner's occupational concerns and his patients' fears of surgery in the early eighteenth century. In addition, they reveal the persistent obstacles that a surgeon and, later, a physician faced in persuading patients to undergo treatment, in protecting his occupational turf, in preserving his own 'professional' reputation, in defending his publicly expressed views, and in advancing himself both professionally and socially.

Establishing a career in the mechanical art of surgery did not prohibit ambitious surgeons like Turner from advancing themselves. Indeed, Turner exemplifies how, through self-education and self-promotion, an individual could advance himself from a tradesman to a professional. As a professional, Turner gained scholarly repute, but he was still unable to gain the respect and recognition of a physician trained by more conventional standards, and he lacked the necessary patronage to become more fully recognized as a gentleman. Despite the increasingly fluid appellation of 'gentleman' in the eighteenth-century, it appears that one's birthright remained a steadfastly limiting factor as to who was recognized as a true gentleman in Enlightenment London. Like most contemporary Londoners, Daniel Turner – surgeon, physician, scholar, and man of letters – died a member of the same social class into which he was born.

Notes

1 D. Turner, *Art of Surgery*, 1725, v. 1, To the Reader.

2 A. Lyell, 'Daniel Turner (1667-1740) LCRP London (1711) M.D. Honorary, Yale (1723) Surgeon, Physician and Pioneer Dermatologist', 164.

3 P.R. Backscheider, *Daniel Defoe*, 21.

4 D. Turner, *Art of Surgery*, vol. 1, To the Reader.

5 Many other contemporaries shared this admiration for Wiseman. Richard Boulton, for instance, offered an explicit 'Abstract' of Wiseman's work in his 1713 *System of Rational and Practical Chirurgery*, viii.

6 D. Turner, *De Morbis Cutaneis*, 1714, 75.

7 Ephraim Chambers, *Cyclopaedia: or, An Universal Dictionary of Arts and Sciences*, vol. I (London: D. Midwinter, J. Senex, R. Gosling, W. Innys and R. Manby, R. Robinson, C. Rivington, A. Ward, J. and P. Knapton, E. Symon, S. Birt, D. Brown, T. Longman, C. Hitch, J. Shuckburgh, A. Millar, J. Pemberton and the Executors of J. Darby, 1738, Chirurgery).

8 Based upon my own sampling of terms. See also John Wiltshire, *Samuel Johnson in the Medical World: The Doctor and the Patient* (Cambridge: Cambridge University Press, 1991), 107-8.

9 J. O. Justamond, *Surgical Tracts* (London: T. Cadell,1789), 43-4. Keith Thomas claimed Wiseman's *Severall Chirurgical Treatises* became popularly known as 'Wiseman's Book of Martyrs' due both the martyr-like torture and mortality associated with surgical operations as well as the renown this work gained. See *Religion and the Decline of Magic* (London: Peregrine Books edition, 1978), 9.

10 D. Turner, *Art of Surgery*, vol. 1, To the Reader.

11 Only five of these were cases in which Turner was specifically involved; the remainder were extracted from earlier authorities. Turner's five cases appear to have been taken from his earlier surgical career.

12 D. Turner, *Art of Surgery*, vol. 1, To the Reader.

13 *Acta Eruditorum*, January 1722, reprinted in D. Turner, *Art of Surgery* (1725), The Booksellers to the Readers.

14 Percival Pott, *Observations on that Disorder of the Corner of the Eye, commonly called Fistula Lachrymalis*, 2nd edn (London: L. Hawes and Co., 1763), 30.

15 Lorenz Heister, *A General System of Surgery* (London: W. Innys, C. Davis, J. Clark, R. Manby, and J. Whiston, 1743), 6.

16 J. Handley, *Colloquia Chyrurgica*, vii.

17 C. Lawrence, 'Democratic, Divine and Heroic', 4.

18 As cited in Mark Noble, *A Biographical History of England,* vol.3 (London: W. Richardson, 1806), 284.

19 T. Aubrey, *The Sea-Surgeon or Guinea Man's Vade Mecum* (London: for John Clark, 1729), dedication. I am grateful to Norris Saakwa-Mante for this reference.

20 See, for example, Joannis Jacobi Magnet, *Bibliotheca Scriptorum Medicorum* (Genevae: Perachon & Cramer, 1731), vol. 4, 403-4; Stephani Hieronymi de Vigilis, *Bibliotheca Chirurgica* (Vindbonae: Joannis Thomae, 1781), vol. 1, 80, 717, and vol. 2, 1596, 1844-5; and Hermanni Boerhaave, *Methodus Studii Medici* (Amsterdami: Jacobi a Westein, 1751), vol. 2, 645, 766, 943.

21 *Memoirs of the Society of Grubstreet*, vol. 1, 36.

22 J. Douglas, *Dissertation on Venereal Disease*, part III, 2.

23 Thomas Bateman, *A Practical Synopsis of Cutaneous Diseases* (London: Longman, Hurst Rees Orme, and Brown, 1813), footnote 148 and 59. See also P.J. Hare, *Our Credulous Countryman.*

24 Alan Lyell noted that Turner's Cerate was found in the *Dispensatory of the USA* through, at least, 1955. See his 'Daniel Turner ... The Man Seen in the Pages of his Book on the Skin', 168.

25 The Daniel Turner Clinic was co-founded by dermatologists Peter W. M. Copeman and Richard Staughton, at St Stephens' Hospital in London in the late 1970s. Upon the closing of this hospital, the clinic was re-established in a state-of-the-art facility at the new Chelsea and Westminster Hospital, Fulham Road, London, with Richard Staughton as Consultant Dermatologist.

Appendix 1
Vernacular Surgical Treatises 1685-1745

Cooke, James. *Mellificum Chirurgiae: or, The Marrow of Chirurgery*, 4th edn, 1685. (4th edn, 1693; 4th edn, 1700; 5th edn, 1704; 6th edn, 1717).

Ryder, Hugh. *New Practical Observations in Surgery*, 1685. (2nd edn, 1693).
_____, *Practical Chirurgery*, 1689.

Muys, Joannes. *A Rational Practice of Surgery*, 1686.

Barbette, Paul. *Thesarus Chirurgiae*, 4th edn, 1687.

Read, Alexander. *Chirurgorum Comes: or, The Whole Practice of Chirurgery*, 1687.

Salmon, William. *Paratepemata: or, Select Physical and Chyrurgical Observations*, 1687 (2nd edn, 1689).
_____, *Ars chirurgica*, 1698 (also 1699).

La Charriere, Joseph de. *New Chyurgical Operacions*, 1694 (also 1695)
_____, *A Treatise of the Operations of Surgery*, 1712, 1722.

Colbatch, John. *Four Treatises of Physic & Chirurgery*, 1698 (2nd edn, 1699; 3rd edn, 1704).
_____, *New Light on Chirurgery*, 1695 (2nd edn, 1704).

La Vauguion, de, *Compleat Body of Chirurgical Operation*, 1699. (2nd edn, 1707; 3rd edn, 1716).

Belloste, Augustin. *The Hospital-Surgeon*, 1701 (2nd edn, 1706; 3rd edn, 1713; 4th edn, 1732-33, 5th edn, 1745).
_____, *The Hospital-Surgeon*, vol. 2, 1729.

Le Clerc, Charles Gabriel. *The Compleat Surgeon*, 1701 (4th edn, 1710; 5th edn, 1714; 6th edn, 1727).
_____, *The Second Part of the Compleat Surgeon*, 1710.

Moyle, John. *Abstractum Chirurgiiae Marinae: or, An Abstract of Sea Syrgery*, 1686.
_____, *Chirurgus Marinus; or, The Sea-Chirurgion*, 1693 (4th edn, 1702).
_____, *The Experienced Chirurgion*, 1703.
_____, *Chyrurgic Memoirs*, 1708.

Wiseman, Richard. *Eight Chirugicall Treatises*, 4th edn, 1705 (5th edn, 1719; 6th edn, 1734).

Handley, James. *Colloquia Chyrurgica: or, The Whole Art of Surgery*,1705. (2nd edn, 1710; 3rd edn, 1721; 4th edn, 1733; 5th edn, 1743).

Purmann, Matthias Gottfried. *Chirurgia Curiosa*, 1706.

Dionis, Pierre. *A Course of Chirurgical Operations*, 1710. (2nd edn, 1733)

Boulton, Richard. *A System of Rational and Practical Chirurgery*, 1713.

Horne, Johannes van. *Micro-Techne: or, A Methodical Introduction to the Art of Chirurgery*, 1717 (2nd edn, 1730)

Douglas, John. *Syllabus of What is to be Perform'd in a Course of Anatomy, Chirurgical Operations, and Bandages*, 1719.
_____, *Syllabus of Chirurgical Operations*, 1727.

Turner, Daniel. *The Art of Surgery*, 1722. (2nd edn, 1725; 3rd edn, 1729; 4th edn, 1732; 5th edn, 1736; 6th edn, 1741-1742).

Garengeot, Rene Jaques Croissant de. *A Treatise of Chirurgical Operations*, 1723.

Dunn, Edward. *A Compendious and New Method of Performing Chirurgical Operations*, 1724.

Atkins, John. *A Treatise of Chirurgical Subjects*, 1729.
_____, *The Navy-Surgeon: or, A Practical System of Surgery*, 1734 (2nd edn, 1737; 3rd edn, 1742).

Smith, George. *Institutiones Chirurgical: or, Principles of Surgery*, 1732.

Stuart, Alexander. *New Discoveries and Improvements in the Most Consideable Branches of Anatomy and Surgery*, 1738.

Le Dran, Henri Francois. *Observations in Surgery*, 1739, (2nd edn, 1740; 3rd edn, 1758; 4th edn, 1771).

Sharp, Samuel. *A Treatise in the Operations of Surgery*, 1739 (2nd edn, 1739; 3rd edn, 1740; 4th edn, 1743; 5th edn, 1747;6th edn, 1751;

7th edn, 1758; 8th edn, 1761; 9th edn, 1769; 10th edn, 1782; New edn, 1788).

Beckett, William. *A Collection of Chirurgical Tracts*, 1740.
_____, *Practical Surgery*, 1740.

Saviard, Barthelemy. *Observations in Surgery*, 1740.

Heister, Lorenz. *A General System of Surgery*, 1743. (2nd edn,1745; 3rd edn, 1748; 4th edn, 1750; 5th edn, 1753; 6th edn, 1757; 7th edn, 1759; 7th edn, 1763; 8th edn,1768).

Appendix 2
Constitution of the Benevolent Society for the Improvement of Chyrurgery, &c. (1704)

I. This society shall consist of Residents and Travellers.

II. There shall be none admitted but Chyrurgeons, who shall be approved by the President, and Four Residing-Members at least, and they not to be Registered till their Second Attendance; and when Registered to pay One Shilling.

III. At the Expiration of half an Hour, the Minutes of the Foregoing Day shall be Read, and during that Sitting, nothing be Treated of but what is Essential to the Society, and that to be gravely Debated by one Voice at a time.

IV. For the Benefit and Improvement of the Society, there shall be Readings on Various Subjects by the Residing-Members.

V. The Travelling Members are advis'd to keep Punctual Journals of their Observations, especially Chyrurgical; which being Communicated to the Society, shall be Registered with the Authors names.

VI. A Scheme of Observations may be given by way of Instruction to any Travelling-Member, adapted to climate, &c they Intend for.

VII. Every Travelling-Member is desired to Establish a Correspondence abroad with qualified Persons, whom we shall Entitle Corresponding-Members.

VIII. Such Corresponding-Members shall be apply'd to by the Society, according to the Circumstances of Time, Place, &c.

IX. Such Journals and Rarities as are presented to the Society, shall be Reposited at their Place of Meeting, and not to be Transferr'd from there without their Consent.

X. Any Members afflicted with Sickness, may (if desired) have the Advice of the Society, and Medicines *gratis*; or if any are taken by Foreign Enemies, or Shipwrack'd, they shall receive such an Exhibition from the Fund of the Society as shall be thought Convenient.

XI. If any Member Travels without taking Leave of the Society, either Personally or by way of Letter, [he] shall be Excluded the aforesaid Benevolence, and likewise pay Five Shillings for his Re-Admittance.

XII. Every Travelling-Member that does not make his Personal Appearance, in the Society within Twenty Days after his Arrival, is subject to the same Penalties.

XIII. No Member shall dare to Expose any of the Society for Errors or Imperfection in Discourse, Practice or Journals delivered in the Society, under Penalty of Expulsion.

XIV. All Laws that are made, shall have the Consent of two Thirds of the Members present, the least Number being Nine, the President, or Vice-President being present.

XV. A Catalogue or Collection may be made of useful Books, Instruments, &c. which may be perus'd by any Member at the Hours of Meeting.

XVI. Every Member shall pay Quarterly One Shilling, and for Non-Appearance the first Meeting-day of each Month Six Pence: sickness or out of Town excepted.

XVII. The Forfitured and quarterly Contributions shall be put into the Common-Stock, which shall be manag'd at the Discretion of the Society.

XVIII. The Place of Meeting shall be near the Royal-Exchange, and not be altered without the Approbation of the Society.

XIX. The Days of Meeting to be Tuesdays and Frydays; and the Time from Two to Four.

XX. To have an Annual Feast on Ladyday, when Four of the Reading-Members shall be elected Officers, viz. Praeses, Treasurer, Register and Conservator of the Rarities.

XXI. These Orders shall be Read by one of the Officers on the First Meetingday of every Month, and also at the Entry of every New Member.

Appendix 3
List of the Books Turner Gave to Yale College

A. Turner's own writings

De Morbis Cutaneis. A Treatise on Diseases Incident to the Skin (London, 1714).

The Art of Surgery, 2 vols. (London, 1722).

Syphilis. A Practical Dissertation on the Venereal Disease (London, 1717).

The Modern Quack or the Physical Imposter Detected (London, 1718).

A Remarkable Case in Surgery (London, 1709).

B. Other medical/surgical writings

Cowper, William. *The Anatomy of Humane Bodies* (Oxford,1698).

Gibson, Thomas. *The Anatomy of Humane Bodies Epitomized*, 6th edn (London, 1703).

Woodward, John. *Naturalis Historia Telluris* (London, 1714).

_______, *The State of Physick and of Diseases* (London, 1718).

C. Religious commentary

White, Samuel. *A Commentary on the Prophet Isaiah* (London,1709).

S[terry], P. *The Appearance of God to Man* (London, 1710).

Mather, Samuel. *The Figures or Types of the Old Testament* (London, 1705).

Hussey, Joseph. *A Warning from the Winds* (London, 1704).

Trapp, Joseph. *A Preservative Against Unsettled Notions and Want of Principles in Religion*, 2 vols. (London, 1722).

Blair, James. *Our Saviour's Divine Sermon on the Mount*, 5 vols. (London, 1722-3).

Fogg, Laurence. *Theologiae Speculativae Schema* (London, 1712).

Limborch, Philippus van. *A Complete System or Body of Divinity*, trans. by W. Jones, 2nd edn (London, 1713).

D. History and geography

Jones, Thomas. *The Rise and Progress of the Most Honorable and Loyal Society of Antient Britons* (London, 1717).

Collins, Arthur. *The Baronettage of England*, 2 vols (London, 1720).

Perry, John. *An Account of the Stopping of Daggenham Breach* (London, 1721).
Traubman, Nathaniel. *Memoirs of the British Fleets and Squadrons in the Mediterranean, Anno 1708 and 1709* (London, 1710).
Walker, Hovenden. *A Journal or Full Account of the Late Expedition to Canada* (London, 1720).
Ashmole, Elias. *The History of the Most Noble Order of the Garter* (London, 1715).

E. Other

Nani Mirabelli, Domenico. *Polyanthea Novissima* (Langius, Francoforti ad Moenum, 1617).
[Wood, William]. *A Survey of Trade* (London, 1718).

Bibliography

Primary Sources

Manuscripts

Barber-Surgeons' Company of London

Court Minutes, vol. 12, MS 5257 (6); vol. 13, MS 5257 (7).

'The Rules, Orders and Ordinances of the Mistery and Commonally [sic] of Barbers and Surgeons of London', 13 January 1708, MS A/2/1.

British Library (London)

Du Plessis, J., 'A Short History of Human Prodigious & Monstrous Births of Dwarfs, Sleepers, Giants, Strong Men, Hermaphrodites, Numerous Births, and Extream Old Age &c.', Sloane MS 5246.

Turner, Daniel, 'Religio Medici Reformata: or, Private Devotion, in 2 parts, conteining certain Forms of Prayer, Thanksgiving &c. To be used in the Times of Health & Sickness. suited to the Authours Occasions', British Library, Additional Manuscripts 14404.

Turner, Daniel, Letters to Sir Hans Sloane, Sloane MSS 4048, f. 135 (1725-6); 4053, f. 3 (1733).

Essex Record Office (Chelmsford)

Holman, William, 'The History of the Parish of Latton', T/P 195/16.

Latton Parish, D/P 344/1/1-4 and T/B 93.

Latton, Transcript of Parish Registers, T/R 26.

Letter (28 Sept. 17_2), T/B93.

Manor of Latton Hall, D/DK M43 (1727-28); D/DK M68 (1600-1768).

Manor of Mark Hall, D/DK M67 (1600-1768); D/DK M69.

Guildhall Library (London)

Index to the Inhabitants of the Parishes of the City of London, which were Assessed in Connection with the Tax on Marriages, Births and Burials, and upon Bachelors and Widowers, 1695, Part 2, *Inhabitants without the Walls* (1938), typescript MS SL 06/2. Printed Works.

Register of Apprenticeship Bindings of the Barber-Surgeons' Company, MS 5266.

Register of Freedom Admissions, Barber-Surgeons' Company, MS 5265.

Russell, Richard, 'Affidavit of Procuring a body from Tyburn', MS 9833, *Miscellaneous Papers of the Barber-Surgeons' Company, 1612-1763.*

Tallow Chandlers Company, Register of Apprenticeship Bindings, MS 6158 (3).

Wright, David, 'An Index of London Surgical Practitioners, 1736-1811, compiled from the Trade Directories in the Guildhall Library, London', MS SL 47 (1989).

Hertfordshire County Record Office (Hertford)

'Articles for Letting Shanlocks from James Harris' [witnessed by Daniel Turner], 80299.

Raffinger End, Datchworth, Lease and Release, and Settlement (19 & 20 Dec. 1727), D/EAS 1610-11.

Turner, Daniel, 'Of the Articles of Agreement before Marriage, that Part Relating to Dower and Thirds', 10 December 1710, D/EAS 1612 (867).

Turner, John, Jr, Land Deed (1688), D/EAS 3131.

Watton Parish Register Book (1737-1812).

Public Record Office, Chancery Lane (London)

Blondel, James, Probated Will (15 October 1734), Prob. 11/667.

Turner, Daniel, Probated Will (16 April 1741), Prob. 11/709.

Turner, John, Probated Will (4 August 1691), Prob. 11/440.

Royal College of Physicians (London)

Annals, vols 8 and 9.

Royal College of Surgeons of England (London)

[Admiralty], Surgeon's Passing Certificates, Navy Board 2952-2963, transcript by R. R. James, 2 vols, MS 129a f.12-13.

Barber-Surgeons' Company Apprenticeship Books, transcript by R. R. James, Book VI (3 July 1683 - 6 August 1689).

Wood, W., [Surgical casebook, 1679-1690], MS Tract A297 (3).

Royal Infirmary (Edinburgh)

Hare, P. J., Personal file, Department of Dermatology.

Royal Society of London

Journal Book, Copy, vol. 8.

T., J. [i.e. Daniel Turner], 'Of a Stone found in the Gall-Bladder of a Woman', Classified Papers 1660-1740, Cl.P. 12(1).38, 81 (6 December 1693).

Turner, Daniel, 'Remarks, taken upon dissecting the Body of A. M. a Maid of about 30 years of Age: who dyed of an Ascites, ye first of August 1689', Classified Papers 1660-1740, Cl.P. 12(1).40, 84 (9 February 1693/94).

Turner, Daniel, 'Observatio Casus non vulgaris de Hydrope intra Uteri Tunicas contento', Classified Papers 1660-1740, Cl.P. 12(1).41, 85.

Turner, Daniel, 'De Morsu venenoso Canis rabidi', Classified Papers 1660-1740, Cl.P. 12(1).41, 85 and 85v.

Turner, Daniel, Letter to Dr Jurin, EL.T.74.

Society of Genealogists

Altham Papers.

Turner Papers.

United Medical and Dental Schools of Guy's and St Thomas's Hospitals, St Thomas's Campus, Medical Library (London)

'Charles Oxley Notebook, Case notes of surgical patients admitted to St Thomas's Hospital, 1725-26', MS S2.a.6.

'Register of Pupils and Dressers', MS 31.d.2.

Published Works

Anonymous, 'The Names of the Governors of St Bartholomew's Hospital' ([London]: s.n., n.d.).

Anonymous, 'The Physician's Reply to the Surgeon's Answer' ([London]: s.n., 1689-90).

Anonymous, 'Short State of the Case Between the Physicians & Surgeons, relating to the Surgeons Bill, now before the Honourable House of Commons' ([London]: s.n., 1690).

Anonymous, *Present State of Physick & Surgery in London* (London: Thos. Speed, 1701).

Anonymous, 'Constitutions of the Benevolent Society for the Improvement of Chyrurgery' ([London]: s.n., 1704).

Anonymous, 'A Bill for the Better Regulating the Practice of Surgery in and About the City of London and Westminster, and the Better Providing Her Majesties Fleet and Army with Skillful and Able Surgeons' (London: Charles Bill & Thomas Newcomb, 1705).

Anonymous, 'Monopoly made a Property; or, The Navy Surgeons Memorial to the Managing Apothecaries in Black-Friars' (London: s.n., 1708).

Anonymous, *The London-Bawd: with her Character and Life*, 4th edn (London: for John Gwillin, 1711).

Anonymous, *A Mechanical Account of the Cause and Cure of a Virulent Gonorrhoea in Both Sexes* (London: for F. Jefferies, 1719).

Anonymous, *Medicina Flagellata: or, The Doctor Scarify'd* (London: J. Bateman & J. Nicks, 1721).

Anonymous, *The True Church of England Man's Companion in the Closet: or, A Complete Manual of Private Devotions* (London: s.n., 1728).

Anonymous, *The Practical Scheme of the Secret Disease* (London: H. Parker, 1730).

Anonymous, *A Letter to a Little Doctor in Scavenger Square, Occasioned by his Curious Dissertation in Latin Concerning a S-rr-v-r-nce Overbaked,*

Addressed to that Great Doctor, Mr Daniel Turner. To Which is Added, The Porter Turned Physician. A Tale (London: for Jacob Ginglymus, 1731).

Anonymous, *London Described, or, The Most Noted Regular Buildings Both Publick and Private with the Views of Several Squares in the Liberties of London & Westminster* (London: Thos & John Bowles, 1731).

Anonymous, *Aristotle's Last Legacy: or, His Golden Cabinet of Secrets*, Part IV of *Aristotle's Works Compleated* (London: The Booksellers, 1733).

Anonymous, *Aristotle's Masterpiece*, in *Aristotle's Works Compleated* (London: The Booksellers, 1733).

Alban, Thomas, *A List of the Royal Society ... with the Places of Abode of Most of its Members* (London: s.n., 1718).

Altham, Roger, *Sermons Preached on Several Occasions*, 2 vols (London: G. Strahan, 1732).

Armstrong, John, *Synopsis of the History and Cure of Venereal Diseases* (London: A. Millar, 1737).

Atkins, John, *The Navy-Surgeon; or, A Practical System of Surgery* (London: C. Ward & R. Chandler, 1734).

Atkyns, Arabella, *The Family Magazine* (London: J. Osborn, 1741).

Aubrey, T., *The Sea-Surgeon o' Guinea Man's Vade Mecum* (London: for John Clark, 1729).

Bate, George, *Pharmacopoeia Bateana; or, Bate's Dispensatory*, 5th edn (London: W. & J. Innys, 1720).

Bateman, Thomas, *A Practical Synopsis of Cutaneous Diseases* (London: Longman, Hurst, Rees, Orme & Brown, 1813).

[Bateman, Thomas], *Delineations of Cutaneous Diseases* (London: Longman, Hurst, Rees, Orme, and Brown, 1817).

Beckett, William, *Free and Impartial Inquiry into the Antiquity and Efficacy of Touching for the Cure of the King's Evil* (London: J. Peele, 1722).

_____, 'An Attempt to Prove the Antiquity of the Venereal Disease, long before the Discovery of the West-Indies', *Philosophical Transactions of the Royal Society of London*, xxx (1717-19), 839-47.

_____, 'A Letter concerning the Antiquity of the Venereal Disease', *Philosophical Transactions of the Royal Society of London*, xxxi (1720-21), 47-65.

_____, 'A Letter to Dr Halley ... in answer to Some Objections made to the History of the Antiquity of the Venereal Disease', *Philosophical Transactions of the Royal Society of London*, xxxi (1720-21), 108-12.

Bellers, John, *An Essay Towards the Improvement of Physick* (London: The Assigns of J. Soule for J. Morphew, 1714).

[Bellet, Isaac], *Letters on the Force of Imagination in Pregnant Women* (London: W. Griffin, 1765).

Belloste, Augustine, *An Essay on Mercury*, translated by J. B., M. B. (Dublin: S. Powell for Phil Crampton, 1733).

_____, *A Treatise on Mercury* (London: Dredge, 1843).

Bianchini, Giovanni Fortunato, *An Essay on the Force of Imagination in Pregnant Women. Addressed to the Ladies* (London: R. Baldwin, 1772).

Bickerstaff, Isaac, 'Dissertation upon Noses', *The Tatler* (London: sold by John Morphew), no. 260, 7 December 1710.

Blackmore, Richard, *Critical Dissertation upon the Spleen* (London: J. Pemberton, 1725).

_____, *Discourses on the Gout, a Rheumatism, and the King's Evil* (London: J. Pemberton, 1727).

Blankaart, Stephen, *The Physical Dictionary*, 5th edn (London: S. Crouch & J. Sprint, 1708).

Blondel, James, *Disputatio Medica Inauguralis de Crisibus* (Leiden: Abraham Elzevier, 1692).

[Blondel, James], *The Strength of Imagination in Pregnant Women Examined* (London: J. Peale, 1727).

_____, *Power of the Mother's Imagination over the Foetus Examined* (London: John Brotherton, 1729).

_____, *Dissertation Physique sur la Force de l'Imagination des Femmes Enceintes sur le Fetus*, translated by Albert Brun (Leyden: Gilbert Langerack and Theodore Lucht, 1737).

_____, *Natuurkundige Verhandeling: Wegens het Vermoogen der Inbeelding van Zwangere Vrouwen op Haar Vrucht*, translated by Jan van der Hulst (Rotterdam: Hermanns Kentlink, 1737).

_____, *Lettres sur le Pouvoir de l'Imagination des Femmes Enceintes* (S.l.: s.n., 1745).

_____, *Drey Merkw Urdige Physikalische Abhandlungen von der Einbildungskraft der Schwangern Weiber, und Derselben Wirkung auf ihre Leibesfrucht* (Strasbourg: Amand Konig, 1756).

_____, *Dissertazione della Forza dell' Immaginazione delle Donne Gravide Sovra il Feto* (Ferrara: Francesco Gardi, 1760).

Boerhaave, Hermanni, *Methodus Studii Medici* (Amsterdami: Jacobi a Westein, 1751).

Boulton, Richard, *A System of Rational and Practical Chirurgery* (London: W. Taylor & W. Innys, 1713).

_____, *An Essay on External Remedies* (London: s.n., 1715).

Boyer, Jean Babtiste de, Marquis d'Argens, *The Jewish Spy*, 4 vols (Dublin: Oli. Nelson and H. Saunders, 1753).

Bradley, Henry, *Physical and Philosophical Remarks on Dr Dover's Late Pamphlet, entitled, The Ancient Physician's Legacy* (London: C. Rivington, 1733).

Brest, Vincent, *An Analytical Inquiry into the Specifick Property of Mercury, Relating to the Cure of Venereal Diseases* (London: J. Nourse, J. Stagg, J. Brindely, and J. Millan, 1732).

B___t, Vint. [i.e. Vincent Brest], *Remarks on the Impositions of Quacks, so much Practiced in this Kingdom* (London: for the author, sold by R. Darre, 1735).

Brookes, Thomas, *London's Lamentations: or, A Serious Discourse Concerning that Late Fiery Dispensation that Turned our (once renowned) City onto a Ruinous Heap* (London: N. Ponder for J. Hancock, 1670).

Brown, James, *The Directory; or List of Principal Traders in London* (London: Henry Kent, 1732).

Brown, Richard, *A Letter from a Physician in London to his Friend in the Country; giving an Account of the Montpellier Practice in Curing the Venereal Disease* (London: J. Roberts, 1730).

Browne, Thomas, *Pseudodoxia Epidemica: or Enquiries into Vulgar and Common Errors* (London: T. H. for E. Dod, 1646).

Buffon, George Louis Leclerc, *Oeuvres completes de Buffon*, edited by M. Flourens (Paris: P. Dumenil, 1835-6).

Bulwer, John, *Anthropometamorphosis: Man Transform'd; or The Artificial Changling* (London: J. Hardesty, 1650).

Burton, John, *Treatise on the Non-Naturals* (London: A. Staples & J. Hildyard, 1738).

Burton, Robert, *Anatomy of Melancholy* (Oxford: John Lichfield and James

Short, 1621).

Cam, Joseph, *A Short Account of the Venereal Disease*, 3rd edn (London: G. Strahan, 1719).

Campbell, R., *The London Tradesman* (London: David & Charles, 1969, 1st edn 1747).

Cantwell, Andrew, 'Pernicious Effects of Crude Mercury Given Inwardly', *Philosophical Transactions of the Royal Society of London*, xl (1737-38), 139-42.

Chamberlayne, Edward, *Magnae Britanniae Notitia: or, The Present State of Great Britain*, 38th edn (London: S. Birt, 1755).

Chambers, Ephraim, *Cyclopaedia: or, An Universal Dictionary of Arts and Sciences*, vol. 1 (London: D. Midwinter, J. Senex, R. Gosling, W. Innys and R. Manby, R. Robinson, C. Rivington, A. Ward, J. and P. Knapton, E. Symon, S. Birt, D. Brown, T. Longman, C. Hitch, J. Shuckburgh, A. Millar, J. Pemberton and the Executors of J. Darby, 1738), 'Chirurgery'.

Chevalier, Thomas, *Observations in Defence of a Bill ... Including a History of Surgery in England* (London: J. Johnson & J. Debrett, 1797).

Cheyne, George, *The Natural Method of Cureing* [sic] *the Diseases of the Body and the Disorders of the Mind* (London: G. Strahan and J. and P. Knapton, 1742).

Chicoyneau, François, *The Practice of Salivating shewn to be of no Use or Efficacy in the Cure of the Venereal Disease*, translated by C. Willoughby (London: J. Roberts, 1723).

Clap, Thomas, *The Annals or History of Yale-College* (New Haven, Connecticut: John Hotchkiss and B. Mecom, 1766).

Clowes, William, *A Briefe and Necessarie Treatise, Touching the Cure of the Disease called Morbus Gallicus* (London: Flesher, 1587).

Clutton, Joseph, *A True and Candid Relation of the Good and Bad Effects of Joshua Ward's Pill and Drop. Exhibited in Sixty-Eight Cases; Quotations from the Writings of Learned Physicians Concerning Arsenick; some Cases of Persons who have Taken it; and Experiments to Shew What are the Component Principles of these Pills. Introduced with Occurances Shewing the Rise and Progress of this Controversy. The Whole Being an Essay to Discover how far this Random Practice of Physick is Really Useful* (London: for the author, 1736).

Coltheart, P., *The Quacks Unmask'd* (London: The Author, 1727).

A Country Physician, *Remarks Upon a Late Scurrilous Pamphlet, entitled, A Review of the Quicksilver Controversy. In which Dr Turner's Character, as a just and impartial Historian in regard to the same, is asserted* (London: H. Whitridge, 1733).

Cowper, William, *The Anatomy of Humane Bodies* (Oxford: for S. Smith & B. Walford, 1698).

C., T., *The Charitable Surgeon, or, The Best Remedies for the Worst Maladies, reveal'd*, 2nd edn (London: Edmund Curll, 1709).

[De Coetlogon, Dennis], *One Physician is e'en Just as Good as t'other, and Surgeons are Not Less Knowing. Apothecaries are as Good as Any; if not Best of All* (London: T. Cooper, 1739).

Defoe, Daniel, *System of Magick* (London: J. Clarke, 1729).

_____, *The Compleat English Gentleman*, Karl D. Bulbring (ed.), (London: David Nutt, 1890).

_____, *A Journal of the Plague Year*, Louis Landa (ed.), (London: Oxford University Press, 1969; 1st edn 1722).

Derham, William, *Physico-Theology: or, A Demonstration of the Being and Attributes of God, from His Works of Creation* (London: W. Innys, 1714).

_____, *Astro-Theology: or, A Demonstration of the Being and Attributes of God, from a Survey of the Heavens* (London: W. Innys, 1715).

Desault, Pierre, *Treatise on the Venereal Distemper*, translated by John Andree (London: printed for John Clarke, 1738).

[Douglas, John], *A Dissertation on the Venereal Disease wherein a Method of Curing ... Without ... Mercurial Drenches, Vomits, ... and ... a Salivation*, 2 parts (London: for the author, 1737).

_____, *A Dissertation on the Venereal Disease, Part III ... in Answer to the ... Invectives, ... Insinuations, and ... Misrepresentations of our Salutary Process ... in a Pamphlet Signed by Dr T[urne]r* (London: for the Author, 1739).

[Dover, T.], *Encomium Argenti Vivi: A Treatise upon the Use and Properties of Quicksilver ... with Some Remarks upon the Animadversions of Dr Turner upon Belloste* (London: for Stephen Austin, sold by J. Roberts, [1733]).

Dover, Thomas, *The Ancient Physician's Legacy*, 6th edn (London: C. Hitch, J. Brotherton, and R. Minors, 1742).

Drake, James, *Anthropologia Nova; or, A New System of Anatomy* (London: Sam Smith and Benjamin Walford, 1707).

Eloy, N., *Dictionnaire Historique de la Medecine: Ancienne et Moderne*, 4 vols (Mons: H. Hoyois, 1778).

The Entertainer, No. 7, 18 December 1717, as reprinted in *The Entertainer*, 3rd edn (London: J. Osborn, 1734).

Erichsen, John E., *Practical Treatise on Diseases of the Scalp* (London: John Churchill, 1842).

Fienus, Thomas, *De Viribus Imaginationis* (Louvain: G. Rivius, 1608).

Floyer, Sir John, *Enquiry into the Right Use and Abuses of the Hot, Cold, and Temperate Baths in England* (London: R. Cland, 1697).

Fog's Weekly Journal (London: printed by J. Wilford, 1728-9).

Fontanus, Nicholas, *The Womans Doctour* (London: J. Blague & S. Howes, 1652).

Freind, John, *The History of Physick: from the Time of Galen, to the Beginning of the Sixteenth Century*, 2 vols (London: J. Walthoe, 1725-26).

_____, *The History of Physick: from the Time of Galen, to the Beginning of the Sixteenth Century*, 2nd edn, corrected (London: J. Walthoe, 1727).

Fuller, Francis, *Medicina Gymnastica: or, A Treatise Concerning the Power of Exercise* (London: J. Matthews for R. Knaplock, 1705).

Fuller, Thomas, *Pharmacopeia Extemporanea* (London: B. Walford, 1710).

Fuller, Thomas (Bishop), *History of the Worthies of England, A new edition*, by John Nichols, 2 vols (London: F. C. and J. Rivington; T. Payne; Wilkie and Robinson; Longman, Hurst, Rees, Orme and Brown; Cadell and Davies; R. H. Evans; J. Mawman; J. Murray; and R. Baldwin, 1811).

Gentleman's Magazine; or, Monthly Intelligencer (London: R. Newton [*et al.*], 1731-1833).

Gibson, Edmund, *The Causes of the Discontents, In Relation to the Plague, and The Provisions Against it, Fairly Stated and Consider'd* (London: J. Roberts, 1721).

Gooch, Benjamin, *Practical Treatise of Wounds and other Chirurgical Subjects to which is Prefixed a Short Historical Account of the Rise and Progress of Surgery and Anatomy* (Norwich: the author, 1767).

Goodall, Charles, *The Royal College of Physicians* (London: M. Flesher for W. Kettilby, 1684).

Grew, N., 'Description and use of the Pores in the Skin of the Hands and Feet', *Philosophical Transactions of the Royal Society of London*, xiv (1684), 566-7.

Guardian, no. 1, 12 March 1713.

Handley, James, *Colloquia Chyrurgia: or, The Whole Art of Surgery Epitomiz'd*, 4th edn (London: A. Bettesworth & C. Hitch, 1733).

Harris, Walter, *Pharmacologia Anti-Empirica; or, A Rational Discourse of Remedies both Chyurgical and Galenical. ... Together with some Remarks on ... the most Notorious Impostures of Diverse Empiricks and Mountebanks* (London: for R. Chiswell, 1683).

Hartley, David, *Observations on Man*, part 1 (London: J. Leake & W. Frederick, 1749).

Harvey, Gideon, *Great Venus Unmask'd*, 2nd edn (London: B. G. for N. Brook, 1672).

Heister, Lorenz, *A General System of Surgery* (London: W. Innys, C. Davis, J. Clark, R. Manby, and J. Whiston, 1743).

Hendley, William, *Loimologia Sacra: or, A Discourse Shewing that the Plague Never Proceeds from any First Natural Cause, but is Sent Immediately From God, and that as a Punishment to a People for their Sins* (London: T. Bickerton, 1721).

Hughes, John, *A Complete History of England* (London: s.n., 1706).

Hutton, Ulrich von, *De Morbo Gallico*, translated by T. Paynell, revised by D. Turner (London: J. Clarke, 1730).

Jackson, Seguin Henry, *Dermato-pathologia; or Practical Observations, from Some New Thoughts on the Pathology and Proximate Causes of Diseases of the True Skin* (London: H. Rynell, 1792).

Jenty, Charles Nicholas, *A Synoptical Exposition of the Parts of the Human Body, as they are Gradually met with in Dissection*, in C. N. Jenty, *Course of Anatomico Physiological Lectures on the Human Structure and Animal Oeconomy* (London: James Rivington and James Fletcher, 1757), vol. 1, clxxxiii-ccxv.

Johnson, Samuel, *Works*, John Hawkins (ed.), (London: J. Buckland, 1787).

_____, *Lives of the English Poets*, 2 vols (London: J. M. Dent & Sons, Everyman's Library Edition, 1925).

Justamond, J. O., *Surgical Tracts* (London: T. Cadell, 1789), *Tract 1, Outlines of the History of Surgery.*

Kennedy, Peter, *An Essay on External Remedies Wherein it is Considered, Whether all the Curable Distempers incident to Human Bodies, may not be Cured by Outward Means* (London: A. Bell, 1715).

Knyveton, John, *The Diary of a Surgeon in the Year 1751-1752*, Ernest Gray (ed. and trans.), (London: D. Appleton-Cent. Co., 1937).

Lemery, N. and Winslow, J. B., *Memories Academie Royale des Sciences*, xxxiii (1733); xxxviii (1738); xl (1740).

Littleton-Costeker, John, *The Fine Gentleman; or, The Compleat Education of a Young Nobleman* (London: J. Roberts, 1732).

Lommius, Jodocus, *A Treatise of Continual Fevers*, translated by T. Dale (London: T. Brotherton, 1732).

[Long, James], *An Enquiry into the Origin of Human Appetites and Affections* (London: W. Wood, 1747).

Lorry, Anne Charles, *Tractatus de Morbis Cutaneis* (Paris: P. G. Cavelier, 1777).

Luisinus, Aloysius, *Aphrodisiacus, Containing a Summary of the Ancient Writers on the Venereal Disease*, translated by Daniel Turner (London: John Clarke, 1736).

Lyser, Michael, *The Art of Dissecting the Human Body* (London: for Joseph Davidson, 1740).

Madden, Dr, 'Account of What was Observ'd upon Opening the Corpse of a Person who had Taken Several Ounces of Crude Mercury Internally', *Philosophical Transactions of the Royal Society of London*, xxxix (1735-36), 291-4.

Magnet, Joannis Jacobi, *Bibliotheca Scriptorum Medicorum* (Genevae: Perachon & Cramer, 1731).

[Mandeville, Bernard], *The Natural Secret History of Both Sexes: or, a Modest Defense of Public Stews*, by Luke Ogle, 4th edn (London: s.n., 1740), in William Beckett, *A Collection of Chirurgical Tracts* (London: E. Curll, 1740).

Marten, John, *A Treatise of the Venereal Disease*, 7th edn (London: for the author, 1711).

Maubray, John, *The Female Physician: The Whole Art of New Improv'd Midwifery* (London: for James Holland, 1724).

Mauclerc, John Henry, *The Power of Imagination in Pregnant Women Discussed* (London: J. Robinson, 1740).
_____, *Dr Blondel Confuted: or, the Ladies Vindicated with Regard to the Power of Imagination in Pregnant Women* (London: M. Cooper, 1747).

Mead, Richard, 'An Abstract of Part of a Letter from D. Bonomo to Signior Redi, Containing Some Observations Concerning the Works of Humane Bodies', *Philosophical Transactions of the Royal Society of London*, xxiii (1702-3), 1296-9.
_____, *A Short Discourse Concerning Pestilential Contagion and the Methods used to Prevent it* (London: S. Buckley and R. Smith, 1720).

Memoirs of the Society of Grubstreet (London: J. Wilford, 1737).

Mercurialis, Hieronymus, *De Morbis Cutaneis et Omnibus Corporis Humani Excrementis Tractatus* (Venice: Paulum & Antonium Meitos, 1572).
_____, *De Decoratione Liber*, 2nd edn (Venice: Junitas, 1601).

Mercurialist, *A Short Review of the Quicksilver Controversy. In a Letter to Dr Dover. Occasioned by the Publication of Dr Turner's late Book* (London: J. Brotherton, A. Bettesworth, and C. Hitch, 1733).

Molière, Jean Baptiste Poquelin de, *The Mock Doctor*, translated by H. Fielding (London: J. Caslon, 1732).

Morgan, T., *Philosophical Principles of Medicine* (London: J. Darby & T. Browne, 1725).
_____, *The Mechanical Practice of Physick* (London: T. Woodward, 1735).

Nigrisoli, Francesco Maria, *Considerazione Intorno alla Generazione de' Viventi* (Ferrara: B. Barbieri, 1712).

Noble, Mark, *A Biographical History of England*, 3 vols (London: W. Richardson, 1806).

Oldmixon, John, *An Essay on Criticism as it Regards Design, Thought, and Expression, in Prose and Verse* (London: for J. Pemberton, 1728).

Packe, Edmund, *An Answer to Dr Turner's Letter to Dr Jurin* (London: J. Roberts, 1735).

Page, John, *Receipts for Preparing and Compounding the Principal Medicines Made use of by the late Mr Ward* (London: Henry Whitridge, 1763).

Pemberton, Henry, *A View of Sir Isaac Newton's Philosophy* (London: s.n., 1728).

Phil-Porney [pseud. of Bernard Mandeville or Charles Ogle], *A Modern Defense of Publick Stews: or, An Essay upon Whoring, as it is now Practis'd in these Kingdoms* (London: A. Moore, 1724).

Philo-Chymicus, *Pillulae Wardearae Dissectio & Examinatio; or Ward's Pill Dissected and Examined, and its True Composition Plainly Discover'd, even to an Ocular Demonstration. In a Latin Epistle to the Ingenious Dr Boerhave, Professor of Physic in the University of Leyden, now translated into English by a Chymist of London* (London: Mr Osborne's, 1736).

[Pitt, Robert], *The Crafts and Frauds of Physick Expos'd*, 3rd edn (London: T. Childe, 1702).

[Poole, Robert], *Physical Vade Mecum: or, Fifth Gift of Theophilus Philanthropos* (London: E. Duncomb, 1741).

Porter, R., *Ad Virum Clarissimum Danielem Turner, M.D. Epistola: Morbi infrequentis Historiam* (London: J. Bettenham, 1731).

Pott, Percival, *Observations on that Disorder of the Corner of the Eye, commonly called Fistula Lachrymalis*, 2nd edn (London: L. Hawes and Co., 1763).

Purmann, Matthias Gottfried, *Chirurgia Curiosa* (London: D. Browne, 1706).

Pye, George, *A Discourse of the Plague; wherein Dr Mead's Notions are Consider'd and Refuted* (London: J. Darby, 1721).

Quincy, John, *Pharmacopoeia Officianalis & Extemporanea; or, A Complete English Dispensatory*, 2nd edn (London: A. Bell, 1719).

——, *Lexicon Physico-medicum; or, A New Physical Dictionary* (London: A. Bell, W. Taylor, and J. Osborn, 1719).

Ramazzini, Bernardino, *A Treatise of the Diseases of Tradesmen* (London: for Andrew Bell, Ralph Smith, Daniel Midwinter, Will. Hawes, Will. Davis, Geo. Straughan, Bern. Linot, Ja. Round, and Jeff Wale, 1705).

Rayer, Pierre François, *Treatise on the Diseases of the Skin*, 2nd edn (London: J. B. Baillière, 1835).

Read, Alexander, *Chirurgorum Comes* (London: E. Jones for C. Wilkinson, 1687).

Richardson, Jonathan, *The Connoisseur: An Essay on the Whole Art of Criticism, as it Relates to Painting*, in J. Richardson, *Two Discourses* (London: W. Churchill, 1719).

_____, *A Discourse on the Dignity, Certainty, Pleasure and Advantage, of the Science of a Connoisseur*, in J. Richardson, *Two Discourses* (London: W. Churchill, 1719).

_____, *An Essay on the Theory of Painting* (Menston, Yorkshire: Scholar Press, 1971, 2nd edn 1725).

Rutty, William, *A Treatise on Urinary Passages* (London: for T. Worrall, 1726).

S., J., *A Mechanical Dissertation upon the Lues Venerea* (London: Richard King, 1731).

Salmon, William, *Ars Chirurgica* (London: J. Dawks, 1698).

Sharp, Samuel, *A Critical Enquiry into the Present State of Surgery* (London: J. & R. Tonson, 1750).

Spectator (London: printed for J. and R. Tonson and S. Draper), no. 559, 25 June 1714.

Spinke, John, *Quackery Unmask'd; or, Reflections on the Sixth Edition of Mr Martin's Treatise of the Venereal Disease* (London: D. Browne, G. Strahan, J. Woodward, B. Barker, and the Author, 1709).

Spooner, Thomas, *A Short Account of the Itch* (London: T. Child, 1714).

Steele, Richard, *Guardian* (London: J. Tonson, 1713), no. 1, 12 March 1713.

Stow, John, *A Survey of the Cities of London and Westminster*, John Strype (ed.) (London: A. Churchill, J. Knapton, R. Knaplock, J. Walthoe, E. Horne, B. Tooke, D. Midwinter, B. Crowse, R. Robinson, T. Ward, 1720, 1st edn 1593).

Superville, Daniel de, 'Some Reflections on Generation and on Monsters', *Philosophical Transactions of the Royal Society of London*, xli (1740), 294 307.

[Swift, Jonathan], *Travels into Several Remote Nations of the World* (London: Benjamin Motte, 1726).

T., J. [i.e. Daniel Turner], 'Of a Stone found in the Gall Bladder of a Woman' (6 December 1693), Royal Society of London, Classified Papers 1660-1740, Cl.P. 12(1).38, 81.

Turner, Daniel, 'Remarks, taken upon Dissecting the Body of A. M. a Maid of about Thirty Years of Age, who dyed of an Ascites', *Philosophical Transactions of the Royal Society of London*, xviii (1693-94), 15-20.

_____, 'Observatio Casus non Vulgaris de Hydrope intra Uteri Tunicas contento [Woman hydropical in the external Coat of the Uterus]', *Philosophical Transactions of the Royal Society of London*, xviii (1693-94), 20-23.

_____, 'De Morsu venenoso Canis rabidi [Observations on a Child bit by a Mad dog, with the sad Effects following therefrom, both from the same hand], *Philosophical Transactions of the Royal Society of London*, xviii (1693-94), 24-25.

[Turner, Daniel], 'Of a Stone found in the Gall-Bladder of a Woman', *Philosophical Transactions of the Royal Society of London*, xviii (1694), 111-12.

_____, *Apologia Chyrurgica: A Vindication of the Noble Art of Surgery* (London: J. Whitlock, 1695).

T., D., *Present State of Chyrurgery, with some short Remarks on the Abuses Committed under a Pretence to the Practice. And Reasons offer'd for Regulating the Same* (London: R. Tookey, 1703).

Turner, Daniel, 'Religio Medici Reformata: or, Private Devotion, in 2 parts, conteining certain Forms of Prayer, Thanksgiving &c. To be used in the Times of Health & Sickness. suited to the Authours Occasions', British Library, Additional Manuscripts, MS 14404.

_____, *A remarkable case in Surgery ... of an uncommon Fracture ... of the Skull* (London: R. Parker, 1709).

_____, 'Of the Articles of Agreement before Marriage, that Part Relating to Dower and Thirds', 10 December 1712, Hertford C. C. Records, MS D/EAS 1612 (867).

_____, *De Morbis Cutaneis: A Treatise of Diseases Incident to the Skin* (London: R. Bonwicke, W. Freeman, T. Goodwin, J. Walthoe, M. Wotton, S. Manship, J. Nicholson, R. Parker, B. Tooke and R. Smith, 1714).

_____, *Syphilis. A Practical Dissertation on the Venereal Disease* (London: R. Bonwicke, Tim. Goodwin, J. Walthoe, M. Wooton, S. Manship, Richard Wilkin, Benj. Tooke, R. Smith, and Thos. Ward, 1717).

[Turner, Daniel], *The Modern Quack, or Medicinal Impostor* (London: J. Roberts, 1718).

_____, 'Catalogue ... of all the Members of the Royal College of Physicians', appended to *The Modern Quack, or Medicinal Imposter* (London: J. Roberts, 1718).

_____, *Art of Surgery* (London: C. Rivington, J. Lacy, and J. Clarke, 1722).

_____, *De Morbis Cutaneis* (London: R. Bonwicke, J. Walthoe, R. Wilkin, T. Ward, and S. Tooke, 1723).

_____, *The Modern Quack, or, Medical Impostor*, 2nd edn (London:

Thomas Warner, 1724).
_____, *Syphilis: A Practical Dissertation on the Venereal Disease* (London: Printed for R. Bonwicke, R. Wilkin, J. Walthoe and T. Ward, 1724).
_____, 'Two cases of Insects voided by the Urinary Passage', *Philosophical Transactions of the Royal Society of London*, xxxiii (1725), 410-11.
_____, *Art of Surgery*, 2nd edn (London: C. Rivington, J. Lacy and J. Clarke, 1725), 2 vols.
_____, 'Some modest Animadversions on Dr Harris's *Dissertationes Medicae*, especially his thirteenth, *de Errotibus Chirugorum*', appended to D. Turner, *Art of Surgery*, 2nd edn (1725), vol. 1, 555-70.
_____, *De Morbis Cutaneis: A Treatise of Diseases Incident to the Skin* (London: R. and J. Bonwicke, J. Walthoe, R. Wilkin, and T. Ward, 1726).
_____, *Syphilis: A Practical Dissertation on the Venereal Disease* (London: J. Walthoe, R. Wilkin, J. and J. Bonwicke, and T. Ward, 1726).
_____, *Remarks upon Dr Willoughby's Translation of Monsieur Chicoyneau's Method of Cure* in D. Turner, *Syphilis* (London: J. Walthoe, R. Wilkin, J. and J. Bonwicke, and T. Ward, 1727), 337-78.
[Turner, Daniel], *Discourse Concerning Fevers* (London: John Oake, 1727).
_____, 'A Short Account of the Pulse and Urine, as Affording Signs Both Diagnostic and Prognostic; as Also of Crises, and Critical Days in Fevers' (London: John Clarke, 1727), in [D. Turner], *Discourses Concerning Fevers* (London: John Oake, 1727).
_____, *The Art of Surgery* (London: C. Rivington, J. Lacy and J. Clarke, 1729).
_____, *Discourse Concerning Gleets* (London: J. Clarke, 1729).
_____, *A Defence of the XIIth Chapter of the First Part of a Treatise De Morbis Cutaneis*, in D. Turner, *Discourse Concerning Gleets* (London: J. Clarke, 1729), 67-162. Also printed under the title *An Answer to a Pamphlet on the Power of Imagination in Pregnant Women.*
_____, 'Prefatory Account of Professor Boerhaave's New Comments on the Venereal Disease; and Some Animadversions thereon', in Daniel Turner, *Discourse Concerning Gleets* (London: John Clarke, 1729), iii-lii.
[Turner, Daniel], *De Morbo Gallico*, by Ulrich von Hutten, translated by T. Paynell, revised by Daniel Turner (London: J. Clarke, 1730).
_____, 'The Force of the Mother's Imagination upon the Foetus in Utero ... by Way of Reply to Dr Blondell's Work' (London: J. Walthoe, etc., 1730).
_____, 'A Letter to Mr James Ferne, Surgeon, Concerning a Very Singular Suppos'd Infection', in Ulrich von Hutten, *De Morbo Gallico*, translated by T. Paynell, revised by Daniel Turner (London: John Clarke, 1730), 103-10.

[Turner, Daniel], *The Modern Quack, or Medicinal Imposter* (London, 1730).
_____, *De Morbis Cutaneis: A Treatise of Diseases Incident to the Skin* (London: J. Walthoe, R. Wilkin, J. and J. Bonwicke, S. Birt, T. Ward, and E. Wickstead, 1731).
_____, *The Art of Surgery* (London: C. Rivington, J. Lacy and J. Clarke, 1732).
_____, *Discourses Concerning Fevers*, 2nd edn (London: J. Clarke, 1732).
_____, *Discourse Concerning Gleets* (London, 1732).
_____, 'A Short Account of the Pulse and Urine, as Affording Signs both Diagnostic and Prognostic; as also of Crises, and Critical Days in Fevers', in D. Turner, *Discourses Concerning Fevers* (London: C. Rivington, J. Lacy and J. Clarke, 1732), Postscript.
_____, *Syphilis: A Practical Dissertation on the Venereal Disease*, 4th edn (London: J. Walthoe, 1732).
_____, *The Ancient Physician's Legacy Impartially Survey'd* (London: John Clarke, 1733).
_____, 'A Discourse on Quicksilver', in D. Turner, *The Ancient Physician's Legacy Impartially Survey'd* (London: J. Clarke, 1733), 'By Way of Postscript', 131-80.
_____, 'Some Historical Memoirs of Quicksilver ['Case of Barton Booth ... as Communicated by Alexander Small'; 'A Particular Account of M. Bellost's Pill Compared with the Author's']', in D. Turner, *The Ancient Physician's Legacy Impartially Survey'd* (London: J. Clarke, 1733), 193-275.
_____, *The Drop and Pill of Mr Ward Consider'd* (London: John Clarke, 1735).
_____, *The Art of Surgery* (London: C. Rivington & J. Clarke, 1736).
_____, *De Morbis Cutaneis: A Treatise of Diseases Incident to the Skin* (London: R. Wilkin, J. and J. Bonwicke, S. Birt, T. Ward, and E. Wicksteed, 1736).
T. D. [i.e. Turner, Daniel], Preface to Aloysius Luisini's *Aphrodisiacus, Containing a Summary of the Ancient Writers on the Venereal Disease ... with a Large Preface by Daniel Turner* (London: J. Clarke, 1736).
Turner, Daniel, *Siphylis* [sic]*: A Practical Dissertation on the Venereal Disease*, 5th edn (London: Printed for R. Wilkin, J. and J. Bonwicke, S. Birt, T. Ward, J. Clarke, and E. Wicksteed, 1737).
[Turner, Daniel], *De Morbo Gallico*, by Ulrich von Hutten, translated by T. Paynell, revised by Daniel Turner (London: J. Clarke, 1739).
_____, *Discourse Concerning Fevers* (London: John Clarke, 1739).
_____, 'The Force of the Mother's Imagination upon the Foetus in Utero ... by Way of Reply to Dr Blondel's Work' (London: J. Clarke, 1739).
_____, *The Modern Quack, or Medicinal Imposter* (London: J. Clarke, 1739).

_____, *Syphilis. The Second Part* (London: J. Clarke, 1739).
_____, *The Art of Surgery* (London: C. Rivington & J. Clarke, 1741-42).
_____, Probated Will (16 April 1741), Public Record Office, Chancery Lane, Prob. 11/709.
_____, *Traité des Maladies de la Peau en General; avec un Court Appendix sur l'Efficacité des Remedes Topiques dans les Maladies Internes, & leur Maniere d'Agir sur le Corps Humain* (Paris: J. Barois Fils, 1743).
_____, *Syphilis; oder, Practische Abhandlung von der Venus- seuche, in zweyen Theilen* (Zelle: s.n., 1754).
_____, *Abhandlung von den Krankheiten der Haut: nebst einem kurzen Anhang von den ausserlichen Mitteln, und der Art, wie sie wirken* (Altenburg: In der Richterischen Buchhandlung, 1766).
_____, *Dissertation sur les maladies venerienne* (Paris: P.-F. Didot le jeune, 1767).

Vari, Ignazio, *Disscussione 'Ragionamento del Sig. Dottore Ignazio Vari ... al Sig. Dottor Lucio Bonaccioli'* in J. Blondel, *Dissertazione della Forza dell' Immaginazione delle Donne Gravide Sovra il Feto* (Ferrara: Francesco Gardi, 1760), 175-212.

Vigiliis, Stephani Hieronymi de, *Bibliotheca Chirurgica* (Vindobonae: Joannis Thomae, 1781).

Vincent, T., *God's Terrible Voice in the City* ([London]: s.n., 1667).

Wainewright, Jeremiah, *A Mechanical Account of the Non-Naturals* (London: R. Smith, 1707).
_____, *An Anatomical Treatise of the Liver, with the Diseases Incident to it* (London: J. Clarke, 1737).

Walpole, Horace, *Anecdotes of Painting* (Strawberry Hill: for Thos. Farmer, 1762-71).

Ward, Ned, *The London Spy* (London: Folio Society, 1955; 1st edn 1706).

Warren, G., *A New Method of Curing, without Internal Medicines, that Degree of Venereal Disease, call'd A Gonorrhoea or Clap*, 2nd edn (London: J. Baker, 1711).

Willan, Robert, *Description and Treatment for Cutaneous Diseases* (London: J. Johnson, 1798-1808).

Wiseman, Richard, *Eight Chirurgical Treatises*, 5th edn (London: for B. Tooke, J. Knapton, T. Horne, R. Knaplock, J. Wyat, D. Midwinter, R. Robinson, W. Taylor, J. Bowyer, H. Clements, W. Mears, R. Gosling, W. and J. Innys, W. Churchill, and B. Cowse, 1719).

_____, *Of Wounds, Of Gun-shot Wounds, Of Fractures and Luxations* (1676; reprint, Bath: Kingsmead Press, 1977).

Secondary Sources

Anonymous, *Index to the Anatomical, Medical, Chirurgical and Physiological Papers contained in the Transactions of the Royal Society of London* (London: for J. Callow, 1818).

Anonymous, 'Archaeologica Medica. XIX: Mary Tofts, the Rabbit Breeder', *British Medical Journal*, ii (1896), 209-10.

Anonymous, 'Some Althams of Mark Hall in the 17th Century', *The Essex Review*, xvii (1908), 74-89, 134-46; xviii (1909), 91-100.

Abernathy, Charles M. and Hamm, Robert M., *Surgical Intuition: What It Is and How To Get It* (Philadelphia: Hanley & Belfus, Inc., 1995).

Ackerknecht, Erwin H., *Therapeutics from the Primitives to the 20th Century* (New York: Hafner Press, 1973).

Addy, John, *Sin and Society in the Seventeenth Century* (London: Routledge, 1989).

Allbutt, T. C., *The Historical Relation of Medicine and Surgery to the End of the Sixteenth Century* (London: Macmillan, 1905).

Allen, Elizabeth, Turk, J.L., Murley, Sir Reginald (eds), *The Case Books of John Hunter, FRS* (London: Royal Society of Medicine Services Ltd, 1993).

Alsop, J. D., 'The Publication of Benjamin Gooch's Surgical Works, 1765-74', *Publishing History*, xxv (1989), 13-26.

Altick, Richard, *The Shows of London* (Cambridge, Mass.: Harvard University Press, 1978).

Anderson, Charles M., *Richard Seltzer and the Rhetoric of Surgery* (Carbondale: Southern Illinois University Press, 1989).

Andreski, Stanislav, *Syphilis, Puritanism and Witch Hunts: Historical Explanations in the Light of Medicine and Psychoanalysis with a Forecast about Aids* (Basingstoke: Macmillan, 1989).

Apple, Rima D. (ed.), *Women, Health, and Medicine in America* (New York: Garland Publishing, Inc., 1990).

Appleby, John H., 'New Light on John Woodall, Surgeon and Adventurer', *Medical History*, xxv (1981), 251-68.

Archibald, E. H. H., *The Fighting Ship in the Royal Navy A.D. 897-1984* (Dorset: Blandford Press, 1984).

Armytage, W. H. G., *Four Hundred Years of English Education* (Cambridge: Cambridge University Press, 1970).

Arrizabalaga, Jon, Henderson, John, and French, Roger, *Before Syphilis: The French Disease in Renaissance Europe* (New Haven: Yale University Press, 1996).

Axtell, J. L., 'Education and Status in Stuart England: The London Physician', *History of Education Quarterly*, x (1970), 141-59.

Backsheider, Paula R., *Daniel Defoe: his Life* (Baltimore: Johns Hopkins University Press, 1989).

Baldwin, Martha R., 'Toads and Plague: Amulet Therapy in Seventeenth-Century Medicine', *Bulletin of the History of Medicine*, lxvii (1993), 227-47.

Balin, Arthur K. and Balin, Loretta Pratt, *The Life of the Skin* (New York: Bantam, 1997).

Ballantine, J. W., *Manual of Antenatal Pathology and Hygiene, vol. 2: The Embryo* (Edinburgh: W. Green and Sons, 1904).

Bannerman, Bruce, *The Register of St Helen's, Bishopgate, London* (London: Harleian Society, 1904).

Barnet, Margaret C., 'The Barber-Surgeons of York', *Medical History*, xii (1968), 19-30.

Bastian, F., *Defoe's Early Life* (Towanda, New Jersey: Barnes & Noble Books, 1981).

Bates, Donald, 'Sydenham and the Medical Meaning of "Method"', *Bulletin of the History of Medicine*, li (1977), 324-38.

Bauer, George C., *The Education of a Gentleman: Theories of Gentlemanly Education in England: 1660-1775* (New York: Bookman Associates, 1959).

Beck, R. Theodore, *The Cutting Edge: Early History of the Surgeons of London* (London: Lund Humphries, 1974).

Bedford, John, *London's Burning* (London: Abelard-Schuman, 1966).

Beekman, Fenwick, 'The Rise of British Surgery in the Eighteenth Century', *Annals of Medical History*, n.s. ix (1937), 549-66.

Beier, A.L., and Finlay, Roger, *London 1500-1700: The Making of the Metropolis* (Harlow, Essex: Longman Group Ltd, 1986), 1-33.

Beier, Lucinda McCray, *Sufferers & Healers: The Experience of Illness in Seventeenth-Century England* (London: Routledge & Kegan Paul, 1987).

_____, 'Seventeenth-century English Surgery: The Casebook of Joseph Binns', in Christopher Lawrence (ed.), *Surgical Theory, Medical Practice: Studies in the History of Surgery* (London: Routledge, 1992), 48-84.

Belanger, Terry, '"Booksellers" Trade Sales, 1718-1768', *Library*, 5th ser., xxx (1975), 281-302.

Bell, Shannon, *Reading, Writing, and Rewriting the Prostitute Body* (Bloomington, Indiana: Indiana University Press, 1994).

Benedek, Thomas G., 'The Influence of Ulrich von Hutten's Medical Descriptions and Metaphorical Use of Medicine', *Bulletin of the History of Medicine*, lxvi (1992), 355-75.

Benjamin, Marina, 'Medicine, Morality and the Politics of Berkeley's Tar-Water', in A. Cunningham and R. French (eds), *The Medical Enlightenment of the Eighteenth Century* (Cambridge: Cambridge University Press, 1990), 165-93.

Bennett, G. V., 'Conflict in the Church', in G. Holmes (ed.), *Britain After the Glorious Revolution*, 5th edn (London: Macmillan, 1984), 155-75.

Bennett, H. Selfe, 'Joshua Ward, 1685-1761', *Proceedings of the Royal Society of Medicine. Section of the History of Medicine*, ix (1916), 100-12.

Berry, George, *Taverns and Tokens of Pepys's London* (London: Seaby, 1978).

Berry, William, *Pedigree of the Families in the County of Kent* (London: Sherwood, Gilbert, and Piper, 1830).

Billings, John Shaw, 'The History and Literature of Surgery', in Frederick S. Denis (ed.), *System of Surgery* (Philadelphia: Lea Brothers, 1895), vol. 1, 17-44.

Biography, Granta 41 (New York: Penguin, 1992).

Birken, William, 'Dissenting Tradition in English Medicine of the Seventeenth and Eighteenth Centuries', *Medical History*, xxxix (1995), 197-218.

Bishop, W. J., *The Early History of Surgery* (London: Robert Hale, 1960).

Black, Jeremy, *The British and the Grand Tour* (London: Croom Helm, 1985).

_____, *Natural and Necessary Enemies: Anglo-French Relations in the Eighteenth Century* (London: Duckworth, 1986).

Blackman, Janet, 'Popular Theories of Generation: The Evolution of Aristotle's Works, the Study of an Anachronism', in J. Woodward and D. Richards (eds), *Health Care and Popular Medicine in Nineteenth Century England* (New York: Holmes and Meier, 1977), 56-88.

Bloom, J. H., and James, R. R., *Medical Practitioners in the Diocese of London, Licensed under the Act of 3 Henry VIII, c.II. An Annotated List 1529-1725* (Cambridge: Cambridge University Press, 1935).

Bodemer, Charles W., 'Embryological Thought in Seventeenth Century England', in Charles W. Bodemer and Lester S. King, *Medical Investigation in Seventeenth Century England* (Los Angeles: William Andrews Clark Memorial Library, University of California, 1968), 3-25.

_____, 'Developmental Phenomena in Seventeenth Century Mechanistic Psychophysiology, with Special Reference to the Psychological Theory of Nicolas Malebranche', *Episteme*, vi (1972), 233-46.

Bonfield, Lloyd, *Marriage Settlements, 1601-1740: The Development of the Strict Settlement* (Cambridge: Cambridge University Press, 1983).

Boucé, P-G. (ed.), *Sexuality in Eighteenth-Century Britain* (Manchester: Manchester University Press, 1982), 74-94.

_____, 'Imagination, Pregnant Women, and Monsters in Eighteenth Century England and France', in G. S. Rousseau and R. Porter (eds), *Sexual Underworlds of the Enlightenment* (Manchester: Manchester University Press, 1988), 86-100.

Bowler, P., 'Preformation and Pre-existence in the Seventeenth Century: A Brief Analysis', *Journal of the History of Biology*, iv (1971), 221-44.

Bowles, Geoffrey, 'Physical, Human, and Divine Attraction in the Life and Thoughts of George Cheyne', *Annals of Science*, xxxi (1974), 473-88.

Bradley, James E., *Religion, Revolution, and English Radicalism: Nonconformity in Eighteenth-Century Politics and Society* (Cambridge: Cambridge University Press, 1990).

Brandt, Allan M., *No Magic Bullet: A Social History of Venereal Disease in the United States since 1880* (New York: Oxford University Press, 1985).

Brauer, George C., Jr, *The Education of a Gentleman: Theories of*

Gentlemanly Education in England, 1660-1775 (New York: Bookman Associates, 1959).

Brewer, John, *Sinews of Power: War Money and the English State, 1688-1783* (London: Unwin Hyman, 1989).

Brieger, Gert, 'The Development of Surgery: Historical Aspects Important in the Origin and Development of Modern Surgical Science', in D. C. Sabiston (ed.), *Christopher's Textbook of Surgery*, 10th edition (Philadelphia: W. B. Saunders Co., 1972), 1-25.

Briggs, Ward W. and Paulshock, Bernadine Z., '"Lively Lustre, Kindly Dew:" William Heberden's "Of Perspiration"', *Journal of the History of Medicine and Allied Sciences*, xvi (1986), 463-81.

Brockliss, L. W. B., 'The Embryological Revolution in the France of Louis XIV: The Dominance of Ideology', in G. R. Dunstan (ed.), *The Human Embryo: Aristotle and the Arabic and European Tradition* (Exeter: University of Exeter Press, 1990), 158-86.

Bronson, Edward Bennet, 'The Classification of Skin Diseases', *Journal of Cutaneous Diseases*, v (1887), 371-81, 427-33.

Brooke, John Hedley, *Science and Religion: Some Historical Perspectives* (Cambridge: Cambridge University Press, 1991).

Brown, John, 'Notes and Observations on Maternal Impressions' (M.D. thesis, Glasgow, 1887-88).

Brown, Theodore M., 'The Mechanical Philosophy and the "Animal Oeconomy": A Study of the Development of English Physiology in the Seventeenth and Early Eighteenth Century' (Ph.D. thesis, Princeton University, 1968).

_____, 'The College of Physicians and the Acceptance of Iatromechanism in England', *Bulletin of the History of Medicine*, xliv (1970), 12-30.

_____, 'From Mechanism to Vitalism in Eighteenth-Century English Physiology', *Journal of the History of Biology*, vii (1974), 179-216.

_____, 'Medicine in the Shadow of the *Principia*', *Journal of the History of Ideas*, xli (1987), 629-48.

Buckman, Robert F. and Futrell, J. William, 'William Cowper', *Surgery*, ic (1986), 582-90.

Bullough, Vern, 'Prostitution and Reform in Eighteenth-Century England', *Eighteenth-Century Life*, ix, n.s. 3 (1985), 61-74.

_____, and Bullough, Bonnie, *Women and Prostitution: A Social History* (Buffalo, New York: Prometheus Books, 1987).

Bundy, M.W., *The Theory of Imagination in Classical and Medieval Thought* (Urbana, Illinois: University of Illinois Press, 1927).

Buret, F., *Syphilis in the Middle Ages and in Modern Times*, 3 vols (Philadelphia: F. A. Davis, 1895).

Burford, E.J., *The Orrible Synne: A Look at London Lechery from Roman to Cromwellian Times* (London: Calder & Boyers, 1973).

_____, *Wits, Wenchers and Wantons: London's Low Life: Covent Garden in the Eighteenth Century* (London: Robert Hale, 1986).

Burgess, Renate, *Portraits of Doctors & Scientists in the Wellcome Institute for the History of Medicine* (London: Wellcome Institute for the History of Medicine, 1973).

Burke, Edmund T., *The Venereal Problem: a Description of the Venereal Diseases, their History, their Prevalence in Great Britain, their Effect upon the National Life, the Factors Causing their Propagation and Spread, and a Discussion of Methods for their Control and Eradication* (London: H. Kimpton, 1919).

Byatt, A. S., *Possession* (London: Vintage, 1991).

Bynum, Caroline Walker, *The Resurrection of the Body in Western Christianity* (New York: Columbia University Press, 1995).

Bynum, W. F., 'The Anatomical Method, Natural Theology, and the Functions of the Brain', *Isis*, lxiv (1973), 445-68.

_____, 'Health, Disease and Medical Care', in G. S. Rousseau and Roy Porter (eds), *The Ferment of Knowledge: Studies in the Historiography of Eighteenth-Century Science* (Cambridge: Cambridge University Press, 1980), 211-53.

_____, 'Treating the Wages of Sin: Venereal Disease and Specialism in Eighteenth-Century Britain', in W. F. Bynum and Roy Porter (eds), *Medical Fringe and Medical Orthodoxy 1750-1850* (London: Croom Helm, 1987), 5-28.

Campbell, W. A., 'Portrait of a Quack: Joshua Ward (1685-1761)', *University of Newcastle Medical Gazette*, (June 1964), 118-22.

Cartwright, Fredrick F., *The Development of Modern Surgery* (London: Arthur Baker Ltd, 1967).

Castronovo, David, *The English Gentleman: Images and Ideas in Literature and Society* (New York: Ungar, 1987).

Channell, David F., *The Vital Machine: A Study of Technology and Organic*

Life (Oxford: Oxford University Press, 1991).

Churchill, Frederick B., 'The History of Embryology as Intellectual History', *Journal of the History of Biology*, iii (1970), 155-81.

Clair, Colin, *Human Curiosities* (London: Abelard-Schuman, 1968).

Clarke, J. R., 'The Royal Society and Early Grand Lodge Freemasonry', *Ars Quatuor Coronatorum*, lxxx (1967), 110-19.

_____, 'The Medical Profession and Early Freemasonry', *Ars Quatuor Coronatorum*, lxxxv (1972), 298-311.

Cleugh, James, *Secret Enemy: the Story of a Disease* (London: Thames and Hudson, 1954).

Clutterbuck, Robert, *The History and Antiquities of the County of Hertfordshire*, 2 vols (London: John Nicholson, 1821).

Cody, Lisa, 'The Doctor's in Labour; or a New Whim Wham from Guilford', *Gender & History*, iv (1992), 175-96.

Cohen, Estelle, 'The Body as a Historical Category: Science and Imagination, 1660-1760', in Mary G. Winkler and Letha B. Cole, (eds), *The Good Body. Asceticism in Contemporary Culture* (New Haven: Yale University Press, 1994), 67-90.

Cole, F. J., *Early Theories of Sexual Generation* (Oxford: Clarendon Press, 1930).

Coleman, D. C., 'Gentlemen and Players', *Economic History Review*, 2nd series, xxvi (1973), 92-116.

Coleman, William, 'Mechanistic Philosophy and Hypothetical Physiology', *Texas Quarterly*, x (1967), 259-69.

Colyer-Fergusson, T. C. (ed.), *The Registers of the French Church, Threadneedle Street, London* (Aberdeen: Huguenot Society, 1906).

Cook, Harold J., *The Decline of the Old Medical Regime in Stuart London* (Ithaca and London: Cornell University Press, 1986).

_____, 'Medical Innovation or Medical Malpractice?: Or, A Dutch Physician in London: Joannes Groenevelt, 1694-1700', *Tractrix*, ii (1990), 63-91.

_____, 'The Rose Case Reconsidered: Physicians, Apothecaries and the Law in Augustan England', *Journal of the History of Medicine*, xlv (1990), 527-55.

_____, 'Sir John Colbatch and Augustan Medicine: Experimentalism, Character and Entrepreneurialism', *Annals of Science*, xlvii (1990),

475-505.

_____, *Trials of an Ordinary Doctor: Joannes Groenevelt in Seventeenth-Century London* (Baltimore: Johns Hopkins University Press, 1994).

_____, 'Good Advice and Little Medicine: The Professional Authority of Early Modern English Physicians', *Journal of British Studies*, 33 (January 1994), 1-31.

Cooter, Roger, 'Bones of Contention? Orthodox Medicine and the Mystery of the Bone-Setter's Craft', in W. F. Bynum and Roy Porter (eds), *Medical Fringe and Medical Orthodoxy 1750-1850* (London: Croom Helm, 1987), 158-73.

_____, *Surgery and Society in Peace and War: Orthopaedics and the Organization of Modern Medicine* (Houndmills, Basingstoke, Hampshire: Macmillan Press, Ltd., 1993).

Cope, Sir Zachary, *William Cheselden* (Edinburgh: E. & S. Livingstone, 1953).

Copeman, P. W. M., and Copeman, W. S. C., 'Dermatology in Tudor and Early Stuart England', *British Journal of Dermatology*, lxxxii (1970), 3-31.

Corporation of London Records Office, *London Inhabitants within the Walls, 1695*, introduction by D. V. Glass (Leicester: London Record Society, 1966).

Cowley, Geoffrey, 'Replacement Parts', *Newsweek*, cxxix (27 January 1997), 66-9.

Cowley, Robert L. S., *Marriage A-la-Mode* (Manchester: Manchester University Press, 1983).

Cox, J. Stevens, *An Illustrated Dictionary of Hairdressing & Wigmaking* (London: Batsford Academic and Educational, 1984).

Cox, John Edmund, *The Annals of St Helen's, Bishopgate* (London: Tinslag Bros., 1876).

Crawford, Catherine, 'Malpractice and Bad Manners: Disputes over Professional Conduct in Eighteenth-Century England', paper delivered at 'History of Medical Ethics', Wellcome Symposium on the History of Medicine (London), 1 December 1989.

Crissey, John Thorne, and Parish, Lawrence Charles, *The Dermatology and Syphilology of the Nineteenth Century* (New York: Praeger, 1981).

Crosby, Alfred, *The Columbian Exchange: Biological and Cultural Consequences of 1492* (Westport, Connecticut: Greenwood Pub. Co.,

1972).

Cunningham, Andrew, *The Anatomical Renaissance. The Resurrection of the Anatomical Projects of the Ancients* (Aldershot, Hampshire: Scolar Press, 1997), 7.

_____, 'The Kinds of Anatomy', *Medical History*, xix (1975), 1-19.

_____, 'Thomas Sydenham: Epidemics, Experiment and the "Good Old Cause"', in R. French and A. Wear (eds), *The Medical Revolution of the Seventeenth Century* (Cambridge: Cambridge University Press, 1989), 164-90.

Cunningham, Phillis, and Lucas, Catherine, *Occupational Costume in England from the Eleventh Century to 1914* (London: Adam & Charles Black, 1967).

Curtis, T. C. and Speck, W. A., 'The Societies for the Reformation of Manners: A Case Study in the Theory and Practice of Moral Reform', *Literature & History*, no. 3 (1976), 45-64.

Cussans, John Edwin, *History of Hertfordshire* (Wakefield, Yorkshire: E P Pub. Ltd., 1972; 1st edn 1870-81).

Dally, Ann, *Women under the Knife: A History of Surgery* (London: Hutchinson Radius, 1991).

_____, *1880-1930: With Special Reference to Sir William Arbuthnot Lane* (Amsterdam: Rodopi, 1996).

Darlington, Anne Carol, 'The Royal Academy of Arts and its Anatomical Teachings; with an Examination of the Art-Anatomy Practices During the Eighteenth and Early Nineteenth Centuries in Britain', 2 vols (Ph.D. thesis, University of London, 1990).

Darnton, Robert, *The Kiss of Lamourette: Reflections in Cultural History* (London: Faber and Faber, 1990).

Davenport-Hines, R. P. T., *Sex, Death and Punishment: Attitudes to Sex and Sexuality in Britain since the Renaissance* (London: Collins, 1990).

Davies, Tony, 'The Ark in the Flames: Science, Language and Education in Seventeenth-Century England', in A. E. Benjamin, G. N. Cantor and J. R. R. Christie (eds), *The Figural and the Literal: Problems of Language in the History of Science and Philosophy, 1630-1800* (Manchester: Manchester University Press, 1987), 83-102.

Davis, Ralph, *Aleppo and Devonshire Square: English Traders in the Levant in the Eighteenth Century* (London: Macmillan, 1967).

Debus, Allen, *The English Paracelsians* (New York: Franklin Watts, 1966).

Deleyiannis, Frederic W.-B., 'The United Company of Barbers and Surgeons of London, 1540-1745: Union and Disintegration' (M.A. thesis, University of Cambridge, 1990).

DeJean, Joan, *Ancients Against Moderns: Culture Wars and the Making of Fin de Siècle* (Chicago: University of Chicago Press, 1997).

De Moulin, Daniel, *A History of Surgery with Emphasis on the Netherlands* (Dordrecht: Martinus Nijhoff, 1988).

Dewhurst, Kenneth, *The Quicksilver Doctor: The Life and Times of Thomas Dover Physician and Adventurer* (Bristol: John Wright, 1957).

_____, *Dr Thomas Sydenham (1624-1689): His Life and Original Writings* (London: The Wellcome Historical Medical Library, 1966).

Dexter, Franklin Bowditch, *Biographical Sketches of the Graduates of Yale College with Annals of the College History October, 1701-May, 1745* (New York: Henry Holt & Co., 1885).

_____ (ed.), *Documentary History of Yale University under the Original Charter of the Collegiate School of Connecticut 1701-1745* (New Haven, Connecticut: Yale University Press, 1916).

Dezeimeris, Ollivier, and Dezeimeris, Raige-Delorme, *Dictionnaire Historique de la Médecine* (Paris: Bechet Jeune, 1828).

Dibben, A. A., *Title Deeds* (London: The Historical Association, 1990).

Digby, Anne, *Making A Medical Living: Doctors and Patients in the English Market for Medicine, 1720-1911* (Cambridge, Massachusetts: Cambridge University Press, 1994).

Dobson, Jessie, 'The Training of a Surgeon', *Annals of the Royal College of Surgeons of England*, xxxiv (1964), 1-36.

Dobson, Jessie, and Walker, R. Milnes, *Barbers and Barber-Surgeons of London* (Oxford: Blackwell Scientific Publications, 1979).

Doherty, Francis, 'The Anodyne Necklace: A Quack Remedy and its Promotion', *Medical History*, xxxiv (1990), 268-93.

_____, *A Study in 18th-Century Advertising Methods: The Anodyne Necklace* (Lewiston, New York: Edwin Mellen, 1992).

Donnison, Jean, *Midwives and Medical Men: A History of the Struggle for the Control of Childbirth*, 2nd edn (New Barnet, Hertfordshire: Historical Publications, Ltd., 1988).

Douglas, Aileen, *Uneasy Sensation. Smollett and the Body* (Chicago: University of Chicago Press, 1995).

DuCille, Ann, *Skin Trade* (Cambridge, Massachusetts: Harvard University Press, 1996).

Duden, Barbara, *The Woman beneath the Skin: A Doctor's Patients in Eighteenth-Century Germany*, trans. Thomas Dunlap (Cambridge, Massachussetts: Harvard University Press, 1991).

Earle, Peter, *The World of Defoe* (Newton Abbot: Reader's Union Limited Edition, 1976).

_____, *The Making of the English Middle Class: Business, Society and Family Life in London, 1660-1730* (London: Methuen, 1989).

Eco, Umberto, *The Search for the Perfect Language* (Oxford: Blackwell Publishers, 1998).

Edel, Leon, *Writing Lines: Principia Biographica* (New York: W. W. Norton, 1984).

Edmunds, Jonathan, *A History of Latton* (Ware, Herts.: Herts. Display Co. for the Church of St Mary-at-Latton, 1980).

Ehring, Franz, *Hautkrankheiten. 5 Jahrhunderte wissenschaftlicher Illustration* (Stuttgart: Gustav Fischer Verlag, 1989).

Elmen, Paul, 'Richard Allestree and The Whole Duty of Man', *The Library*, 5th series, vi (1951-52), 19-27.

Emch-Deriaz, Antoinette, 'The Non-naturals Made Easy', in R. Porter (ed.), *The Popularization of Medicine 1650-1850* (London and New York: Routledge, 1992), 134-59.

Engel, J., *The Creative Imagination: Enlightenment to Romanticism* (Cambridge, Mass.: Harvard University Press, 1981).

English, Christine (compiler), 'Dr William Hunter and "maternal impressions"' (London: Wellcome Institute for the History of Medicine Library, 6 December 1983), RQ no. 817b.

Erickson, Robert A., 'The Books of Generation: Some Observations on the Style of the British Midwife Books, 1671-1764', in P.-G. Boucé (ed.), *Sexuality in Eighteenth-Century Britain* (Totowa, New Jersey: Manchester University Press; Barnes & Noble Books, 1982), 74-92.

Everitt, Graham, *Doctors and Doctors: Some Curious Chapters in Medical History and Quackery* (London: S. Sonnenschein, Lowrey & Co., 1888).

Faber, Knud, *Nosography in Modern Internal Medicine* (New York: Paul Hoeber, 1923).

Fara, Patricia, *Sympathetic Attractions: Magnetic Practices, Beliefs, and Symbolism in Eighteenth-Century England* (Princeton: Princeton University Press, 1996).

Favazza, Armando R., *Bodies Under Siege: Self-Mutilation and Body Modification in Culture and Psychiatry* (Baltimore: Johns Hopkins University Press, 2nd edn, 1996).

Fessler, A., 'Skin Diseases in 17th and 18th Century Lancashire Local History Documents', *Bulletin of the History of Medicine*, xxvii (1953), 414-19.

Fisher, John L., *The Deanery of Harlow: A Small Contribution to the History of the Church in Essex* (Colchester: Benham and Company, Ltd., 1922).

Fissell, Mary, 'Gender and Generation: Representing Reproduction in Early Modern England', *Gender & History*, vii (1995), 432-56.

Fleck, Ludwig, *Genesis and Development of a Scientific Fact* (Chicago: University of Chicago Press, 1979).

Flynn, Carol Houlihan, *The Body in Swift and Defoe* (Cambridge: Cambridge University Press, 1990).

Forbes, Thomas, *The Midwife and the Witch* (New Haven: Yale University Press, 1966).

_____, 'A Note on the Procurement of Bodies for Dissection at the Royal College of Physicians of London in 1694 and 1710', *Journal of the History of Medicine*, xxix (1974), 332-4.

_____, 'Apprentices in Trouble: Some Problems in the Training of Surgeons and Apothecaries in Seventeenth-Century London', *Yale Journal of Biology and Medicine*, lii (1979), 227-37.

Fouke, D. C., 'Mechanical and "Organical" Models in Seventeenth-Century Explanations of Biological Reproduction', *Science in Context*, iii (1989), 365-81.

Foxon, David, *Pope and the Early Eighteenth-Century Book Trade*, revised by James McLaverty (Oxford: Clarendon Press, 1991).

Frank, Robert G., Jr, 'Thomas Willis and His Circle: Brain and Mind in Seventeenth-Century Medicine', in G. S. Rousseau (ed.), *The Languages of Psyche: Mind and Brain in Enlightenment Thought*

(Berkeley: University of California Press, 1990), 107-46.

French, R. K., 'Sauvages, Whytt & the Motion of the Heart: Aspects of Eighteenth-Century Animism', *Clio Medica*, vii (1972), 35-54.

_____, 'Surgery and Scrophula', in C. Lawrence (ed.), *Surgical Theory, Medical Practice: Studies in the History of Surgery* (London: Routledge, 1992), 85-100.

Garrison, Fielding, 'The Skin as a Functional Organ of the Body', *Bulletin of the New York Academy of Medicine*, ix (1933), 417-32.

Gascoigne, John, 'Anglican Latitudinarianism, Rational Dissent and Political Radicalism in the late Eighteenth Century', in Knud Haakonssen (ed.), *Enlightenment and Religion: Rational Dissent in Eighteenth-Century Britain* (Cambridge: Cambridge University Press, 1996), 219-40.

Gaskings, E., *Investigations into Generation, 1651-1828* (London: Hutchinson & Co., 1967).

Gelfand, Toby, *Professionalizing Modern Medicine: Paris Surgeons and Medical Science and Institutions in the Eighteenth Century* (Westport, Connecticut: Greenwood Press, 1980).

George, M. Dorothy, *London Life in the Eighteenth Century* (London: Penguin Books, 1965).

Gibbons, Peter, 'The Medical Projectors, 1640-1720', *Journal of the History of Medicine and Allied Sciences*, xxiv (1969), 247-71.

Gittings, C., *Death, Burial and the Individual in Early Modern England* (London: Croom Helm, 1984).

Glacken, Clarence, *Traces of the Rhodian Shore: Nature and Culture in Western Thought from Ancient Times to the End of the Eighteenth-Century* (Berkeley: University of California Press, 1976).

Goldgar, Bertrand A., 'The Grub Street Journal', in Alvin Sullivan (ed.), *British Literary Magazines. Vol. 1: The Augustan Age and the Age of Johnson, 1698-1788* (Westport, Connecticut: Greenwood Press, 1983), 144-9.

Goldwater, Leonard J., *Mercury: A History of Quicksilver* (Baltimore, Maryland: York Press, 1972).

Gooding, David, Pinch, Trevor, and Schaffer, Simon (eds), *The Uses of Experiment: Studies in the Natural Sciences* (Cambridge: Cambridge University Press, 1988).

Goodman, Herman, *Notable Contributions to the Knowledge of Dermatology* (New York: Medical Lay Press, 1953).

Graham, Harvey (pseud. for Flack, Isaac Harvey), 'Rabbits and Quacks', in Harvey Graham (pseud.), *Eternal Eve* (Altrincham: William Heinemann, 1950), 334-74.

Graham, John, 'Lavater's "Physiognomy" in England', *Journal of the History of Ideas*, xxii (1961), 561-72.

Granger, J., continued by Noble, Mark (ed.), *Biographical History of England, from the Revolution to the End of George I's Reign* ..., 3 vols (London: W. Richardson, Darton and Harvey, W. Bayner, 1806).

Gray, Sir Archibald, 'Dermatology from the Time of Harvey', *Lancet*, ii (1951), 795-802.

Guerrini, Anita, 'James Keill, George Cheyne, and Newtonian Physiology, 1690-1740', *Journal of the History of Biology*, xviii (1985), 247-66.

_____, 'The Tory Newtonians: Gregory, Pitcairne and their Circle', *Journal of British Studies*, xxv (1986), 288-311.

_____, 'Archibald Pitcairne and Newtonian Medicine', *Medical History*, xxxi (1987), 70-83.

_____, 'Isaac Newton, George Cheyne and the "Principia Medicinae"', in R. French and A. Wear (eds), *The Medical Revolution of the Seventeenth Century* (Cambridge: Cambridge University Press, 1989), 222-45.

_____, '"A Club of Little Villains": Rhetoric, Professional Identity and Medical Pamphlet Wars', in Marie Mulvey Roberts and Roy Porter (eds), *Literature and Medicine during the Eighteenth Century* (London: Routledge, 1993), 226-44.

_____, 'Newtonianism, Medicine and Religion' in Ole Peter Grell and Andrew Cunningham (eds), *Religio Medici: Medicine and Religion in Seventeenth-Century England* (Aldershot, Hampshire: Scolar Press, 1996), 293-312.

Guy, John R., 'The Episcopal Licensing of Physicians, Surgeons, and Midwives', *Bulletin of the History of Medicine*, lvi (1982), 528-42.

Gywnn, Robin D., *Huguenot Heritage: The History and Contribution of the Huguenots in Britain* (London: Routledge & Kegan Paul, 1985).

Haeger, Knut, *The Illustrated History of Surgery* (New York: Bell, 1988).

Haiken, Elizabeth, *Venus Envy: A History of Cosmetic Surgery* (Baltimore:

Johns Hopkins University Press, 1997).

Halberstam, Judith, and Livingston, Ira (eds), *Posthuman Bodies* (Bloomington, Indiana: Indiana University Press, 1995).

Hambridge, R., 'Empiricomany, or an Infatuation in Favour of Empiricism or Quackery: The Socio-economics of Eighteenth-Century Quackery', in S. Soupel and R. Hambridge, *Literature and Science and Medicine* (Los Angeles: University of California Press, 1982), 47-102.

Hamilton, Ian, *Keepers of the Flame: Literary Estates and the Rise of Biography* (London: Pimlico, 1993), vii.

Hankins, Thomas L., 'The Influence of Malebranche on the Science of Mechanics during the Eighteenth Century', *Journal of the History of Ideas*, xxviii (1967), 193-210.

_____, 'In Defence of Biography: The Use of Biography in the History of Science', *History of Science*, xvii (1979), 1-16.

Harding, Richard, *The Evolution of the Sailing Navy, 1509-1815* (London: Macmillan Press, 1995).

Hare, P. J., 'Daniel Turner (1667-1741)', *British Journal of Dermatology*, lxxix (1967), 657-61.

_____, *Our Credulous Countryman* (Edinburgh: Constable Publications, 1968).

Harley, David, 'Honour and Property: the Structure of Professional Disputes in Eighteenth-Century English Medicine', in A. Cunningham and R. French (eds), *The Medical Enlightenment of the Eighteenth Century* (Cambridge: Cambridge University Press, 1990), 138-64.

Harris, Michael, *London Newspapers in the Age of Walpole: A Study of the Origins of the Modern English Press* (Rutherford: Assoc. Univ. Presses, 1987).

Harrison, Peter, *Religion and the 'Religious' in the English Enlightenment* (Cambridge: Cambridge University Press, 1990).

Haslam, Fiona, *From Hogarth to Rowlandson: Medicine in Art in Eighteenth Century Britain* (Liverpool: Liverpool University Press, 1996).

Henning, Aloy, *Die Affare Hillmer: Ein Okkulist aus Berlin in Petersburg 1751* (Frankfurt am Main: Peter Lang, 1987).

_____, 'A German oculist in Russia', *Documenta Ophthalmologica*, lxxvii

(1991), 277-93.

Henriques, Fernando, *Prostitution in Europe and the New World* (London: Macgibbon & Kee, 1963).

Hillhouse, James T., *The Grub-Street Journal* (Durham, North Carolina: Duke University Press, 1928; New York: Benjamin Blom, 1967 reissue).

Hirschauer, Stefan, 'The Manufacture of Bodies in Surgery', *Social Studies of Science*, xxi (1991), 279-319.

Historical Manuscripts Commission, *Manuscripts of the Earl of Egmont. Vol. 2: Diary of the First Earl of Egmont (Viscount Perceval)* (London: HMSO, 1923).

Hof, Ulrich Im, *The Enlightenment* (Oxford: Blackwell Publishers, 1997).

Holmes, Geoffrey, 'Science, Reason and Religion in the Age of Newton', *British Journal for the History of Science*, xi (1978), 164-71.

_____, 'The Professions and Social Change in England, 1680-1730', *Proceedings of the British Academy*, lxv (1979), 313-54.

_____, *Augustan England: Professions, State and Society, 1680-1730* (London: George Allen & Unwin, 1982).

Holmes, Richard, *Footsteps. Adventures of a Romantic Biographer* (New York, Penguin, 1985).

Huet, Marie-Hèléne, *Monstrous Imagination* (Cambridge, Massachussetts: Harvard University Press, 1993).

Hughes, J. Trevor, *Thomas Willis 1621-1675. His Life and Work* (London: Royal Society of Medicine Services Ltd, 1991).

Hulpian, Chantal, 'Le Metier des Chirurgiens-barbiers à Namur, au XVIIIe siècle', *Annales de la Societe Belge d'Histoire des Hopitaux*, xxiii-xxiv (1985-86), 33-47.

Humphry-Smith, C. R. (ed.), *The Phillimore Atlas & Index of Parish Registers* (Chichester: Phillimore, 1984).

Hunt, Lynn (ed.), *Eroticism and the Body Politic* (Baltimore: Johns Hopkins University Press, 1991).

Hunt, Tony, *The Medieval Surgeon* (Woodbridge: The Boydell Press, 1992).

Hunter, Michael, *Science and Society in Restoration England* (Cambridge: Cambridge University Press, 1981).

_____, *The Royal Society and its Fellows 1660-1700* (Buckinghamshire:

British Society for the History of Science, 1982).

_____, 'The Problem of "Atheism" in Early Modern England', *Transactions of the Royal Historical Society*, 5th series xxxv (1985), 135-57.

_____, *Establishing the New Science: The Experience of the Early Royal Society* (Woodbridge: Boydell Press, 1989).

Hunter, Michael, and Wootton, David (eds), *Atheism from the Reformation to the Enlightenment* (Oxford: Clarendon Press, 1992).

Hunter, Richard and Macalpine, Ida, *Three Hundred Years of Psychiatry, 1535-1860* (Hartsdale, New York: Carlisle Publishing Co., 1982).

Hunter, W. B., 'The Seventeenth Century Doctrine of Plastic Nature', *Harvard Theological Review*, xliii (1950), 197-213.

Hutchinson, Keith, 'Supernaturalism and the Mechanical Philosophy', *History of Science*, xxi (1983), 297-333.

Hutton, Ronald, *Charles the Second: King of England, Scotland and Ireland* (Oxford: Clarendon Press, 1989).

Jackson, S. W., 'The Imagination and Psychological Healing', *Journal of the History of Behavioral Sciences*, xxvi (1990), 345-58.

Jacob, James R., and Jacob, Margaret C., 'The Anglican Origins of Modern Science: the Metaphysical Foundations of the Whig Constitution', *Isis*, lxxi (1980), 251-67.

Jacob, Margaret C., *The Newtonians and the English Revolution* (Hassocks, Sussex: Harvester Press, 1976).

_____, *The Radical Enlightenment: Pantheists, Freemasons and Republicans* (London: George Allen & Unwin, 1981).

_____, *Living the Enlightenment: Freemasonry and Politics in Eighteenth-Century Europe* (Oxford: Oxford University Press, 1992).

Jacyna, L. S., 'Images of John Hunter in the Nineteenth Century', *History of Science*, xxi (1983), 85-108.

James, R. R., 'Licences to Practice Medicine and Surgery Issued by the Archbishops of Canterbury', *Janus*, xli (1936), 97-106.

_____, 'Apprentice books at Barber-Surgeons' Hall', *British Medical Journal*, ii (1944), 288.

Jameson, Eric, *The Natural History of Quackery* (London: Michael Joseph, 1971).

Jenner, Mark, 'Quackery and Enthusiasm, or Why Drinking Water Cured the Plague', in Ole Peter Grell and Andrew Cunningham (eds), *Religio Medici: Medicine and Religion in Seventeenth-Century England* (Aldershot, Hampshire: Scolar Press, 1996), 313-39.

Jewson, N. D., 'Medical Knowledge and the Patronage System in Eighteenth-Century England', *Sociology*, viii (1974), 369-85.

Johnson, Allen, and Malone, Dumas, *Dictionary of American Biography* (London: Humphrey Milford, 1930).

Jones, D. W., 'London Merchants and the Crisis of the 1690's', in P. Clark and P. Slack (eds), *Crisis and Order in English Towns, 1500-1700* (London: Routledge & Kegan Paul, 1972), 311-55.

Jones, J. H., *Bad Blood: The Tuskegee Syphilis Experiment* (New York: Free Press, 1981).

Jordanova, Ludmilla, *Sexual Visions: Images of Gender in Science and Medicine Between the Eighteenth and Twentieth Centuries* (Madison: University of Wisconsin Press, 1989).

Jutte, Robert, 'A Seventeenth-Century German Barber-Surgeon and his Patients', *Medical History*, xxxiii (1989), 184-98.

Kantha, Sachi Sri, *Prostitutes in Medical Literature: An Annotated Bibliography* (Westport, Connecticut: Greenwood Press, 1991).

Keevil, John, 'Coffeehouse Cures', *Journal of the History of Medicine*, ix (1954), 191-5.

_____, *Medicine and the Navy 1200-1900. Vol. 2: 1649-1714* (Edinburgh: E. & S. Livingstone, 1958).

Kellett, J. R., 'The Breakdown of Gild and Corporation Control over the Handicraft and Retail Trade in London', *Economic Historical Review*, x (1958), 388-94.

Keogh, Andrew, 'The Growth of the University Library', *Yale University Library Gazette*, v (1931), 129-35.

_____, 'Bishop Berkeley's Gift of Books in 1733', *The Yale University Library Gazette*, viii (1934), 16.

Kerslake, John, *Early Georgian Portraits* (London: National Portrait Gallery, HMSO, 1977).

King, Lester S., 'Some Problems of Causality in Eighteenth Century Medicine', *Bulletin of the History of Medicine*, xxxvii (1963), 15-24.

_____, 'Stahl and Hoffmann: A Study in Eighteenth-Century Animism', *Journal of the History of Medicine*, xix (1964), 118-30.

_____, *The Road to Medical Enlightenment, 1650-1695* (London: Macdonald & Co.; New York: American Elsevier, 1970).
_____, *The Philosophy of Medicine: The Early Eighteenth Century* (Cambridge, Massachussetts: Harvard University Press, 1978).

Kirkup, J. R., 'The Tercentenary of Richard Wiseman's "Several Chirurgicall Treatises"', *Annals of the Royal College of Surgeons of England*, ilx (1977), 271-83.

Kottek, Samuel, 'La Force de l'Imagination chez les Femmes Enceintes: A Propos d'un Texte Biblique Apporté par J. Blondel en Illustration à ce Théme Controversé', *Revue d'Histoire de la Médecine Hebraique*, xxvii (1974), 43-8.

Kruck, William E., *Looking for Dr Condom* (American Dialectic Society, Publication No. 66) (University, Alabama: University of Alabama Press, 1981).

Kubrin, David, 'Providence and the Mechanical Philosophy: The Creation and Dissolution of the World in Newtonian Thought. A Study of Relations of Science and Religion in Seventeenth Century England' (Ph.D. thesis, Cornell University, 1968).

Kuhn, A. J., 'Hutchinson vs. Newton', *Journal of the History of Ideas*, xxii (1961), 303-22.

LaCasce, S., 'Swift on Medical Extremism', *Journal of the History of Ideas*, xxxi (1970), 599-606.

Landers, John, 'Mortality and Metropolis: the Case of London 1675-1825', *Population Studies*, xli (1987), 59-76.
_____ and Mouzas, Anastasia, 'Burial Seasonality and Causes of Death in London 1670-1819', *Population Studies*, xlii (1988), 59-83.
_____, 'Age Patterns of Mortality in London during the "Long Eighteenth Century": A Test of the "High Potential" Model of Metropolitan Mortality', *Social History of Medicine*, iii (1990), 27-60.

Lane, Joan, 'The Role of Apprenticeship in Eighteenth-Century Medical Education in England', in W. F. Bynum and Roy Porter (eds), *William Hunter and the Eighteenth-Century Medical World* (Cambridge: Cambridge University Press, 1985), 57-103.
_____, 'Eighteenth-Century Medical Practice: A Case Study of Bradford Wilmer, Surgeon of Coventry', *Social History of Medicine*, iii (1990), 369-86.
_____, and Tarver, Anne, 'Henry Fogg (1707-1750) and his Patients: The Practice of an Eighteenth-Century Staffordshire Apothecary',

Medical History, xxxvii (1993), 187-96.

Lane, John E., 'Daniel Turner and the First Degree of Doctor of Medicine Conferred in the English Colonies of North America by Yale College in 1723', *Annals of Medical History*, 2nd series, ii (1919), 367-80.

_____, 'A Note on the Prophylaxis of Syphilis from the Writings of Daniel Turner, M.D. (Honorary), Yale, 1723', *Archives of Dermatology and Syphilology*, vii (1923), 800-4.

_____, 'The Medical Books in the 1742 Yale College Library', *Yale University Library Gazette*, vi (1936), 84-8.

Langford, Paul, *A Polite and Commercial People: England, 1727-1783* (Oxford: Oxford University Press, 1989).

Lappe, Marc, *The Body's Edge: Our Cultural Obsession with Skin* (New York: Holt, 1996).

Lawrence, C. J., 'The Nervous System and Society in the Scottish Enlightenment', in B. Barnes and S. Shapin (eds), *Natural Order: Historical Studies of Scientific Culture* (London: Sage Publications, 1979), 19-40.

_____, 'Democratic, Divine and Heroic: The History and Historiography of Surgery', in C. Lawrence (ed.), *Surgical Theory, Medical Practice: Studies in the History of Surgery* (London: Routledge, 1992), 1-47.

_____ (ed.), *Surgical Theory, Medical Practice: Studies in the History of Surgery* (London: Routledge, 1992).

Lawrence, Ghislane, 'Surgery (Traditional)', in W.F. Bynum and Roy Porter (eds), *Companion Encyclopedia of the History of Medicine* (London: Routledge), vol. 2, 961-83.

Lawrence, Susan Catherine, 'Science and Medicine at the London Hospitals: The Development of Teaching and Research, 1750-1815' (Ph.D. thesis, University of Toronto, 1985).

_____, *Charitable Knowledge: Hospital Pupils and Practitioners in Eighteenth-Century London* (Cambridge, Massachusetts: Cambridge University Press, 1996).

Leder, Drew., *The Absent Body* (Chicago: University of Chicago Press, 1990).

LeFanu, William R., 'The Lost Half-Century in English Medicine, 1700-1750', *Bulletin of the History of Medicine*, xlvi (1972), 319-48.

Lehman, Bruce, 'Physicians and Politics in the Jacobite Era', in Eveline Cruickshanks and Jeremy Black (eds), *The Jacobite Challenge* (Edinburgh: John Donald, 1988), 74-91.

Leslie, Glennda, 'Cheat and Imposter: Debate Following the Case of the Rabbit Breeder', *The Eighteenth Century*, xxvii (1986), 269-86.

Lett, Hugh, 'Anatomy at the Barber Surgeons' Hall', *The British Journal of Surgery*, xxxi (1943), 101-11.

Levin, David Michael, *The Body's Recollection of Being: Phenomenologica Psychology and the Deconstruction of Nihilism* (London: Routledge & Kegan Paul, 1985).

Levine, Joseph M., *Dr Woodward's Shield: History, Science and Satire in Augustan England* (Berkeley: University of California Press, 1977).

_____, 'Ancients and Moderns Reconsidered', *Eighteenth Century Studies*, xv (1981), 72-89.

_____, *The Battle of the Books: History and Literature in the Augustan Age* (Ithaca: Cornell University Press, 1991).

Liggett, John, *The Human Face* (London: Constable & Co., 1974).

Lillywhite, Bryant, *London Coffee Houses: A Reference Book of Coffee Houses of the Seventeenth, Eighteenth, and Nineteenth Centuries* (London: George Allen & Unwin, 1963).

Lindeboom, G. A., *Herman Boerhaave, the Man and his Work* (London: Methuen & Co., 1968).

Lindsay, Jack, *The Monster City: Defoe's London 1688-1730* (London: Hart-Davis, MacGibbon, 1978).

Linebaugh, Peter, 'The Tyburn Riot Against the Surgeons', in Douglas Hay, Peter Linebaugh, John G. Rule, E. P. Thompson, and Cal Winslow, *Albion's Fatal Tree: Crime and Society in Eighteenth-Century England* (London: Allen Lane, 1975), 65-117.

Lingo, Alison Klairmont, 'Empirics and Charlatans in Early Modern France: The Genesis of the Classification of the "other" in Medical Practice', *Journal of Social History*, xxx (1996-97), 583-603.

Longmore, Sir Thomas, *Richard Wiseman, Surgeon and Sergeant-Surgeon to Charles II: A Bibliographical Study* (London: Longmans, 1891).

Longo, Lawrence D., 'The Rise and Fall of Battey's Operation [bilateral oophorectomy]: A Fashion in Surgery', *Bulletin of the History of Medicine*, liii (1979), 244-67.

Lowe, N. F., 'Hogarth, Beauty Spots, and Sexually Transmitted Diseases', *British Journal for Eighteenth-Century Studies*, xv (1992), 71-9.

_____, 'The Meaning of Venereal Disease in Hogarth's Graphic Art', in

Linda E. Merians (ed.), *The Secret Malady: Venereal Disease in Eighteenth-Century Britain and France* (Lexington, Kentucky: The University Press of Kentucky, 1996) 168-82.

Lowenthal, L. J. A., 'Daniel Turner and "De Morbis Cutaneis"', *Archives of Dermatology*, lxxxv (1962), 517-23.

Lupton, Deborah, *Medicine as Culture: Illness, Disease and the Body in Western Societies* (London: SAGE Publications, 1994).

Lyell, Alan, 'Daniel Turner (1667-1740) LRCP London (1711) M.D. Honorary, Yale (1723) Surgeon, Physician and Pioneer Dermatologist: The Man Seen in the Pages of his Book on the Skin', *International Journal of Dermatology*, xxi (1982), 162-70.

_____, 'Daniel Turner, and the First Controlled Therapeutic Trial in Dermatology', *Clinical and Experimental Dermatology*, xi (1986), 191-4.

Lyons, H. G., 'Biographical Notes', *Notes and Records of the Royal Society*, iii (1939), 88-96.

_____, *The Royal Society 1660-1940: A History of its Administration under its Charters* (Cambridge: The University Press, 1944).

McGuire, J. E., 'Force, Active Principles, and Newton's Invisible Realm', *Ambix*, xv (1968), 154-208.

McHugh, Paul, *Prostitution and Victorian Social Reform* (London: Croom Helm, 1980).

MacIntosh, J. J., 'Perception and Imagination in Descartes, Boyle, and Hooke', *Canadian Journal of Philosophy*, iii (1983), 327-57.

McKendrick, Neil, Brewer, John, and Plumb, J. H., *The Birth of a Consumer Society: The Commercialization of Eighteenth-Century England* (London: Europa Publications Ltd, 1982).

McLaren, A., 'Quackery and Control of Fertility in Eighteenth-Century England', in A. McLaren, *Birth Control in Nineteenth-Century England* (London: Croom Helm, 1978), 19-39.

McLynn, Frank, *Crime & Punishment in Eighteenth-Century England* (Oxford: Oxford University Press, 1991).

McMahon, C., 'Images as Motives and Motivators: A Historical Perspective', *American Journal of Psychology*, lxxxvi (1973), 465-90.

_____, 'The Role of Imagination in the Disease Process: Pre-Cartesian History', *Psychological Medicine*, vi (1976), 179-84.

_____, and Hastrup, J. L., 'The Role of Imagination in the Disease Process: Post-Cartesian History', *Journal of Behavioral Medicine*, iii (1980), 205-17.

Maehle, Andreas-Holger, 'Pharmacological Experimentation with Opium in the Eighteenth Century', in R. Porter and M. Teich (eds), *Drugs and Narcotics in History* (Cambridge: Cambridge University Press, 1995), 52-76.

Magli, Patrizia, 'The Face and the Soul', in Michael Feher (ed.), *Fragments for a History of the Human Body* (New York: Zone,1989), Part 2, 86-127.

Magner, Lois, *Doctors, Nurses, and Medical Practitioners: A Bio-Bibliographical Sourcebook* (Westport, Connecticut: Greenwood Press, 1997).

Malacrida, Lorenzo Marri, and Panconesi, Emiliano, *Vincenzio Chiarugi, I Suoi Tempi, Il Suo Libro Su le Malattie Cutanee Sordide : Vincenzio Chiarugi, His Times, and his Book on Sordid Cutaneous Diseases* (Firenze: Edizioni Riviste Scientifiche, 1989).

Mann, Ruth J., 'Daniel Turner, the First British Dermatologist', *Mayo Clinic Proceedings*, li (1976), 62-6.

Martin, Julian, 'Sauvages's Nosology: Medical Enlightenment in Montpellier', in A. Cunningham and R. French (eds), *The Medical Enlightenment of the Eighteenth Century* (Cambridge: Cambridge University Press, 1990), 111-37.

Martin, R. J. J., 'Explaining John Freind's *History of Physic*', *Studies in History and Philosophy of Science*, xix (1988), 399-418.

Mascia-Lees, Frances E., and Sharpe, Patricia, *Tattoo, Torture, Mutilation and Adornment. The Denaturalization of the Body* (Albany: State University of New York Press, 1992).

_____, 'The Marked and the Un(re)marked: Tattoo and Gender in Theory and Narrative', in Frances E. Mascia-Lees and Patricia Sharpe (eds), *Tattoo, Torture, Mutilation and Adornment. The Denaturalization of the Body in Culture and Text* (Albany: State University of New York Press, 1992), 145-69.

Matsushita, Masaaki, 'The Body as Visible Mind', a paper presented at the 22nd Tangiuchi Symposium on the Comparative History of Medicine East and West in Autumn 1997.

Matusak, Susan (compiler), *Bibliography of the Eighteenth-Century Holdings of the Institute for Sex Research Library* (Bloomington, Indiana:

Institute for Sex Research, 1975).

Mead, Kate Campbell Hurd, *A History of Women in Medicine from the Earliest Times to the Beginning of the Nineteenth Century* (Haddam, Connecticut: Haddam Press, 1938).

Meier, Richard Y., '"Sympathy" in the Neurophysiology of Thomas Willis', *Clio Medica*, xvii (1982), 95-111.

Merians, Linda E., 'The London Lock Hospital and the Lock Asylum for Women', in Linda E. Merians (ed.), *The Secret Malady: Venereal Disease in Eighteenth-Century Britain and France* (Lexington, Kentucky: The University Press of Kentucky, 1996), 128-45.

Meyer, Alfred and Heirons, Raymond, 'On Thomas Willis's Concepts of Neurophysiology', *Medical History*, ix (1965), 1-15, 142-55.

Meynell, G. G., *Materials for a Biography of Thomas Sydenham (1624-1689): a New Survey of Public and Private Archives* (Folkestone, [England]: Winterdown, 1988).

Michael, E. and Michael, F. S., 'Two Early Modern Concepts of Mind: Reflecting Substance vs. Thinking Substance', *Journal of the History of Philosophy*, xxvii (1989), 29-48.

_____ and _____, 'Corporeal Ideas in Seventeenth-Century Psychology', *Journal of the History of Ideas*, l (1989), 31-48.

Millburn, John R., 'Benjamin Martin and the Royal Society', *Notes and Records of the Royal Society of London*, xxviii (1973), 15-23.

Miller, Genevieve, *The Adoption of Inoculation for Smallpox in England and France* (Philadelphia: University of Pennsylvania Press, 1957).

Minet, W. and Minet, S. (eds), *Livre des Temoigrages, 1669-1719 De L'Eglise de Threadneedle Street* (London: For the Huguenot Society, 1909).

Mischel, T., '"Emotion" and "Motivation" in the Development of English Psychology: D. Hartley, James Mill, A. Bain', *Journal of the History of Behavioral Sciences*, ii (1966), 124-9.

Montagu, M. F. Ashley, *Edward Tyson, M.D., F.R.S., 1650-1708: and the Rise of Human and Comparative Anatomy in England; A Study in the History of Science* (Philadelphia: American Philosophical Society, 1943).

Morantz-Sanchez, Regina Markell, *Sympathy and Science: Women Physicians in American Medicine* (New York: Oxford University Press, 1985).

_____, 'Making It in a Man's World: The Late-Nineteenth-Century

Surgical Career of Mary Amanda Dixon Jones', *Bulletin of the History of Medicine*, lxix (1995), 542-68.

Morgan, Sir Clifford Naunton, 'Surgery and Surgeons in 18th-Century London', *Annals of the Royal College of Surgeons of England*, xlii (1968), 1-37.

Morton, R. S., 'Dr Thomas ('Quicksilver') Dover, 1660-1742', *British Journal of Venereal Disease*, xliv (1968), 342-6.

_____, 'Syphilis in Art: An Entertainment in Four Parts. Part 3', *Genitourinary Medicine*, lxvi (1990), 208-21.

Moscucci, Ornella, *The Science of Woman: Gynaecology and Gender in England, 1800-1920* (Cambridge: Cambridge University Press, 1990).

Mullett, Charles F., *Public Baths and Health in England, 16th-18th Century* (Baltimore: Johns Hopkins University Press, 1946).

Munby, Lionel M., *The Hertfordshire Landscape* (London: Hodder & Stoughton, 1977).

Munger, Robert S., 'Guaiacum: the Holy Wood from the New World', *Journal of the History of Medicine*, iv (1949), 196-229.

Munk, William, *Roll of the Royal College of Physicians of London*, 2nd edn (London: The College, 1878).

Nash, Stanley Dana, 'Social Attitudes towards Prostitutes in London from 1752-1829' (Ph.D. thesis, New York University, 1980).

Needham, Joseph, 'Limiting Factors in the Advancement of Science as Observed in the History of Embryology', *Yale Journal of Biology and Medicine*, viii (1935), 1-18.

Nicolson, Malcolm, 'The Metastatic Theory of Pathogenesis and the Professional Interests of the Eighteenth-Century Physician', *Medical History*, xxxii (1988), 277-300.

Nicolson, Marjorie H., 'Ward's "Pill and Drop" and Men of Letters', *Journal of the History of Ideas*, xxix (1968), 177-96.

_____, 'The Scientific Background of Swift's "Voyage to Laputa"', in *idem*, *Science and the Imagination* (Hamden, Connecticut: Archon Books, 1976), 110-54.

Norberg, Kathryn, 'From Courtesan to Prostitute: Mercenary Sex and Venereal Disease, 1730-1802', in Linda E. Merians (ed.), *The Secret Malady: Venereal Disease in Eighteenth-Century Britain and France* (Lexington, Kentucky: The University Press of Kentucky, 1996),

34-50.

Norman, H. J., 'John Bulwer and his *Anthropometamorphosis*', in E. A. Underwood (ed.), *Science, Medicine and History* (London: Oxford University Press, 1953), vol. 2, 89-95.

Novarr, David, *The Lines of Life: Theories of Biography, 1880-1970* (West Lafayette, Indiana: Purdue University Press, 1986).

Nuland, Sherwin B., *How We Die: Reflections on Life's Final Chapter* (New York: Knopf, 1993).

_____, *Doctors: the Biography of Medicine* (New York: Random House, 1995).

Nutton, Vivian, 'Humanist Surgery', in A. Wear, R. K. French and I. M. Lonie (eds), *The Medical Renaissance of the Sixteenth Century* (Cambridge: Cambridge University Press, 1985), 75-99.

O'Connor, Ulrick, *Biographers and the Art of Biography* (Dublin: Wolfhound Press, 1991).

Olby, R., Cantor, G. N., Christie, J. R. R., and Hodge, M. J. S. (eds), *Companion to the History of Modern Science* (London: Routledge, 1990).

Oldham, J. B., 'Two Eighteenth Century Liverpool Surgeons – Park and Alanson', *Proceedings of the Royal Society of Medicine*, xlvii (1954), 1056-8.

Olson, Richard, 'Tory-High Church Opposition to Science and Scientism in the Eighteenth Century: the Works of John Arbuthnot, Jonathan Swift, and Samuel Johnson', in John G. Burke (ed.), *The Uses of Science in the Age of Newton* (Berkeley: University of California Press, 1983), 171-204.

Oviatt, Edwin, *The Beginnings of Yale (1701-1726)* (New Haven: Yale University Press, 1916).

Packer, John W., *The Transformation of Anglicanism 1643-1660, with Special Reference to Henry Hammond* (Manchester: Manchester University Press, 1969).

Parish, Lawrence Charles, Holloway, Lisabeth M., Ashby, Susan and Rovner, Jack L., 'Bibliography of Secondary Sources on the History of Dermatology I. Journal Articles in English', *Archives of Dermatology*, cviii (1973), 351-66.

_____, _____, _____, Soifer, Betsy E., and Rovner, Jack L., 'Bibliography of Secondary Sources on the History of Dermatology II. Obituaries and Biographies in English Journals Before 1973: A Through L',

Archives of Dermatology, cxi (1975), 1036-48.

_____, _____, _____, _____, and _____, 'Bibliography of Secondary Sources on the History of Dermatology II. Obituaries and Biographies in English Journals Before 1973: M Through Z', *Archives of Dermatology*, cxi (1975), 1188-99.

Park, Katherine, 'Healing the Poor: Hospitals and Medical Assistance in Renaissance Florence', in Jonathan Barry and Colin Jones (eds), *Medicine and Charity before the Welfare State* (London and New York: Routledge, 1991), 26-45.

Park, Katherine and Daston, Lorraine J., 'Unnatural Conceptions: The Study of Monsters in Sixteenth- and Seventeenth-Century France and England', *Past and Present*, xcii (1981), 46-51.

Parker, George, *The Early History of Surgery in Great Britain, its Organization and Development* (London: A. & C. Beach, 1920).

Parsons, F. G., *The History of St Thomas's Hospital* (London: Methuen, 1934).

Payne, Lynda, '"To Lose Foolish Tenderness": Clinical Detachment and its Origins Among Medical Men in Early-Modern England', (Ph.D. thesis, University of California, Davis, 1997).

Peachey, George C., *A Memoir of William & John Hunter* (Plymouth: William Brendon & Son, 1924).

Pelling, Margaret, 'Occupational Diversity: Barber-Surgeons and the Trades of Norwich, 1550-1640', *Bulletin of the History of Medicine*, lvi (1982), 484-511.

_____, 'Appearance and Reality: Barber-Surgeons, The Body and Disease', in A. L. Beier and Roger Finlay (eds), *London 1500-1700: The Making of the Metropolis* (London: Longman, 1986), 82-112.

_____, 'Medical Practice in Early Modern England: Trade or Profession', in W. Prest (ed.), *The Professions in Early Modern England* (London: Croom Helm, 1987), 90-128.

_____, and Webster, Charles, 'Medical Practitioners', in Charles Webster (ed.), *Health, Medicine and Mortality in the Sixteenth Century* (Cambridge: Cambridge University Press, 1979), 165-235.

Peltier, Leonard F., *Fractures: A History and Iconography of their Treatment* (San Francisco: Norman Pub., 1990).

Perett, D. B., 'Ethics and Error: The Dispute between Ricord and Auzias-Turenne over Syphilization, 1845-70' (Ph.D. thesis, Stanford

University, 1977).

Perkin, Harold, *The Origins of Modern English Society, 1780-1880* (London: Routledge, Kegan Paul, 1969).

Pettigrew, T. J., 'History of the Barber-Surgeons of London', *British Journal of Archaeology*, viii (1852), 95-130.

Phear, D. N., 'Thomas Dover 1662-1742, Physician, Privateering Captain, and Inventor of Dover's Powder', *Journal of the History of Medicine and Allied Sciences*, ix (1954), 139-56.

Picard, Liza, *Restoration London* (London: Weidenfeld & Nicolson, 1997).

Pinto-Correia, Clara, *The Ovary of Eve: Egg and Sperm and Preformation* (Chicago: University of Chicago Press, 1997).

Piper, David, *The English Face* (London: Thames and Hudson, 1957).

Plarr, Victor G., *Catalogue of Manuscripts in the Library of the Royal College of Surgeons of England* ([London]: s.n., 1928).

Plomer, Henry R., *A Dictionary of the Printers and Booksellers Who Were at Work in England, Scotland, and Ireland, from 1668-1725* ([Oxford]: printed for the Bibliographical Society at the Oxford University Press, 1922).

_____, *Dictionaries of the Printers and Booksellers who were at Work in England, Scotland, and Ireland, 1557-1775* ([London]: Bibliographical Society, 1977).

Pointon, Marcia, *Hanging the Head. Portraiture and Social Formation in Eighteenth-Century England* (New Haven and London: Yale University Press, 1993).

Porter, Roy, 'Was there a Medical Enlightenment in Eighteenth-Century England?', *British Journal for Eighteenth-Century Studies*, v (1982), 49-63.

_____, *English Society in the Eighteenth Century* (Harmondsworth, Middlesex; New York: Penguin Books, 1982).

_____, 'William Hunter: a Surgeon and a Gentleman', in W. F. Bynum and Roy Porter (eds), *William Hunter and the Eighteenth-Century Medical World* (Cambridge: Cambridge University Press, 1985), 7-34.

_____, 'Making Faces: Physiognomy and Fashion in Eighteenth-Century England', *Etudes Anglaises*, xviii (1985), 185-96.

_____, 'Laymen, Doctors, and Medical Knowledge in the Eighteenth Century: the Evidence of the *Gentleman's Magazine*', in R. Porter (ed.), *Patients and Practitioners* (Cambridge: Cambridge University

Press, 1985), 283-314.

_____, '"The Secrets of Generation Display'd": *Aristotle's Master-piece* in Eighteenth-Century England', in R. P. Maccubbin (ed.), *'Tis Nature's Fault: Unauthorized Sexuality During the Enlightenment* (Cambridge: Cambridge University Press, 1987), 7-21.

_____, 'The Language of Quackery in England, 1660-1800', in Peter Burke and Roy Porter (eds), *The Social History of Language* (Cambridge: Cambridge University Press, 1987) (Cambridge Studies in Oral and Literate Culture 12), 73-103.

_____, 'Before the Fringe: Quackery and the Eighteenth-Century Medical Market', in R. Cooter (ed.), *Studies in the History of Alternative Medicine* (Basingstoke: Macmillan Press, 1988), 1-26.

_____, 'Death and the Doctors in Georgian England', in Ralph Houlbrooke (ed.), *Death, Ritual, and Bereavement* (London and New York: Routledge, 1989), 77-93.

_____, *Health for Sale: Quackery in England 1660-1850* (Manchester: Manchester University Press, 1989).

_____, 'Female Quacks in the Consumer Society', *History of Nursing Journal*, iii (1990), 1-25.

_____, 'Bodies of Thought: Thoughts about the Body in Eighteenth-Century England', in Joan H. Pittock and Andrew Wear (eds), *Interpretation and Cultural History* (New York: St Martin's, 1991), 82-108.

_____, *Doctor of Society: Thomas Beddoes and the Sick Trade in Late-Enlightenment England* (London: Routledge, 1992).

_____, '"Laying Aside Any Private Advantage", John Marten and Venereal Disease', in Linda E. Merians (ed.), *The Secret Malady: Venereal Disease in Eighteenth-Century Britain and France* (Lexington, Kentucky: The University Press of Kentucky, 1996), 51-67.

_____, 'Accidents in the Eighteenth Century' in Roger Cooter and Bill Luckin (eds), *Accidents in History: Injuries, Fatalities and Social Relations* (Amsterdam: Rodopi, 1997), 90-106.

_____, and Porter, Dorothy, *In Sickness and In Health: The British Experience 1650-1850* (London: Fourth Estate Ltd, 1988).

_____, and _____, *Patient's Progress: Doctors and Doctoring in Eighteenth-Century England* (Cambridge: Polity Press, 1989).

Pouchelle, Marie-Christine, *The Body and Surgery in the Middle Ages*, translated by Rosemary Morris (Cambridge: Polity Press, 1990).

Powell, W. R., *Victorian History of the Counties of England, A History of Essex, Vol. 8* (Oxford: Oxford University Press for the Institute of Historical Research, 1983).

Power, Sir D'Arcy, *Selected Writings 1877-1930* (Oxford: Clarendon Press, 1931).

Poynter, F. N. L., *The Journal of James Yonge (1647-1721), Plymouth Surgeon* (London: Longmans, Green & Co., 1963).

Pratt, Anne Stokely, 'The Books sent from England by Jeremiah Dummer to Yale College', in *Papers in Honor of Andrew Keogh* (New Haven, Connecticut: Yale University Press, 1938), 7-44.

_____ and Keogh, Andrew, 'The Yale Library of 1742', *Yale University Library Gazette*, xv (1940), 29-40.

Prendergast, William J., 'The First Honorary Degree of Doctor of Medicine was Granted in New Haven in 1723', *Sunday Pictorial*, 13 November 1966.

Prest, Wilfrid, 'Introduction: The Professions and Society in Early Modern England', in W. Prest (ed.), *The Professions in Early Modern England* (London: Croom Helm, 1987), 1-24.

Preston, Thomas R., 'Biblical Criticism, Literature, and the Eighteenth-Century Reader', in Isabel Rivers (ed.), *Books and their Readers in Eighteenth-Century England* (Leicester: Leicester University Press; New York: St Martin's Press, 1982), 97-126.

Proksch, J. K., *Die Litteratur uber die venerischen Krankheiten*, 3 vols in 5 (Bonn: P. Hanstein, 1889-1900).

_____, *Die Geschichte der venerischen Krankheiten*, 2 vols in 1 (Bonn: P. Hanstein, 1895-1900).

Purdon, H. S., 'Brief Historical Sketch of Dermatology, Classification of Skin Diseases, General Remarks on the Anatomy of the Skin', *Journal of Cutaneous Medicine*, iv (1871), 203-7.

Pusey, Wm. Allen, *The History of Dermatology* (Springfield, Illinois; Baltimore: Charles C. Thomas, 1933).

Quetel, Claude, *History of Syphilis*, translated by J. Braddock and B. Pike (Cambridge: Polity Press, 1990).

Rather, L. J., 'Thomas Fienus' (1567-1631) Dialectical Investigation of the Imagination as Cause and Cure of Bodily Disease', *Bulletin of the History of Medicine*, xli (1967), 349-67.

Rayer, P. F. O., *Theoretical and Practical Treatise on the Diseases of the Skin*, 2nd edn (London: J. B. Baillière, 1835).

Reddaway, T. F., *The Rebuilding of London after the Great Fire* (London:

Jonathan Cape, 1940).

Rees, Abraham, *The Cyclopaedia; or, Universal Dictionary of Arts, Sciences, and Literature* (London: Printed for Longman, Hurst, Rees, Orme, & Brown, 1819).

Reeve, M. D., 'Conceptions', *Proceedings of the Cambridge Philosophical Society*, No. 215, n.s. No. 35 (1989), 81-112.

Reilly, Philip R., *The Surgical Solution. A History of Involuntary Sterilization in the United States* (Baltimore: John Hopkins University Press, 1991).

Reiss, Frederick, 'Percutaneous Absorption, A Critical and Historical Review', *American Journal of Medical Science*, cclii (1966), 588-602.

Renbourn, E. T., 'The History of Sweat and the Sweat Rash From Earliest Times to the End of the 18th Century', *Journal of the History of Medicine*, ivx (1959), 202-27.

_____, 'The Natural History of Insensible Perspiration: A Forgotten Doctrine of Health and Disease', *Medical History*, iv (1960), 135-52.

Rey, Roselyn, *History of Pain*, trans., Louise Elliot Wallace and J.A. & S.W. Cadden (Paris: Editions La Decouverte, 1993).

Ribeiro, Aileen and Cumming, Valerie, *The Visual History of Costume* (London: B. T. Batsford Ltd, 1989).

Richardson, Ruth, *Death, Dissection and the Destitute: A Political History of the Human Corpse* (London: Routledge & Kegan Paul, 1987).

Riha, Ortrun, 'Surgical Case Records as an Historical Source: Limits and Perspectives', *Social History of Medicine*, viii (1995), 271-83.

Risse, Guenter, *Hospital Life in Enlightenment Scotland: Care and Teaching at the Royal Infirmary of Edinburgh* (Cambridge: Cambridge University Press, 1986).

_____, 'The History of Therapeutics', *Clio Medica*, xxii (Amsterdam: Rodopi, 1991), 3-11.

_____, and Warner, John Harley, 'Reconstructing Clinical Activities: Patient Records in Medical History', *Social History of Medicine*, v (1992), 183-205.

Robinson, F. J. G., Auerley, G., Esslemont, D. R., and Wallis, P. J. (compilers), *Eighteenth-Century British Books: An Author Union Catalogue*, 5 vols (Folkestone, Kent: Wm. Dawson and Sons, 1981).

_____, and Wallis, P. J., *Book Subscriptions Lists: A Revised Guide*, supplements 1-4 (Newcastle upon Tyne: Harold Hill & Sons Ltd,

1975-81; new edition 1989).

Robinson, H. W., 'Gleanings from the Library-I. A Note on the Early Minutes', *Notes and Records of the Royal Society*, i (1938), 92-4.

Robinson, Victor, 'Anatomical Dissection in the 18th Century', *Ciba Symposium*, iii (1941), 845-53.

Rodger, N. A. M., *The Wooden World: An Anatomy of the Georgian Navy* (Glasgow: William Collins Sons & Co., 1986).

Roe, S. A., *Matter, Life, and Generation: 18th Century Embryology and the Haller–Wolff Debate* (Cambridge: Cambridge University Press, 1981).

Rogers, Pat, *Grub Street: Studies in Subculture* (London: Methuen & Co., Ltd., 1972).

_____, (ed.), *The Eighteenth Century* (Cambridge: Cambridge University Press, 1978).

Rolleston, Humphry, 'I. The Early History of the Teaching of Human Anatomy in London', *Annals of Medical History*, 3rd series, i (1939), 203-16.

Rose, John C., and Corn, Milton, 'Dr E. and Other Patients: New Lessons from Old Case Reports', *Journal of the History of Medicine*, xxxix (1984), 3-32.

Rousseau, G. S., 'Science and the Discovery of the Imagination in Enlightened England', *Eighteenth Century Studies*, iii (1969), 108-35.

_____, 'Pineapples, Pregnancy, Pica, and *Peregrine Pickle*', in G. S. Rousseau and P.-G. Boucé (eds), *Tobias Smollett: Bicentennial Essays* (New York: Oxford University Press, 1971), 79-109.

_____, 'Science', in P. Rogers (ed.), *The Eighteenth Century* (The Context of English Literature) (London: Methuen & Co., 1978), 153-207.

Russell, Colin A., *Science and Social Change 1700-1900* (London: Macmillan Press, 1983).

Russell, K. F., *British Anatomy 1525-1800*, 2nd edn (London: St Paul's Bibliographies, 1987).

Ryan, Michael, *Manual of Midwifery*, First American edition (Burlington: Smith and Harrington, 1835).

Samuel, Raphael, *Theatres of Memory. Volume 1: Past and Present in Contemporary Culture* (London: Verso, 1994), 4.

Sassen, F. L. R., 'The Intellectual Climate in Leiden in Boerhaave's Time', in G. Lindeboom (ed.), *Boerhaave and his Times* (Leiden: E. J. Brill, 1970), 1-16.

Saunders, J. W., *The Profession of English Letters* (London: Routledge and Kegan Paul, 1964).

Sawday, Jonathan, *The Body Emblazoned: Dissection and the Human Body in Renaissance Culture* (London: Routledge, 1995).

Schaffer, Simon, 'Godly Men and Mechanical Philosophers: Souls and Spirits in Restoration Natural Philosophy', *Science in Context*, i (1987), 55-86.

_____, 'Newtonianism', in Olby, R. C., Cantor, G. N., Christie, J. R. R., and Hodge, M. J. S. (eds), *Companion to the History of Modern Science* (London: Routledge, 1990), 610-26.

Schalick, Walton O., 'Add One Part Pharmacy to One Part Surgery and One Part Medicine: Jean de Saint-Armand and the Development of Medieval Medical Pharmacology' (Ph.D. thesis, The Johns Hopkins University, 1997).

Schiebinger, Londa, *The Mind Has No Sex?: Women in the Origins of Modern Science* (Cambridge, Massachusetts: Harvard University Press, 1989).

Schwartz, Hillel, *The French Prophets: the History of a Millenarian Group in Eighteenth-Century England* (Berkeley: University of California Press, 1980).

Seligman, S. A., 'Mary Toft: the Rabbit Breeder', *Medical History*, v (1961), 349-60.

Sewell, Jane Eliot, 'Bountiful Bodies: Spencer Wells, Lawson Tait, and the Birth of British Gynaecology' (Ph.D. thesis, Johns Hopkins University, 1991).

Shapin, Steven, 'Social Uses of Science', in G. S. Rousseau and Roy Porter (eds), *The Ferment of Knowledge: Studies in the Historiography of Eighteenth-Century Science* (Cambridge: Cambridge University Press, 1980), 93-139.

_____, '"A Scholar and a Gentleman": The Problematic Identity of the Scientific Practitioner in Early Modern England', *History of Science*, xxix (1991), 279-327.

Shaw, W. A. (ed.), *Letters of Denization and Acts of Naturalization for Aliens in England and Ireland, 1603-1700* (Lymington: for the Huguenot Society, 1911).

Shaw-Taylor, Desmond, *The Georgians: Eighteenth-Century Portraiture & Society* (London: Barrie & Jenkins, 1990).

Sheets-Pyenson, Susan, 'New Directions for Scientific Biography: The Case of Sir William Dawson', *History of Science*, xxviii (1990), 399-410.

Shelton-Jones, Eric, 'The Barber-Surgeons Company of London and Medical Education 1540-1660' (M.Phil. thesis, University of London, 1981).

Shephard, Alan, 'The Literature of a Medical Hoax: The Case of Mary Toft, "The Pretende Rabbet-Breeder"', *Eighteenth-Century Life*, xix (1995), 59-77.

Sherwood, Joan, 'Treating Syphilis: The Wetnurse as Technology in an Eighteenth-Century Parisian Hospital', *Journal of the History of Medicine and Allied Sciences*, l (1995), 315-39.

Shorr, Philip, *Science and Superstition in the Eighteenth Century: A Study of the Treatment of Science in Two Encyclopedias of 1725-1750* (New York: Columbia University Press, 1932).

Shortland, Michael, and Yeo, Richard, *Telling Lives in Science: Essays on Scientific Biography* (Cambridge: Cambridge University Press, 1996).

Silvette, Herbert, *The Doctor on the Stage: Medicine and Medical Men in Seventeenth-Century England* (Knoxville: University of Kentucky Press, 1976).

Siraisi, Nancy G., *Medieval and Early Renaissance Medicine: An Introduction to Knowledge and Practice* (Chicago: University of Chicago Press, 1990).

Smith, Alan DeForest, 'Richard Wiseman: His Contributions to English Surgery', *Bulletin of the New York Academy of Medicine*, xlvi (1970), 167-82.

Smith, Dale C. 'Appendicitis, Appendectomy, and the Surgeon', *Bulletin of the History of Medicine*, lxx (1996), 414-41.

Smith, Steven R., 'The Social and Geographical Origins of the London Apprentices, 1630-1660', *The Guildhall Miscellany*, iv (1973), 195-206.

Smith, Virginia Sarah, 'Cleanliness: the Development of Idea and Practice in Britain, 1770-1850' (Ph.D. thesis, University of London, 1985).

South, J. Flint, *Memorial of the Craft of Surgery in England* (London: Cassell & Co. Ltd, 1886).

Speck, W. A., 'Politicians, Peers, and Publication by Subscription 1700-50', in Isabel Rivers (ed.), *Books and their Readers in Eighteenth-Century England* (Leicester: Leicester University Press; New York: St Martin's Press, 1982), 47-68.

Spellman, W.M., *The Latitudinarians and the Church of England* (Athens, Georgia: University of Georgia Press, 1993).

Sponger, Mary, *Feminizing Venereal Disease: The Body of the Prostitute in Nineteenth-Century Medical Discourse* (New York: New York University Press, 1997).

Spurr, John, '"Latitudinarians" and the Restoration Church', *The Historical Journal*, xxxi (1981), 61-82.

_____, *The Restoration Church of England, 1646-1689* (New Haven, Connecticut: Yale University Press, 1992).

Stafford, Barbara Maria, 'One Face of Beauty, One Picture of Health: The Hidden Aesthetic of Medical Practice', *Journal of Medical Philosophy*, xiv (1989), 213-30.

_____, *Body Criticism: Imaging the Unseen in Enlightenment Art and Medicine* (Cambridge, Massachussetts: MIT Press, 1991).

Stephen, Leslie, *English Literature and Society in the Eighteenth Century* (London: Duckworth & Co., 1904).

_____ and Lee, Sidney (eds), *Dictionary of National Biography*, 22 vols (London: Smith, Elder, & Co., 1908-9).

Stevenson, Ian, 'The Mother's Possible Influence in Birthmarks in Causes of the Reincarnation Type', paper presented at 'Parapsychology: A State-of-the-Art Conference' (New York), 22 January 1989.

_____, *Reincarnation and Biology: A Contribution to the Etiology of Birthmarks and Birth Defects*, 2 vols, (London: Praeger Publishers, 1997).

Stevenson, John, *Popular Disturbances in England 1700-1870* (London and New York: Longman, 1979).

Stevenson, Lloyd G., 'A Note on the Relation of Military Service to Licensing in the History of British Surgery', *Bulletin of the History of Medicine*, xxvii (1953), 420-7.

Stewart, Mary Margaret, '"And blights with plagues the Marriage hearse": Syphilis and Wives', in Linda E. Merians (ed.), *The Secret Malady: Venereal Disease in Eighteenth-Century Britain and France* (Lexington, Kentucky: The University Press of Kentucky, 1996), 103-13.

Stoll, David M., *A Woman's Skin* (New Brunswick: Rutgers University Press, 1994).

Stone, Lawrence, 'Social Mobility in England, 1500-1700', *Past and Present*, xxxiii (1966), 16-55.

Stonehill, Charles A., Jr, Block, Andrew, and Stonehill, H. Winthrop, *Anonyma and Pseudonyma* (London: C. A. Stonehill, Jr., 1926).

Strong, L. A. G., *Dr Quicksilver 1660-1745: The Life and Times of Thomas Dover, MD* (London: Andrew Melrose, 1955).

Sutton, Richard L., 'Diseases of the Skin: Mercurialis, 1572', *Archives of Dermatology*, xciv (1966), 763-72.

_____, *Sixteenth Century Physician and His Methods: Mercurialis on Diseases of the Skin: The First Book on the Subject (1572)* (Kansas City, Missouri: Lowell Press, 1986).

Suzuki, Akihito, 'Soul Lost and Regained: British Iatromathematicians, 1690-1730', paper presented at the 'Day of Enlightenment' workshop, London Centre for the History of Science, Medicine and Technology (Imperial College, London), 1 March 1991.

Tamny, Marin, 'Atomism and the Mechanical Philosophy', in R. C. Olby, G. N. Cantor, J. R. R. Christie, and M. J. S. Hodge (eds), *Companion to the History of Science* (London: Routledge, 1990), 597-609.

Temkin, Owsei, 'The Role of Surgery in the Rise of Modern Medical Thought', *Bulletin of the History of Medicine*, xxv (1951), 248-59.

_____, 'Fernel, Joubert, and Erastus on the Specificity of Cathartic Drugs', in A. G. Debus (ed.), *Science, Medicine, and Society in the Renaissance* (New York: Science History Publications, 1972), vol. 1, 61-68.

Thomas, James H., 'Hampshire and the Company of Barber-Surgeons, 1658-1720', *Hampshire Family Historian*, x (1983), 15-18.

Thomas, K. Bryn, *James Douglas of the Pouch and his Pupil William Hunter* (London: Pitman Medical Publishing Co., 1964).

Thomas, Keith, *Religion and the Decline of Magic: Studies in Popular Beliefs in Sixteenth and Seventeenth Century England* (Harmondsworth: Penguin Books, 1978).

Thompson, C. J. S., *The Mystery and Lore of Monsters* (London: Williams & Norgate, 1930).

Thompson, E. P., 'Eighteenth Century English Society: Class Struggle Without Class?', *Social History*, iii (1978), 133-65.

Thompson, Rosemaire Garland (ed.), *Freakery: Cultural Spectacles of the Extraordinary Body* (New York: New York University Press, 1996).

Todd, Dennis, *Imagining Monsters: Miscreations of the Self in Eighteenth-Century England* (Chicago: The Chicago University Press, 1995).

Toner, Joseph M., *Contributions to the Annals of Medicine and Medical Education in the United States Before and During the War of Independence* (Washington, D.C.: Government Printing Office, 1874).

Tröhler, Ulrich, 'Quantification in British Medicine and Surgery, 1750-1830: With Special Reference to its Introduction into Therapeutics' (Ph.D. thesis, University of London, 1978).

_____, 'Surgery (Modern)', in W.F. Bynum and Roy Porter (eds), *Companion Encyclopedia of the History of Medicine* (London: Routledge), vol. 2, 984-1029.

Turner, M. L., 'The Minute Book of the Patrons in the Grub Street Journal [with transcription]', *Publishing History*, iv (1978), 49-94.

Tytler, Graeme, *Physiognomy in the European Novel: Faces and Fortunes* (Princeton, New Jersey: Princeton University Press, 1982).

Urdang, George, 'The Early Chemical and Pharmaceutical History of Calomel', *Chymia: Annual Studies in the History of Chemistry*, i (1948), 93-108.

Wadd, William, *Nugae Chirurgicae; or a Biographical Miscellany* (London: J. Nichols, 1824).

[Wadd, William], *Nugae Conorae; or Epitaphian Momentos* (London: J. B. Nichols, 1827).

Wagner, Anthony, *Heralds of England: A History of the Office and College of Arms* (London: HMSO, 1967).

Wagner, Peter, *Eros Revived: Erotica of the Enlightenment in England and America* (London: Paladin Grafton Books, 1988).

Wall, Cecil, *History of the Surgeons' Company 1745-1800* (London: Hutchinsons, 1937).

Wall, L. Lewis, 'The Strange Case of Mary Toft (Who was Delivered of Sixteen Rabbits and a Tabby Cat in 1726)', *Medical Heritage*, i (1985), 199-212.

Wallis, P. J. and Wallis, R. V., *Eighteenth-Century Medics* (Newcastle upon Tyne: Project for Historical Biobibliography, 1988).

Walsh, James J., *Cures: the Story of Cures that Fail* (New York: D. Appleton, 1923).

Wangensteen, Owen H., and Wangensteen, Sarah D., *The Rise of Surgery: From Empiric Craft to Scientific Discipline* (Folkestone, Kent: William Dawson & Sons, 1978).

Watson, Foster, *The English Grammar Schools to 1660: Their Curriculum and Practice* (Cambridge: Cambridge University Press, 1908).

Waugh, M. A., 'Attitudes of Hospitals in London to Venereal Disease in the 18th and 19th Centuries', *British Journal of Venereal Disease*, xlvii (1971), 146-50.

Wear, Andrew, 'Medical Practice in Late Seventeenth- and Early Eighteenth-Century England: Continuity and Change', in R. French and A. Wear (eds), *The Medical Revolution of the Seventeenth Century* (Cambridge: Cambridge University Press, 1989), 294-320.

_____, 'Religious Beliefs and Medicine in Early Modern England', in Hilary Marland and Margaret Pelling (eds), *The Task of Healing: Medicine Religion and Gender in England and the Netherlands, 1450-1800* (Rotterdam: Erasmus Press, 1996) 145-69.

Wendorf, Richard, 'Ut Pictura Biographia: Biography and Portrait Painting as Sister Arts', in R. Wendorf (ed.), *Articulate Images: The Sister Arts from Hogarth to Tennyson* (Minneapolis: University of Minnesota Press, 1983), 98-124.

_____, *The Elements of Life: Biography and Portrait-Painting in Stuart and Georgian London* (Oxford: Clarendon Press, 1990).

West, Shearer, 'Patronage and Power: the Role of the Portrait in Eighteenth-Century England', in: Jeremy Black and Jeremy Gregory (eds), *Culture, Politics and Society in Britain, 1660-1800* (Manchester and New York: Manchester University Press, 1991), 131-53.

Wilde, C. B., 'Hutchinsonianism, Natural Philosophy and Religious Controversy in Eighteenth Century Britain', *History of Science*, xvii (1980), 1-24.

Wilks, Samuel, and Bettany, G. T., *A Biographical History of Guy's Hospital* (London: Ward, Lock, Bowden & Co., 1892).

Williams, Glyndwr, '"The Inexhaustible Fountain of Gold": English Projects and Ventures in the South Seas, 1670-1750', in John E. Flint and Glyndwr Williams (eds), *Perspectives of Empire: Essays Presented to Gerald S. Graham* (New York: Barnes & Noble, 1973), 27-53.

Williamson, Raymond, 'John Martyn and the Grub-Street Journal, with Particular Reference to his Attacks on Richard Bentley, Richard

Bradley and William Cheselden', *Medical History*, v (1961), 361-74.

Wilson, Adrian, 'The Politics of Medical Improvement in Early Hanoverian London', in A. Cunningham and R. French (eds), *The Medical Enlightenment of the Eighteenth Century* (Cambridge: Cambridge University Press, 1990), 4-39.

Wilson, Dudley, *Signs and Portents: Monstrous births from the Middle Ages to the Enlightenment*, (London: Routledge, 1993).

Wilson, Philip K., '"Out of Sight, Out of Mind?": The Daniel Turner-James Blondel Debate over Maternal Impressions', (M.A. thesis, The Johns Hopkins University, 1987).

_____, 'Surgeon "Turned" Physician: The Career and Writings of Daniel Turner (1667- 1741)' (Ph.D. thesis, University of London, 1992).

_____, 'Acquiring Surgical Know-How: Occupational and Lay Instruction in Early Eighteenth-Century London', in Roy Porter (ed.), *The Popularization of Medicine 1650-1850* (London: Routledge, 1992), 42-71.

_____, '"Out of Sight, Out of Mind?": The Daniel Turner–James Blondel Dispute Over the Power of the Maternal Imagination', *Annals of Science*, xlix (1992), 63-85.

_____, '"Sacred Sanctuaries for the Sick": Surgery at St Thomas's Hospital (1725-26)', *The London Journal*, xvii (1992), 49-66.

_____, 'William Cowper's Anatomy of Human Skin', *International Journal of Dermatology*, xxxi, no. 5 (1992), 361-3.

_____, 'Vernacularisation vs. Vulgarisation of Early Eighteenth-Century English Surgical Writings', *Transactions of the Eighth International Congress on the Enlightenment* (Oxford: Voltaire Foundation, 1993), vol 7.

_____, 'Daniel Turner and the *Art of Surgery* in early eighteenth-century London', *Journal of the Royal Society of Medicine*, lxxxvii (1994), 781-85.

_____, 'An Enlightenment Science?: Surgery and the Royal Society' in Roy Porter (ed.) *Medicine and the Enlightenment* (Amsterdam: Rodopi, 1995), 360-86.

_____, 'Reading A Man Through His Gifts: Daniel Turner's 1722 Book Donation to Yale College' *Yale University Library Gazette*, lxix (1995), 129-48.

_____, (ed.), *Childbirth. Changing Ideas and Practices in Britain and America, 1600 to the Present* (New York: Garland Publishing, 1996).

_____, 'Exposing the "Secret Disease": Recognizing and Treating Syphilis in Daniel Turner's London', in Linda E. Merians (ed.), *The Secret*

Malady. Venereal Disease in Eighteenth-Century France and Great Britain (Lexington, Kentucky: University Press of Kentucky, 1996), 253-66.

_____, 'Healers in History', in Roy Porter (ed.), *Medicine: A History of Healing. Ancient Traditions to Modern Practices* (New York: Marlowe & Co., 1997), 168-95.

_____, 'Imaging the Human Body: A Surgical Perspective of Skin in Enlightenment London', in Shigehisa Kuriyama and Shizu Sakai (eds), *Medicine and the History of the Body: Proceedings of the 20th, 21st and 22nd International Symposia on the Comparative History of Medicine – East and West* (Tokyo: Ishiyaku EuroAmerica Inc., in press).

Wiltshire, John, *Samuel Johnson in the Medical World: The Doctor and the Patient* (Cambridge: Cambridge University Press, 1991).

Wing, Donald (compiler), *Short-Title Catalogue of Books Printed in England, Scotland, Ireland, Wales and British America, and of English Books Printed in Other Countries 1641-1700*, 2nd edn, 3 vols (New York: Index Committee of Modern Language Association, 1972-1988).

Winslow, Donald J., 'Glossary of Terms in Life Writing Part I', *Biography* i (1978), 61-78.

Woodforde, John, *The Strange Story of False Hair* (London: Routledge & Kegan Paul, 1971).

Wrigley, E. A., and Schofield, R. S., *Population History of England 1541-1871: A Reconstruction* (London: Edward Arnold, 1981).

_____, and _____, *The Population History of England, 1541-1871* (Cambridge: Cambridge University Press, 1989).

Wyman, A. L., 'The Surgeoness: The Female Practitioner of Surgery 1400-1800', *Medical History*, xxviii (1984), 22-41.

Yale University, *Catalogue of the Officers and Graduates of Yale University in New Haven, Connecticut, 1701-1924* (New Haven: The University, 1924).

Young, Sidney, *Annals of the Barber-Surgeons of London* (London: Blades, East, & Blades, 1890).

Zimbardo, Rose A., 'Satiric Representation of Venereal Disease: The Restoration versus the Eighteenth-Century Model', in Linda E. Merians (ed.), *The Secret Malady: Venereal Disease in Eighteenth-Century Britain and France* (Lexington, Kentucky: The University

Press of Kentucky, 1996), 183-95.

Zimmerman, E. L., 'Early Collections of Syphilogic Works: Aloysius Luisinus and His Influence on Syphilology', *Bulletin of the History of Medicine*, iv (1936), 582-99.

Zimmerman, Leo M., 'Surgery', in Allen G. Debus (ed.), *Medicine in Seventeenth-Century England* (Berkeley: University of California Press, 1974), 49-69.

Zuckerman, Arnold, 'Dr Richard Mead (1673-1754): A Biographical Study', (Ph.D. thesis, University of Illinois, 1965).

_____, 'Disease and Ventilation in the Royal Navy: The Woodenship Years', *Eighteenth-Century Life*, xi, n.s. 3 (1987), 77-89.

INDEX

M

N

O

P